The Suicidal Crisis

The Suicidal Crisis

Clinical Guide to the Assessment of Imminent Suicide Risk

Igor Galynker, MD, PhD

Professor of Psychiatry, the Icahn School of Medicine
at Mount Sinai, New York, NY 10029, USA
Director of Research, Department of Psychiatry at
Mount Sinai Beth Israel, New York, NY 10003, USA
Director of the Richard and Cynthia Zirinsky Center
for Bipolar Disorder, Mount Sinai Beth Israel,
New York, NY 10003, USA
Director, Suicide Research Laboratory,
Mount Sinai Beth Israel, New York, NY 10003, USA

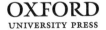

OXFORD
UNIVERSITY PRESS

OXFORD
UNIVERSITY PRESS

Oxford University Press is a department of the University of Oxford. It furthers
the University's objective of excellence in research, scholarship, and education
by publishing worldwide. Oxford is a registered trade mark of Oxford University
Press in the UK and certain other countries.

Published in the United States of America by Oxford University Press
198 Madison Avenue, New York, NY 10016, United States of America.

CIP data is on file at the Library of Congress
ISBN 978-0-19-026085-9

1 3 5 7 9 8 6 4 2
Printed by Webcom, Inc., Canada

To Cynthia Zirinsky.

Contents

Foreword

The possibility of suicide begins with agency. Suicide is its end, often driven by an impression of its impossibility. Being social animals, generally, our agency resides in a social matrix that both regulates it and thereby also gives it much of its meaning. This social entanglement, long recognized in the study of suicide (Emile Durkheim's (1897/1951) sociological study being perhaps the most notable example), is, however, easily obscured in much contemporary medical thought that implicitly conceptualizes suicide as merely a sometime symptom of various mental disorders—disease processes that are inherent in the individual.

Nonetheless, the structuring relationship between the social and the individual is reciprocal; whereas societies and, with them, social forces may change, other features of our humanity are less mutable. Thus, the Hippocratic texts, comprising actually the work of multiple authors, generally dating to the end of the 5th century BCE, describe many sources of morbidity still common today, including suicide (Hippocrates, Flemming, & Hanson, 1998). The text that discusses suicide, "Diseases of Young Girls," begins with a condensed description of extreme, possibly psychotic, agitation, fear, and possible sleep disturbance in association with "the sacred disease"—what would today be called a seizure disorder, including perhaps psychogenic non-epileptic seizures; the outcome is suicide by hanging—a highly lethal means. The text goes on immediately to an epidemiological observation that this is more prevalent among women than men. The first paragraph concludes with the explanation of this observation by the further observation that "female nature is weaker and more troublesome." Given the much higher rates of suicide attempt among women than men today, the contemporary reader should be doubly troubled by this 2,400-year-old observation. If one conceives of "female nature" as socially constructed, and thus reflecting not merely the essential qualities of women but also the social conditions in which they find themselves, "weaker" might be retranslated as "more vulnerable," whereas "troublesome" may be read as describing lives rather than persons.

The text goes on to tell a medical story interweaving life narrative, symptomatic description, and pathophysiology. Whereas the narrative and symptomatic accounts are liable to still ring true, the pathophysiological account may be met with greater skepticism, although the overarching phenomenon is described as an inflammatory process—a domain that still remains active in biological suicide research. The implicit life narratives become clearer, however, when discussion of movements and stagnations of the blood are trimmed away: A young woman who has gone through puberty and could be married remains unmarried. Then, something happens (described in the text as a closure of the vagina), resulting in a cession of menses. The woman becomes lethargic, then full of rage and terror, and then restless and suicidal. Although never mentioned, rape and/or the prospect of single motherhood seem to loom large behind this account. This impression may be reinforced by the recommended treatment—marriage and pregnancy "as quickly as possible." The efficacy of such an intervention may have lain in shifting the young woman's untenable social position to a tenable one.

Contemporary medical thought does not only tend to treat suicide as a manifestation of individual illness, however. It also tends to consider suicide as a discrete action rather than as a process. This tendency has a number of consequences.

First, it drives our attention away from altering the process in favor of halting the action. A narrow focus on halting the action rather than altering the process of which it is a part bears an uncanny resemblance to the mode of operation that may lead an individual to suicide in the first place. This is not to say that it is ineffective; our greatest successes in suicide reduction appear to have come through means restriction. Thus, halting the action may often achieve a change in the process. Failure to attend to the process, however, may, like the suicide attempter, give the future short shrift. Indeed, half of suicide deaths have followed previous attempts, and suicide rates shortly following psychiatric hospitalization are elevated by two orders of magnitude compared to those 1 year later.

Second, it tempts us to think in terms of risk calculation, tabulating factors, rather than in terms of developmental trajectory, following implications. Although it is not a logical consequence of such an approach, a psychological consequence to the risk-centric approach, reducing patients to a single metric, is a loss of appreciation for the variety of ways in which a patient might be at high risk for imminent suicide. With this is lost an ear for the gestalt of individuals viewing death as their immediate best option. These gestalts are the narrative patterns, the stories, clinicians experienced in work with suicidal patients (such as the author of the Hippocratic text on young girls, perhaps) have learned to recognize.

Stories are the tools by which we grasp processes, understand other people, and understand ourselves. Stories, like other artworks, also orchestrate emotions, elaborating names for the motions our emotions induce. In short, they may be both the most efficient descriptions of the patterns we learn to recognize in evaluating suicide risk and the keys to defusing it.

Although this book has many virtues, including comprehensive reviews of current models of suicidal behavior, clinically meaningful interpretation of actuarial and clinical risk factors for suicide, and a detailed examination of the acute states in which suicide may be imminent, perhaps its greatest value is as a detailed description of a narrative and process-oriented approach to understanding suicide. Furthermore, this approach is distinctively illuminated by its marriage to an examination of how the clinician operates within it as a diagnostic sensor and as a healer, for not only do clinicians hear the story of the patient but also they participate as characters and authors.

Zimri Yaseen

Acknowledgments

I am grateful to Oxford University Press for believing that imminent suicide risk is a topic worthy of a book and to my editors, Andrea Knobloch, Allison Pratt, and Saranyaa Moureharry, for their support throughout the writing process. Without their appreciation for the fact that no printed book has addressed the desperate need for a guide to help clinicians assess imminent suicide risk in high-risk individuals, this book would never have been written.

I thank the American Foundation for Suicide Prevention for its support of research in acute suicidal states and in short-term suicide risk. In particular, I thank Dr. Jill Harkavy-Friedman for her dedication to the cause of suicide prevention; for her generosity with her time and her ideas; for her belief in the importance of developing clinical approaches to suicide prevention; and for her grace, wit, and good humor.

This book would not have been possible without the work of my long-time collaborator Dr. Zimri Yaseen. During our many years of trying to solve the puzzle of the psychological processes that make suicide possible, I benefited greatly from Zimri's intellectual voracity, unparalleled scientific mind, and unique kindness and generosity. All the work leading to the discovery of the suicide crisis syndrome, the formulation of the narrative crisis model of suicidal behavior, and the innovative work on clinicians' emotional responses to suicidal patients has resulted from our joint research and clinical effort.

I also thank my collaborators from the Suicide Research Group and from the Richard and Cynthia Zirinsky Center for Bipolar Disorder at the Mount Sinai Beth Israel Department of Psychiatry. Their contribution to *The Suicidal Crisis* lies in many stimulating and lively discussions we have had during our research meetings and clinical work rounds. I am particularly grateful to Dr. Lisa Cohen, Irina Kopeykina, Jessica Briggs, Deimante McClure, Zhanetta Gerlovina, Shira Barzilay, Mariah Hawes, Farouz Ardalan, and HaeJoon Kim for their dedication to suicide research and their hard work on making our studies run as smoothly as they have been.

The Suicidal Crisis would not have been completed without the support and encouragement of our department chairman, Dr. Arnold Winston. Arnold's steady leadership, ability to foster collegiality, and mutual respect for his colleagues have helped me and my work and have shaped my leadership style throughout the years. I also thank our research group's many volunteers for their enthusiasm, willingness to learn, and particularly for their help with the book editing. I am most grateful to my co-authors of Chapters 3, 4, and 9—Shoshana Linzer, Adina Chesir, Tal Ginsburg, Raquel Rose, Nicolette Molina, and Olivia Varas.

I consider being a psychiatrist a great privilege, and deciding to become one was the best career decision I have ever made. Writing this book gave me an opportunity to share many aspects of my 30 years of clinical experience as an inpatient and outpatient psychiatrist. In this book, the names and identifiers of individual patients and their family members have been changed to protect their privacy. I remember all of them, and I am deeply grateful for their trust in my skill and judgment.

Finally, I thank my wife Asya for her love, kindness, and infinite patience. *The Suicidal Crisis* was written afterhours and ate mercilessly into our time together. We'll catch up, and the time was not lost, I promise.

Introduction

OUR INABILITY TO PREDICT IMMINENT SUICIDE

One of the most difficult determinations a psychiatrist makes is whether the chronically suicidal patient is at risk for imminent suicide. Although some clinicians rarely work with suicidal patients, whereas others assess them daily, all clinicians will face this challenge at least once. Hence, one of the aspirational goals of the National Alliance for Suicide Prevention's Research Prioritization Task Force is to find ways to assess who is at risk for attempting suicide in the immediate future.

Already, there has been debate regarding the terminology that should be used to refer to this high-risk period. The dictionary definition of the word "imminent" is "about to happen." It is also a legal term that, when applied to suicide risk, implies that suicide will happen so soon that immediate clinical intervention is required to prevent it. The term "risk for suicide in the immediate future" was chosen by the task force instead of "imminent risk" because the latter may imply (incorrectly) that mental health professionals have the ability to predict precisely when an impending suicidal act is going to take place (Claassen, Harvilchuck-Laurenson, & Fawcett, 2014). The more accurate terms "near-term" and "short-term" suicide risk refer to a defined time period, such as 1 month, that could be used in suicide research studies. However, these terms obscure the urgency of the life-and-death decisions made daily by frontline clinicians.

To underscore the pressure experienced by psychiatrists in their daily risk assessments, I chose to retain the term "imminent suicide risk." In this guide, it is used interchangeably with the aforementioned more research-oriented terms and with the intuitive clinical term "acute risk." In this guide, the term imminent suicide implies a time interval from the moment the patient parts with the psychiatrist until the next appointment. Imminent suicide defined in this manner implies that unless action is taken, the patient *will* attempt suicide prior to his or her next clinical visit. The length of this "imminent" time period can vary from hours for the same-day post-discharge outpatient appointment to months, as is the case for a regular outpatient visit for medication management.

Most often, however, "imminent" or "immediate future" means several days, reflecting the regular interval between care appointments post-hospital discharge or while in weekly or biweekly therapy. Regardless of the duration of this interval, however, in the eyes of the patient's loved ones, the medical profession, and the law, during this time it is the clinician who last saw the patient alive who bears the responsibility for the suicide, should it occur.

Currently, there is no guide that can help a clinician accurately evaluate the risk of imminent suicide. The scope of the problem is staggering. In 2014, 42,773 people in the United States died by suicide (Centers for Disease Control and Prevention [CDC], 2015a; McIntosh & Drapeau, 2014). It is estimated that for each completed suicide, 25 people attempt suicide and 100 people think about suicide. At the current rates, it is estimated that in 2016, 400,000 people will have attempted suicide and 4 million people will have considered it (American Foundation for Suicide Prevention [AFSP], 2016).

The 1:100 ratio of suicides completed to suicides considered means that 1.5% of the US population should be evaluated for suicide risk at some point in their lives. Indeed, in 2008, an estimated 678,000 US citizens were treated for a suicide attempt, confirming that the aforementioned official numbers may an underestimation (Claassen et al., 2014).

Whereas the suicide rate in the United States has been increasing, in other industrialized countries, such as Great Britain, suicide rates have been steadier (Office for National Statistics, 2016). In the United States, however, suicide is currently the 10th leading cause of death overall and the second leading cause of death in adolescents and young adults aged 10–34 years (AFSP, 2016; CDC, 2014). Given the scope of the problem, health professionals and even laypersons need a reliable, systematic approach to accurately identify those who are about to take actual steps toward ending their lives. If we succeed in developing such a tool, thousands of lives could be saved by timely interventions.

LONG-TERM AND IMMINENT SUICIDE RISK

Unfortunately, at present, our ability to identify those at imminent risk for suicide in emergency departments, outpatient offices, and inpatient units is close to chance (Large, Sharma, Cannon, Ryan, & Nielssen, 2011). However, although the current clinical reality may be disheartening, recent advances in the field of suicidology have resulted in new, promising approaches to assessing short-term suicide risk. One such new development is the recent attention toward the distinction between long- and short-term risk for suicide. The difference between the two was first described by Fawcett, Scheftner, and Clark (1987), who, in a prospective study, discovered that risk factors for suicide attempts in the first year were different from those in years 2–10 (Table 1).

Table 1 Long-Term Versus Short-Term Risk Factors for Suicide

Short Term (<1 Year)	Long Term (1–5 Years)
Anhedonia	Hopelessness
Panic attacks	Helplessness
Psychic anxiety	Suicidal ideation
Insomnia	Past suicide attempts
Moderate alcohol abuse	

In Fawcett et al.'s (1987) study, the well-known risk factors for suicide—depression, hopelessness, helplessness, and suicidal ideation—were associated only with eventual risk for suicidal behavior. The short-term risk factors were the anxiety-related factors: anxiety, panic attacks, insomnia, agitation, and anhedonia. The latter finding has since been confirmed by multiple epidemiological and clinical studies (Katz, Yaseen, Mojtabai, Cohen, & Galynker, 2011; Rappaport, Moskowitz, Galynker, & Yaseen, 2014; Weissman, Klerman, Markowitz, & Ouellette, 1989; Yaseen, Chartrand, Mojtabai, Bolton, & Galynker, 2013).

Another recent development in suicide research is the appreciation of the difference between risk factors and warning signs of suicide and of the need to identify the latter. Conceptually, this is based on research distinguishing risk factors and warning signs of cardiovascular disease. The ongoing Framingham study has shown that cardiovascular long-term risk factors include hypertension, obesity, diabetes, lack of exercise, and high cholesterol (Hajar, 2016). These factors predict who may have a myocardial infarction during the next decades but not tomorrow. An imminent heart attack is predicted by warning signs that reflect lack of myocardial perfusion or ischemia: crushing chest pain, shortness of breath, and diaphoresis.

The third important development in the imminent risk assessment is the growing appreciation for the "suicidal crisis syndrome"—a unique negative affective state that may precede suicide attempts. To continue the cardiovascular disease analogy, a history of mental illness and suicide attempt, depression, hopelessness, helplessness, and suicidal ideation are associated with the lifetime risk for suicidal behavior. The suicide crisis syndrome (SCS) is similar to myocardial ischemia in that warning signs of suicide resemble the signs and symptoms of unstable angina and signify short-term suicide risk. Although the suicide crisis–myocardial infarction analogy is not literal, it is a useful parallel to keep in mind when assessing imminent suicide risk.

LACK OF TESTS FOR SUICIDE PREDICTION

The suicide assessment instruments currently in use do not distinguish between long-term risk factors for eventual suicide and short-term risk factors for imminent suicide. Moreover, the majority of these scales rely on consensus opinion or on psychological autopsies and past suicide attempts, which may not be predictive of future suicidal behavior. Indeed, when tested for prediction of completed suicide and suicide attempt, these instruments were not predictive short term.

An example of a consensus-derived, widely used scale that was never validated is the SAD PERSONS scale (see Chapter 8). In a large-scale retrospective study, the SAD PERSONS scale was not predictive of suicide attempts and suicides in the immediate future (6 months) (Bolton, Spiwak, & Sareen, 2012). Another large study showed that 60% of persons who completed suicide within 1 year after psychiatric discharge were judged "low suicide risk" by this scale (Large et al., 2011).

Even the best validated instruments, such as the Beck Suicide Intent Scale, the Beck Depression Inventory, and the Beck Hopelessness Scale, are only predictive long term during a period of 5–10 years (Table 2). As a result, some of the recent opinion papers have proposed that no currently available assessment methods can predict who

Table 2 Prospective Studies Examining Suicidal Outcomes

Predictor	Studies	Attempt	Completion	Time of Follow-Up
Beck Depression Inventory (BDI)	Oquendo et al. (2004)	X	X	2 years
Beck Hopelessness Scale (BHS)	Beck, Steer, Kovacs, and Garrison (1985); Beck, Brown, and Steer (1989)		X	5–10 years
Suicide Intent Scale (SIS)	Harriss and Hawton (2005)		X	5 years
Physical Anhedonia Scale (PAS)	Loas (2007)		X	6.5 years
Implicit Association Task (IAT)	Nock et al. (2010)	X		0.5 years
SKA-2	Guintivano, Brown, and Newcomer (2014)	X		0.5 years
Suicide Trigger Scale (STS)	Yaseen et al. (2014)	X		0.5 years
Suicide Stroop	Cha, Najmi, Park, Finn, and Nock (2010)	X		0.5 years

will and who will not attempt suicide in the near future (Miller, Azrael, & Hemenway, 2006). Others have suggested that suicide attempts are inherently unpredictable (Large & Nielssen, 2012). In fact, the British Department of Health explicitly recommended against clinical use of scales designed to assess and stratify suicide risk, instead suggesting that we rely on clinical judgment.

CLINICAL APPROACH TO THE ASSESSMENT OF IMMINENT RISK

Thus, currently, imminent suicide risk assessment remains difficult, requiring a clinician to organize often disjointed bits of information into a coherent and subjective clinical opinion. In the absence of diagnostic tests, clinicians must rely on patients' truthful answers to explicit questions about their suicidal history and intent. Discouragingly, even an honest self-report of suicidal ideation can be unhelpful in risk assessment (see Chapter 6).

Research shows that of patients seen in the emergency department for a serious suicide attempt, only 39% had persistent suicidal ideation, whereas the rest had either fleeting thoughts about suicide or none at all (Paykel, Myers, Lindenthal, & Tanner, 1974). Thus, patients may not have suicidal ideation or a plan until immediately prior to their attempt. On the other hand, those who are determined to end their lives often hide their suicide intent (Horesh & Apter, 2006; Horesh, Zalsman, & Apter, 2004). Therefore, posing the question, "Have you been thinking about killing yourself" to somebody who will attempt suicide imminently is often likely to provoke a negative response.

Thus, we cannot rely on self-report of suicidal intent and must instead evaluate imminent suicide risk indirectly through the clinical history and current mental state. Parts of this assessment are empirical; others are based on the suicide theories discussed in Chapter 1. Unfortunately, like most of the assessment scales, most theories have not yet been tested by prospective studies.

The most recognized suicide risk assessment models are Beck's cognitive diathesis stress model (Wenzel & Beck, 2008) and Mann's biological vulnerability diathesis stress model (Mann & Arango, 1992). Beck's model postulates the existence of long-standing maladaptive cognitive style traits, whereas Mann's theory suggests that low levels of serotonin and norepinephrine associated with impulsivity and depression predispose people to suicidal behavior under stress. Neither model discusses the SCS or mental processes leading to the emergence of the suicidal crisis (see Chapter 1).

Some of the newer theories integrate suicide traits with acute interpersonal and psychodynamic constructs reflective of the events and mental status that often immediately precede suicide (suicide states). The most recognized of these are Thomas Joiner's (Joiner et al., 2010) interpersonal theory of suicide and Rory O'Connor's (2011) integrated motivational–volitional theory of suicide.

Joiner's theory posits that suicidal behavior requires both suicidal desire and the capability to act on that desire. Suicidal desire stems from "thwarted belongingness" and "perceived burdensomeness," whereas the capability for suicide arises through habituation to physically painful or frightening experiences (Joiner et al., 2010). The integrated motivational–volitional model of suicide incorporates elements of the stress–diathesis models of suicidality in the premotivational phase and considers the suicidal process as moving along a timeline during the motivational phase, before resulting in suicidal action (O'Connor, 2011).

O'Connor's model is valuable in that it uses the stress–diathesis model as the starting point for the development of a dynamic suicidal process leading to a suicidal behavior. This is similar to our proposed narrative crisis model of suicide, which goes a step further and postulates that the suicide narrative is a dynamic psychological process that allows for evolution of trait suicidality into SCS. To date, data suggest that the magnitude of SCS is predictive of near-term suicidal behavior (Galynker et al., 2016; also see Chapter 2). The overall imminent suicide risk is determined from three factors: trait vulnerability to suicide, the suicidal narrative, and the intensity of the suicidal crisis.

MULTIMODAL ASSESSMENTS

It may come as a surprise that the "in-depth" psychiatric interview may not be the best method of gathering information. According to information theory, when trying to identify a signal over noise, combining information from several independent sources is more powerful than collecting extensive information from a single source (Battauz, Bellio, & Gori, 2007). In psychiatry, the signal is usually a clinical diagnosis, and the noise is symptoms or signs that may or may not be descriptive of the illness being diagnosed.

In simple clinical cases, the signal is so strong that even nonspecialists can see the diagnosis. For example, almost anyone can diagnose a severe psychotic episode in somebody with a known history of schizophrenia or a recent suicide by a self-inflicted gunshot wound when the victim left a suicide note. However, most clinical cases are complicated, and the low signal-to-noise ratio requires much investigative work before definitive diagnosis is reached.

The SCS signal, even when relatively strong, can be difficult to distinguish from the signal of the mental state that leads to a dangerous but nonfatal suicide attempt or gesture. This is because all three conditions often include slightly different mixtures of despair, anxiety, anhedonia, and hopelessness. These are difficult to distinguish when the patient is forthcoming, but they are even more difficult to distinguish when intentionally concealed by a suicidal person (Horesh & Apter, 2006; Horesh et al., 2004). The risk of suicide is further obscured by the dynamic nature of many contributing factors: the presence (or lack) of a specific plan, new hopes or failures at work, or personal and romantic rejections. The resulting tangle of events and intentions makes it difficult for even the most well-trained clinician to decipher.

The signal of imminent suicide is even more difficult to detect than the signal of suicide crisis. This necessitates a modular approach beyond patients' self-reports of their mental state and clinical history, which includes several independent lines of inquiry. In the United States, more than 41,000 people die by suicide each year; therefore, accurate diagnosis of imminent suicide is literally a matter of life and death (CDC, 2015a). If the correct clinical interventions follow the correct diagnosis, hundreds, if not thousands, of lives would be saved.

ONE-INFORMANT VERSUS MULTI-INFORMANT ASSESSMENTS

The natural choice for an independent source of information is another informant. In an emergency room, this is most often a close family member or friend. Indeed, obtaining collateral information about a patient's past history and mental state is an essential part of a clinical assessment. Only recently, however, have researchers realized that this multi-informant evaluation also opens another dimension of clinical evaluation. Not only may the opinions of other independent informants be less subjective than the patient's opinion but also they are subject to informative systematic biases of their own (Reyes, Henry, Tolan, & Wakschlag, 2009).

For example, in a multi-informant study of depression and suicidality in adolescents (Lewis et al., 2014), parents' proxy reporting of adolescent depression and suicidal indices was only weakly correlated with their children's reports. Parents tended to overreport their adolescents' depressive symptoms while underreporting both their suicidal thoughts and behavior.

However, obtaining this collateral information does have challenges, such as obtaining the patient's consent to speak to other informants. The Health Insurance Portability and Accountability Act (HIPAA), although essential for protection of private information, requires separate consents for each informant; a suicidal patient may be unwilling or unable to sign the form(s). Although this law may be bypassed if the clinician believes that the collateral information would be life-saving, this subjective clinical judgment may open the clinician up to potential legal action. Legal considerations frequently present a barrier to a multi-informant patient assessment, even when assessing something as important as acute suicidal risk.

Unfortunately, even multi-informant assessment does not guarantee accuracy in the diagnosis of SCS. Suicide risk assessment is difficult even for trained professionals, and laypeople often miss or misinterpret signs of impending suicide. Survivors of those who commit suicide often state that they had no idea that their loved one was acutely suicidal. Newspaper coverage of suicides by celebrities is full of statements such as "I saw him/her the day before and he/she was laughing as usual." A close friend of model Ruslana Korshunova described their last meeting several hours before Korshunova leaped to her death off the roof of her apartment building in Manhattan as follows (Pomerantsev, 2014):

> We had dinned in Manhattan, at our favorite bistro. We were planning for her to maybe come to Paris in a few days' time. Later that night I took a plane to Paris for a shoot. She texted me when I landed—to see if I had arrived OK . . . and then a few hours later . . . a few hours later I saw on the news she was dead. (p. 144)

Fortunately, many of these limitations do not apply when the independent informants are evaluating clinicians. Indeed, the work of Des Los Reyes and team suggests that in addition to suicidal patients' significant others, the multi-informant approach should also include their clinicians (Reyes, Thomas, Goodman, & Kundey, 2013). This statement may sound paradoxical: Aren't we, the assessing clinicians, already providing another informant's professional opinion on the patient's suicide risk? This is true, but clinicians' professional reports by definition omit their personal opinion about the patient being evaluated. The former is the conclusion reached in accordance with professional training guidelines, whereas the latter is an opinion or a "gut feeling." This personal judgment may be quite different from clinician's objective, fact-based report of suicide risk.

In particular, discrepancies between clinicians' objective assessment and their subjective opinion are often seen in the inpatient setting, prior to discharge of patients admitted for danger to self. In the United States, criteria for psychiatric admission are centered not on severity of psychiatric illness per se but, rather, on the patient's dangerousness to self or to community. Therefore, to be discharged, the patient needs only to be deemed "not dangerous to self and/or others."

For clinicians to feel safe discharging a recently suicidal patient, the latter must deny suicidal intent and must be in control of his or her behavior. This means that during the hospitalization, there must not be suicide attempts or aggressive behavior toward others, and the patient must participate in the unit activities at a level commensurate with his or her illness severity. In most cases, such objective signs of patient improvement are listed in institutional discharge polices, and they make clinicians and hospital administrators feel secure about their discharge plan.

However, even when these criteria are met, a clinician may often feel deep unease and anxiety. Such responses may be reflective of the patient's risk for imminent suicide. Our emotional reactions to suicidal patients can differentiate suicide attempters from ideators and need to be considered as independent and valuable data to be included in a decision-making algorithm.

HOW TO USE *THE SUICIDAL CRISIS*

The Suicidal Crisis: Clinical Guide to the Assessment of Imminent Suicide Risk describes a framework for a systematic and comprehensive assessment of risk for imminent suicide. The guide is designed as a textbook, a reference guide, and a reader.

In an academic setting, the guide can be used as a comprehensive textbook for a dedicated course on the recognition, prevention, and treatment of imminent suicidal behavior. It can also be used as one of the textbooks in broader courses on psychopathology or in specialized seminars on emergency medicine and suicidology. Finally, the guide can be used as an off-the-shelf reference book for mental health professional trainees: psychiatry residents, psychology interns, social workers, and others.

Outside the classroom, the guide can be an educational reader for any clinician wanting to learn how to assess imminent risk for suicide. Whether on the acute psychiatric inpatient unit, a medical/surgical floor, an outpatient clinic, or a private psychiatrist's office, the guide provides interested clinicians with a framework of inquiry into a suicidal state. *Suicidal Narrative* contains more than 50 concise or extended case vignettes illustrating specific aspects of risk-related clinical material, which may be useful when encountering a new and difficult clinical situation.

The guide contains detailed risk assessment interviews, which readers can use as templates for their real-life evaluations. Each aspect of the narrative crisis model is discussed in a separate chapter under a descriptive heading and/or subheading, making finding an answer to a specific clinical question relatively easy. Specifically, the guide contains detailed discussions of each trait vulnerability, each component of the suicidal narrative, and each symptom of SCS.

The examples of risk assessment interviews in Chapters 5–7, which are devoted to specific levels of risk, conclude with summary risk assessment tables. These are intended to help the reader organize the clinical information obtained in the course of each interview and to gauge the degree of suicide risk. The tables are not meant as categorical risk stratification instruments, and to underscore the illustrative and educational purpose of the tables, the complete assessment interviews in Chapter 8 do not include them, encouraging readers to use their clinical judgment as they would in real life.

Chapters 5 and 6 also include "test" interviews and the summary risk assessment table shells to be used for self-assessment; the answer keys are listed at the end of the guide. After reading each chapter and doing the test cases, the reader should have sufficient mastery of the material and a "gestalt" memory of representative cases to make confident clinical judgments in real life. In addition to the test cases, the reader can use the individual case vignettes to practice risk assessment and also to examine his or her own emotional reaction to particular types of suicidal patients.

It cannot be overemphasized that this book is a *guide* to clinical decision-making and not a risk assessment and stratification tool with a training manual. The book does not include a questionnaire to be scored and used to determine an objective level of suicide risk that should automatically trigger a particular action by a clinician (i.e., a hospitalization). Several scales are currently being tested in clinical trials and, it is hoped, will have clinical use in the near future.

A ROADMAP FOR COMPREHENSIVE ASSESSMENT

Suicide is a very complex behavior, which results from a dynamic interplay of trait vulnerabilities, societal factors, cultural trends, stressful life events, the propensity to view one's life as a suicidal narrative, and the acuity of the suicide crisis syndrome. Studying this guide, understanding the narrative crisis model, and doing the test cases should give clinicians the framework for conducting imminent suicide risk assessment with confidence. Following the guide ensures that *all* relevant information, which could be obtained during a clinical interview, was indeed obtained and analyzed appropriately. Regardless of the clinician's risk assessment skills, some suicidal patients will not cooperate with an interview, leaving the clinician perplexed. Finding similarities between the vignettes and real-life cases could help connect the dots when assessing a patient's suicidal narrative or SCS and clarify the case.

Because of its focus on risk assessment, *The Suicidal Crisis* does not include treatment recommendations. Several excellent books are currently available with explicit instructions on how to care for, treat, and, it is hoped, save a person in acute suicidal crisis (Jobes, 2016; Rudd, 2006).

However, books on treatment of acutely suicidal individuals are only useful once clinicians are able to identify those who are at imminent suicide risk. Currently, with very rare exceptions, imminent risk determination is primarily based on the answer to the question, "Are you planning to kill yourself?" As discussed previously and in Chapter 6, the answer to this question is often either inaccurate or intentionally misleading. *The Suicidal Crisis* is intended to help clinicians conduct such identifications with accuracy and confidence in their own assessment skills.

1

Psychological Models of Suicide

With Shira Barzilay and Abbie Cohen

INTRODUCTION

Suicide is a complex set of behaviors that originate from the interplay of biological, psychological, social, and other unknown factors. Suicide is also an endpoint of psychological processes that evolve over time and are poorly understood. A comprehensive model of suicidal processes and behavior is essential for the assessment of imminent risk for suicide and for designing informed interventions.

During the past several decades, researchers have formulated a number of models of suicidal behavior. The early psychodynamic models (Baumeister & Leary, 1995; Shneidman, 1993) were based on clinicians' individual experiences. More recent first-generation models of suicide (Claassen, Harvilchuck-Laurenson, & Fawcett, 2014) went a step further by gaining credibility through consensus opinion and clinical judgment. Although attractive conceptually, these models were never tested experimentally in predicting suicide (Litman, Curphey, Shneidman, Farberow, & Tabachnik, 1963).

Second-generation prognostic models hypothesized that suicide risk was determined by measurable biological and clinical risk factors. These factors were static and long term, and they included biomarkers (i.e., serotonin levels), demographic factors (sex, age, and occupation), clinical factors (diagnosis of mental illness and prior suicide attempt), as well as standardized measures of psychopathology (Hamilton Depression Rating Scale [HAM-D] scores). These models were tested for predictive value and were modestly successful in identifying individuals at long-term suicide risk; however, they were not predictive of imminent suicidal behavior (Pokorny, 1983).

Third-generation models of suicidal behavior focused on *dynamic* risk elements, which appear later in life, change over time, and are operational immediately proximal to suicide. Some of these factors may refer to social stressors, whereas others may describe mental processes or the state of mind of acutely suicidal persons. Some of these models incorporate the second-generation static risk factors (O'Connor, 2011). Aspects of the third-generation models have recently been tested experimentally with encouraging results, but none have yet been reproduced (Dhingra, Boduszek, & O'Connor, 2016). This chapter describes several influential theories of suicidal behavior and provides an assessment of their strengths and limitations.

HISTORICAL PERSPECTIVE

The first theories of suicide originated in psychoanalysis and were formulated by Freud (1922) in his influential work, *Beyond the Pleasure Principle*. Freud posited that life and death drives were opposing basic instincts. The aim of the life drive was to overcome the conflicts associated with survival; the purpose of the death drive was to eliminate the conflicts of life itself. Freud hypothesized that the desire to kill oneself was derived from an earlier repressed desire to destroy others. According to Freud, suicide represented an internalization of this process and a transformation of the external death wish into an internal one.

In 1938, Menninger took Freud's death wish a step further by claiming that every suicide is an inverted homicide. He theorized the existence of a suicidal triad composed of the wish to kill (murder), the wish to be killed (guilt), and the wish to die (depression). Menninger believed that the wish to kill is originally oriented to external objects that are not acceptable for the ego (i.e., loved ones), leading to feelings of guilt. As a result of ego destruction by guilt and self-loathing, depression and hopelessness ensue, leading to the wish to die as punishment for thoughts of killing others. Klein (1935, 1946) further developed this concept and hypothesized that suicide is the result of an unbearable guilt over aggressive fantasies toward internalized objects of envy. As the guilt causes feelings of malice, suicide becomes self-destructive to prevent destructiveness toward others.

The previously discussed psychoanalytical approaches were intuitive rather than experimental and viewed suicide as a philosophical and moral dilemma rather than psychopathology (i.e., psychosis or depression). At that time, society agreed with this view. The work of early psychoanalysts created momentum for a transformation of suicide from a spiritual problem to a manifestation of a psychiatric disorder (Ellis, 2001).

A serious flaw in psychoanalytic theories is that they are nearly impossible to test experimentally. The few studies that attempted to do so obtained mixed results. Baumeister and Scher (1988) studied the concept of self-destructiveness as a biological drive intended to harm the self as punishment for tolerating the disliked part of the self. No experimental evidence was found.

Related to the inherent self-destructiveness concept are the ideas of Apter, Plutchik, and van Praag (1993) and others who hypothesized that suicide is aggression turned inward (Maiuro, O'Sullivan, Michael, & Vitaliano, 1989). To support this, Orbach (1996, 2003a) demonstrated that the relationship between early insecure attachment and suicidal behavior was mediated by negative attitudes toward the body. Maltsberger (2004) found evidence for a psychodynamic explanation of suicide in psychological autopsies of suicide decedents. All these researchers' conclusions, however, were based on descriptions rather than statistical analyses.

SHNEIDMAN'S THEORY OF PSYCHACHE

Shneidman's theory posited that suicide is caused by "psychache" (Shneidman, 1993, p. 51), an intolerable emotional pain for which individuals cannot find relief in any other solution but death. Shneidman postulated two types of individual needs: primary, or biological needs of survival, and secondary, or psychological needs of fulfillment. When the psychological needs, such as love and belonging, positive self-image, and meaningful relationships, are frustrated by career failures, romantic rejections, and losses, psychache develops. In his view, suicide occurs as a means of fulfilling a specific psychodynamic need. Although stemming from psychache, suicide is not only an escape from pain but also an attempt to achieve a goal or fulfill a fantasy, such as impressing a loved one, achieving fame, or gaining love (Figure 1.1).

Shneidman's ideas are at the core of many contemporary models (Jobes & Nelson, 2006), and his conceptualization of suicide as a problem solvent (Shneidman, 1993) influenced other psychological theories of suicide, most notably the escape theory (Baumeister, 1990) and the cry of pain model (Williams, 1997). The theory has received some experimental support in relating psychache to suicidal ideation and past attempts (Troister & Holden, 2010).

However, to date, there has been no research on what defines psychological pain and what cognitive and emotional processes characterize psychache. Furthermore, psychache, depression, and hopelessness are strongly intercorrelated ($r = \sim.80$) (Troister & Holden, 2012) and may or may not be independent. Moreover, the mechanism by which psychache interacts with other risk factors to trigger suicide has not been explored, nor has whether psychache is related to short-term suicide risk or to imminent suicidal behavior.

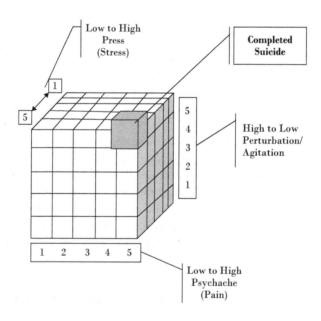

Figure 1.1 Theory of psychache.
Source: Schneidman (1993).

SUICIDE AS ESCAPE FROM SELF

Another psychodynamic model that had a significant influence on the field of suicidology was Baumeister's (1990) concept of suicide as an escape from self. Baumeister noted that escape from an aversive life situation and relief from unbearable mental anguish were the most common goals reported by suicide attempters. He suggested that there are six steps to the suicidal process. The process begins when unrealistically high expectations are created, setting up an objective failure to meet those expectations. Next, the individual interprets the objective failure as a personal defeat. Third, a negative cognitive bias ensues that brings on a distorted and unforgiving comparison of the self with an idealized and unrealizable success. The fourth step is the resulting uncontrolled escalation of emotional pain, which, in the fifth step, brings numbness and cognitive deconstruction. Baumeister hypothesized that in the final step, cognitive deconstruction results in behavioral disinhibition, which allows one to overcome the fear of causing oneself pain through death and to end one's life by suicide.

Baumeister's theory does not consider suicide a self-execution and punishment, nor does it suppose psychodynamic explanations but, rather, views suicide as an escape from unbearable psychological pain. His other assumption is that negative suicidal emotions are experienced as an acute state rather than a prolonged one. Baumeister's theory is consistent with Shneidman's (1993) conceptualization of suicide as an escape from mental pain. The two theories share the concept that self-destructive behaviors are rooted in cognitive distortion.

The escape from self theory found some indirect experimental support (O'Connor & O'Connor, 2003) in that a major disappointment in oneself plays a role in precipitating suicidal behavior (DeWall, Baumeister, & Vohs, 2008). However, there has been no direct evidence linking Baumeister's theory of imminent suicidal behavior with short-term suicide risk. Although the six-stage model is attractive, there has been no research on when and how suicidal thoughts and behaviors emerge and transition from one step to the next, culminating in suicide. Still, the escape theory is compelling, and it has influenced other theoreticians and researchers, including Williams (1997), O'Connor (2011), and the author of this guide.

THE SUICIDE CRISIS SYNDROME

In his seminal work, which differentiated long-term and short-term suicide risk factors, Fawcett (2006) indicated that before a serious suicide attempt, individuals often experience increased anxiety and agitation—a combination of symptoms termed "psychic pain" (Fawcett et al., 1990). This parallels Baumeister's concept of suicide as an acute process and is also similar to Shneidman's construct of psychache and to Hendin's (2001) construct of a "suicide crisis"—an acute, high-intensity, negative affect state that may serve as a trigger for a suicide attempt (Hendin, Maltsberger, Haas, Szanto, & Rabinowicz, 2004) (Figure 1.2).

Building on the work of these theoreticians and researchers, Galynker and Yaseen hypothesized that before attempting suicide, suicidal individuals enter a state of cognitive

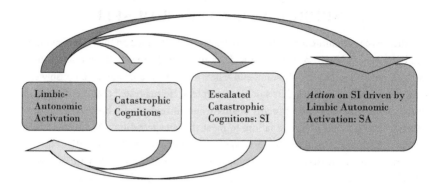

Figure 1.2 Positive feedback model for suicide.

and affective dysregulation, or the acute suicide crisis syndrome (SCS), initially termed the suicide trigger state. The researchers then attempted to establish the exact emotions that constitute SCS and whether it overlaps with the constructs of psychological pain and psychache.

Galynker and Yaseen showed that SCS includes three factors: frantic hopelessness (FH), an affective state of entrapment, dread, and hopelessness; ruminative flooding (RF), a cognitive state of incessant rumination and a sense of one's head bursting with uncontrollable thoughts; and near-psychotic somatization (NPS), a state of strange somatic experiences in the context of severe anxiety and panic (Yaseen et al., 2010, 2014; Yaseen, Gilmer, Modi, Cohen, & Galynker, 2012). Galynker and Yaseen showed that SCS intensity correlated with current and past suicidal ideation and behavior. Moreover, in high-risk psychiatric inpatients, it was also associated with future post-discharge suicidal behavior in the near term (Yaseen et al., 2012). This finding has since been replicated (Yaseen et al., 2014; Galynker et al., 2016), and to date, Galynker and Yaseen's SCS model is the only model that is predictive of imminent suicidal behavior.

Of the symptoms comprising SCS, FH/entrapment is associated with depression and anxiety but, as in Hendin's (Hendin, Maltsberger, & Szanto, 2007) "suicide crisis," differs from simple anxiety and depression by its sense of urgency. For example, one study participant described this sense as "being trapped inside an empty department store after hours and trying to get out, but all the doors are locked." This highlights the nature of FH as a heightened fear response to a perception of being in a dead end with no good options.

The next SCS component, RF, is characterized by an onslaught of automatic and affectively charged negative thoughts, and it is similar to the constructs of ruminations and rigidity proposed by the fluid vulnerability and integrated motivational–volitional (IMV) theories (discussed later). Unlike simple ruminations, RF includes significant negativistic cognitive distortions and paranoia. The nihilistic thought content intrinsic to RF echoes Nock and Kazdin's (2002) finding that negative automatic thoughts are significantly associated with suicidal ideation, suicidal intent, and current suicide attempt. Another distinguishing feature of RF is that it is associated with headaches or head pressure—migraine-like somatic symptoms that confer increased risk of suicidal ideation and coincide with past suicide attempts (Wang, Fuh, Juang, & Lu, 2009).

Near-psychotic somatization is characterized by the experience of somatic symptoms commonly associated with a panic-like dissociative state, such as unfamiliar sensations felt all over the body, especially involving the skin. The inclusion of NPS in SCS is consistent with reports that have linked increased risk for suicide with affectively intense panic attacks (Katz, Yaseen, Mojtabai, Cohen, & Galynker, 2011; Weissman, Klerman, Markowitz, & Ouellette, 1989).

Further exploring the role of panic in SCS, Galynker and Yaseen demonstrated that in depressed individuals with panic attacks, RF-like "catastrophic cognitions"—that is, fear of dying, fear of losing control, or fear of being otherwise irreversibly trapped—were most strongly associated with *past* suicide attempts. Dissociation, trembling, choking, and chest pain were most strongly associated with suicidal ideation. Moreover, only panic attacks with fear of dying were predictive of *future* suicide attempts (Yaseen et al., 2013).

Expanding on Barlow's work on the role of somatic arousal in post-traumatic stress disorder, Galynker and Yaseen proposed that suicidal behavior involves a feedback mechanism between physiologic arousal symptoms and catastrophic ruminative cognitions. Symptoms of a panic attack feed suicidal preoccupation and vice versa in a positive feedback loop between negative cognitions and autonomic–limbic arousal (Katz et al., 2011). According to this model, the emergence of fear of dying in panic attacks may indicate a susceptibility to suicide-related morbid ruminations, such as thoughts of "having no way out." The combination of high arousal and suicidal ideation may drive the transition to suicide attempt. This model is consistent with Deisenhammer et al.'s (2009) finding that the average interval between suicidal ideation and attempt is a mere 10 minutes.

In their most recent work, Galynker and Yaseen showed that in high-risk psychiatric inpatients, fear of dying during panic attacks was predictive of imminent suicidal behavior (Yaseen et al., 2014). According to the authors, another factor of SCS leading to imminent suicidal behavior is the symptom of "emotional pain," which is strongly correlated with anxiety, depression, and the other four factors. However, among all SCS factors, FH/entrapment is most strongly associated with imminent suicidal behavior.

In summary, Galynker and Yaseen proposed and demonstrated the existence of the affective–cognitive suicide crisis syndrome, which describes the mental state of imminently suicidal individuals. To date, SCS severity as measured by Galynker and Yaseen's Suicide Crisis Inventory (SCI) appears to be the most predictive of imminent suicidal behavior. In high-risk psychiatric inpatients, SCS severity as measured by the SCI predicts near-term suicidal behavior within 4–6 weeks after discharge. The strength of the SCS model is its potential clinical utility in assessing imminent risk. Its main drawback is that it focuses on the intensity of SCS exclusively and does not reflect on how trait vulnerability to suicide or recent stressful life events may lead to its emergence.

THE CRY OF PAIN/ARRESTED FLIGHT MODEL

Williams (1997) posited that suicide results from a feeling of defeat in response to humiliation or rejection, which in turn leads to a perception of entrapment. When the latter is combined with a failure to find alternative ways to solve the problem (i.e., cognitive rigidity; Schotte & Clum, 1987), a suicidal person may see no exit out of perceived entrapment but suicide. This model draws upon the concept of arrested flight reported in animal behavior, which has been suggested to account for depression in humans (Gilbert & Allan, 1998). Pollock and Williams (1998, 2001) suggested that when individuals perceive their attempts at solving problems to be unsuccessful, they feel powerless to escape the situation (Figure 1.3).

Specifically, Williams and Pollock's (2001) intuitively titled "cry of pain" or "arrested flight" model of suicidality posits that major alterations in the domains attention, memory, and judgment are related to three components of suicidal behavior: hypersensitivity to signals of defeat, perception of being trapped, and perception of no rescue from the situation.

With regard to hypersensitivity to signals of defeat, Williams and Pollock (2001) argue that depression is a form of yielding behavior that is observed in animals, specifically birds, in the context of ritual agonistic behavior. This analogy can be viewed as a simplified model of human struggles for power and control. Williams and Pollock hypothesize that once defeat or "loser status" is triggered, there is an attentional bias toward signals of defeat. Using the emotional Stroop task, they showed that suicidal individuals had an attentional bias toward words associated with rejection or defeat.

Much like Schotte and Clum (1987), Williams and Pollock (2001) point out impaired problem solving in suicidal individuals, but they argue that the key feature is not the deficit in problem solving itself but, rather, the feeling of being trapped, which arises as a result of this deficit. They argue that suicidal individuals' problem-solving abilities are impaired due to alterations in their memory retrieval. It was observed that when asked to recall a happy time, suicidal patients responded with overgeneralized responses such as "when people give me presents." Williams and Pollock postulate that these patients have "stopped short" of specific memory retrieval in an effort to regulate emotional responses

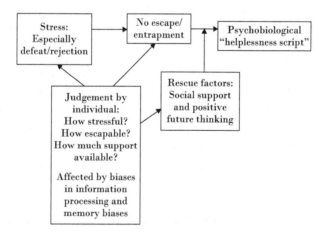

Figure 1.3 The cry of pain model.
Source: Adapted from Williams (2001).

to traumatic memories. This is problematic because specific memories provide more associations, which one can use in any given situation to create varied solutions.

Finally, Williams and Pollock (2001) argue that a crucial factor in suicidality is the lack of rescue. They found that suicidal individuals did not anticipate a greater number of negative lifetime events than controls but, rather, anticipated significantly fewer positive events. Without the anticipation of positive events, hopelessness, a final component of suicidality, sets in.

Although this model incorporates empiric observations of the cognitive processes of suicidal individuals—specifically in terms of memory and attention—the premise of social defeat flattens the human experience into simplistic antagonistic relationships. This model does not account for the possibility of social rescue factors, and modern models of animal behavior that take into account the complexities of interactions aimed at group cohesiveness and survival (Warburton & Lazarus, 1991).

COGNITIVE VULNERABILITY MODEL

Schotte and Clum (1987) propose a stress–diathesis model of suicidality in which cognitive rigidity accounts for the relationship between stress and suicidal behavior. In lay terms, when faced with a difficult life problem, such patients tend to perceive it as impenetrable and are too rigid in their thinking to imagine a viable alternative.

To test this hypothesis, Schotte and Clum (1987) compared 50 psychiatric inpatients who met the criteria of suicidality to 50 subjects who did not. Both groups were given an assessment of interpersonal problem solving, in which participants were presented with situations and desired outcomes and asked to complete the middle of a story to achieve a stated goal (alternative uses test). They were also asked to list problems that led to their hospitalization and generate possible alternative solutions to the problems and to then rate the probability of success of each alternative (modified means-end problem solving [MEPS] test).

Schotte and Clum (1987) found suicidality to positively correlate with life stress, hopelessness, and poor problem-solving skills, but not with depression. On assessments of problem solving, suicidal patients generated 60% fewer options on the alternative uses test compared to nonsuicidal controls, and suicidal patients generated fewer than half as many potential solutions on the modified MEPS. Suicidal subjects anticipated more negative consequences from the possible solutions they generated, and they generated more irrelevant solutions than their nonsuicidal cohorts.

Schotte and Clum (1987) used their study to argue that cognitive rigidity is a key moderator between life stress and suicidal ideation. The implication is that cognitive rigidity forms the diathesis of the stress–diathesis model, setting the stage for suicidal ideation when an individual has difficulty finding solutions to problems. Of note, the authors acknowledged that problem-solving deficits might be state dependent—activated by significant life stress, rather than an intrinsic trait—and proposed further examination of cognitive rigidity over time.

Although this model is elegant in its simplicity and in drawing attention to the cognitive aspect of suicidal behavior, it is limited in its focus on problem-solving ability, thus restricting possible interventions.

FLUID VULNERABILITY MODEL

To explain the suicidal process, Rudd (2006) proposed the fluid vulnerability theory, which assumes that suicidal episodes are time-limited and triggered by factors that change over time and with an individual's mental state. Rudd posited that each person has a set baseline vulnerability to suicide with three main contributing factors: cognitive susceptibility (attentional bias and inability to recall specific memories), biological susceptibility (physiological or major psychiatric symptoms [i.e., psychosis]), and behavioral susceptibility (deficient interpersonal skills and impaired affect regulation). According to this theory, long-term suicide risk is determined by the magnitude of the susceptibility factors (Figure 1.4).

The near-term risk is determined by the presence of constellations of internal and external stimuli, interpreted by an individual through cognitive, emotional, behavioral, and other themes, forming a "suicide mode." The main cognitive themes that can activate the suicide mode are the notion of being unloved, the thought that one is a burden to others, and feelings of helplessness. The constellation of unique themes that comprise a particular person's suicide mode recur and may define that person's vulnerability to a suicide crisis and the probable triggers.

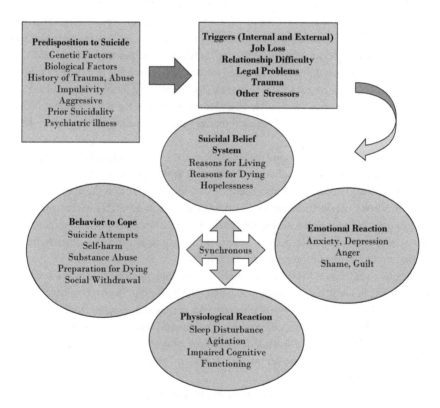

Figure 1.4 The fluid vulnerability model.
Source: Rudd (2016).

Repeated activation of a suicide mode lowers the threshold for future activation, creating a unique vulnerability. Similar to Beck (1996), Rudd, Rajab, and Dahm (1994) suggested that the suicide mode is a combination of a suicidal belief system, physiological–affective symptoms, and associated behaviors and motivations. According to the theory, individuals with a sensitized suicidal belief system will have recurrent crises, with each crisis building vulnerability for future ones.

The fluid vulnerability theory is supported by studies suggesting that rumination (Surrence, Miranda, Marroquín, & Chan, 2009) and cognitive inflexibility (Miranda, Gallagher, Bauchner, Vaysman, & Marroquín, 2012) are predictive of suicidal ideation. Barzilay and Apter (2014) suggested that this model best combines acute risk factors, primarily current suicidal ideation, and chronic risk factors. The theory, however, is vague about the triggers of suicidal behavior, and the hypothesis that cognitive vulnerabilities increase suicide risk has not been tested prospectively.

BECK'S DIATHESIS–STRESS MODEL

Behavioral theorists Wenzel and Beck (2008) proposed a cognitive model of suicidal behavior based on attempts to distinguish long-term and short-term suicide risk by separating dispositional vulnerability factors (diathesis) and distorted cognitive processes that characterize the suicide crisis. If suicide diathesis is present, life stress can activate a maladaptive cognitive response, with increased attention paid to suicide-related stimuli. This distorted cognition narrows attention on the suicidal act and creates a scenario in which suicide appears to be the only solution.

The dispositional vulnerability factors postulated by Beck's model are long-standing stress vulnerability factors (traits), which are not specific for suicide but make one susceptible to suicide crises even with low levels of stress. Beck defined five main dispositional vulnerability factors: impulsivity, deficits in problem solving, an overgeneral memory style, a maladaptive cognitive style, and personality (Figure 1.5).

Beck distinguishes between two types of *impulsivity*: lack of planning versus failure to inhibit responses, the latter being more prominent in suicidal patients. Beck is in agreement with Brent and Mann (2005, 2006), who report that impulsive aggression is heritable, making it more likely that an individual will act on suicidal thoughts. Although evidence is mixed regarding the way that *problem-solving* deficits may mediate suicidal behavior, Beck notes that suicidal patients generate fewer possible solutions to problems, and he posits that cognitive rigidity may prompt feelings of hopelessness in high-stress situations.

Beck also agrees with Williams et al. (2007) that an *overgeneral memory* exacerbates hopelessness because individuals have difficulty judging specific situations and perceive no escape from their distress. Beck notes a trait-like *maladaptive cognitive style*, characterized by cognitive distortions including "black and white" thinking and jumping to conclusions, which form a chronic pattern of thought and exacerbate stressors. Finally, he notes that a great deal of literature has examined *personality* traits among suicidal individuals, including perfectionism and socially prescribed perfectionism, defined as an interpersonal dimension involving perceptions of one's need and ability to meet the standards and expectations imposed by others (Hewitt, Flett, Sherry, & Caelian, 2006).

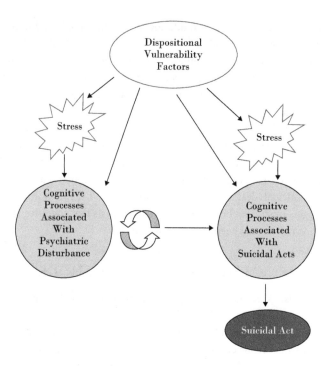

Figure 1.5 Diathesis–stress model.
Source: Wenzel and Beck (2008).

Other personality traits related to suicidal risk were psychoticism, introversion, self-criticalness, novelty seeking, harm avoidance, cynicism, sensitivity, dependency, and the decreased tendency to be warm and experience positive emotions.

In the context of vulnerability factors, stress activates maladaptive cognitive processes, including more generalized cognitive processes associated with psychiatric disturbances and specific cognitive processes associated with suicidal acts. According to Beck's (2005, p. 953) cognitive model, "the processing of external events or internal stimuli is biased and therefore systematically distorts the individual's construction of his or her experiences, leading to a variety of cognitive errors."

Information is processed according to an individual's schema, defined as "relatively enduring internal structures" used to organize new information, or as a highly ingrained "lens" through which one views the world. For example, a depressive schema contains negative attitudes about loss and failure. Depressed individuals will place greater emphasis on processing negative than positive information. Beck asserts that hopelessness may form the core of a suicide schema, noting evidence that patients with recent suicide attempts showed attentional biases toward suicide-related stimuli (Becker, Strohbach, & Rinck, 1999). Beck posits that this attention to suicide-related stimuli encourages a suicidal crisis when an individual is experiencing hopelessness, and it creates difficulty disengaging from these stimuli and thoughts.

There is evidence that patients describe cognitive disorientation, racing thoughts, acute restlessness, and "tunnel vision" during a suicide crisis. Beck describes these phenomena as *attentional fixation*, or narrowing on suicide as a solution. In the context of hopelessness, he proposes that attentional fixation can lead to a downward spiral in which suicide is identified as the only solution to one's problems.

Beck suggests that cognitive–behavioral therapy (CBT) interventions can be used to modify dispositional factors, cognitive processes, and a suicide schema. Treatment occurs in phases. The emphasis in the *early phase* is placed on engaging patients in treatment and conveying a sense of hope, particularly because patients may feel hopeless about the perceived treatment benefits. Clinicians perform a risk assessment and create a safety plan including identifying crisis signs, examining coping strategies, and creating a list of contacts to whom the patient can turn for support. One technique targets overgeneral memories by creating a "hope kit"—a memory aid that includes meaningful texts and objects that can anchor the patient in times of crisis. In the *intermediate phase*, the clinician helps the patient develop cognitive and behavioral strategies to manage suicidal ideation. In the *late phase*, they prepare for termination of treatment, including a relapse prevention protocol in which the patient is led through guided imagery to revisit the suicide crisis and identify learned coping strategies that reduce distress.

In summary, Beck's diathesis–stress model posits that long-standing chronic vulnerabilities can amplify the impact of life stressors. These stressors are then processed and distorted by a patient's maladaptive schema, leading to a fixation on suicide in which a patient's cognition is biased toward suicide-associated stimuli. Therefore, overwhelmed by suicidal thoughts, suicide appears to become an attractive solution to stressors. Beck's theory is strong in its attention to how life story influences the suicidal crisis and its suggested interventions through CBT. Its main drawback is its insufficient attention to the emotional side of the suicidal crisis.

MANN'S STRESS–DIATHESIS MODEL

The stress–diathesis clinical model suggested by Mann's team (Mann et al., 2005) is similar to Beck's model (Wenzel & Beck, 2008) in that it suggests that life stressors lead to suicide only when combined with vulnerability. Mann broadly defines stressors as either psychiatric illness or psychosocial factors, while positing that diathesis lies in low levels of serotonin and norepinephrine. The model is based on the clinical phenomenon of impulsive aggression, which is a propensity to react impulsively to frustrations with anger and aggression (Apter et al., 1991) (Figure 1.6).

The common feature of suicidal behavior, impulsive aggression, is a mediator between psychopathology and suicidal actions, and it is subserved by low serotonergic activity. Brent and Mann (2006) proposed that the vulnerability to suicidal behavior is biological with a strong familial component, both genetic and environmental. The genetic component is rooted in parental mood disorder and/or impulsivity and aggression, whereas childhood abuse and neglect add the environmental component.

The stress–diathesis model has generated voluminous research on the neurochemical and neuroanatomical pathways underlying both the diathesis and the stress-activated susceptibility to suicidal behavior (Mann et al., 2009). Many studies suggest a link between impulsivity and suicide (Mann, Waternaux, Haas, & Malone, 1999) as well as

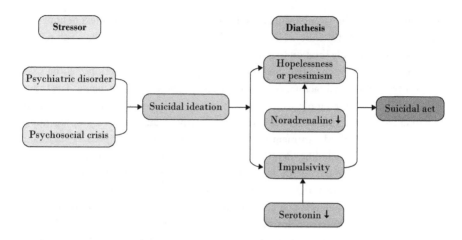

Figure 1.6 Stress–diathesis model.
Source: Mann & Arango, 1992.

evidence that impulsive suicide is more common among young attempters and completers (Brent & Mann, 2005, 2006).

The theory, however, does not explain suicidal behavior, and other studies did not find a significant association between impulsivity and suicidal behavior (Horesh, 2001). Witte et al. (2008) reported that less than one-fourth of attempters did so without planning, consistent with the view that suicide is not necessarily an impulsive act. Furthermore, patients who made impulsive suicide attempts appeared to have the same level of impulsivity as patients who had planned their attempts (Baca-Garcia et al., 2005).

Although Mann and colleagues found a correlation between aggression, impulsivity, and suicidal ideation, the model was not useful in identifying those *currently* at risk for future suicidal behaviors. In retrospective studies, rates of lifetime aggression and impulsivity were higher in attempters, as were rates of borderline personality disorder, smoking, past substance use disorder, family history of suicidal acts, head injury, and childhood abuse. It is possible that Mann's model identifies a general psychopathological trait not specific enough to distinguish those at risk for near-term suicide.

JOINER'S INTERPERSONAL MODEL

Joiner's interpersonal theory of suicide has generated a substantial body of research. The theory posits that suicidal behavior requires a combination of suicidal desire and the acquired capability to act on that desire. Suicidal desire is framed by two simultaneous interpersonal constructs: "thwarted belongingness" and "perceived burdensomeness." Because lethal means of suicide are fear-inducing and painful, an additional step of acquired capability must develop before an individual engages in suicidal behavior. This capability arises through "habituation" and "opponent processes" in response to physically painful and/or fear-inducing experiences (Figure 1.7).

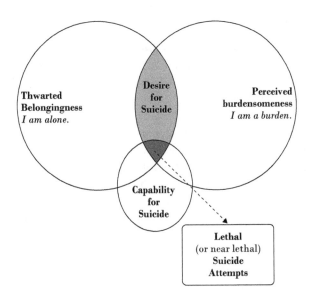

Figure 1.7 Interpersonal model of suicide.
Source: Van Orden et al. (2010).

Joiner notes that social isolation is one of the most reliable predictors of suicidal behavior. Per Baumeister and Leary (1995), humans have a fundamental "need to belong." When this need is unmet, a state of *thwarted belongingness* emerges, and a desire for death or passive suicidal ideation develops. Baumeister and Leary further conceive of thwarted belongingness as having two facets: loneliness—"an affectively laden cognition that one has too few social connections"—and the absence of reciprocally caring relationships. Joiner's group (Joiner & Van Orden, 2010, p. 10) found a linear relationship between thwarted belongingness and suicidal ideation, but only among participants who also reported high levels of *perceived burdensomeness.*

Suicidal individuals often perceive themselves as burdens to family and loved ones, feeling that people around them would be better off without them. Joiner cites Woznica and Shapiro's (1990) study, which found a positive correlation between adolescents' perceptions of their own expendability within their family structures and suicidal behavior. Joiner's own work (Joiner et al., 2010) examined suicide notes by individuals who made lethal and nonlethal attempts and found that the notes of those who died were characterized by a high degree of perceived burdensomeness. Among those who died, greater perceptions of burdensomeness predicted more lethal means of suicide. In Joiner's theory, perceived burdensomeness has two dimensions—a perception that the self is so flawed as to be a liability to others and affectively laden self-loathing.

Once thwarted belongingness and perceived burdensomeness come together to promote suicidal ideation, an individual still must overcome the fear of pain and death. Joiner notes Öhman and Mineka's (2001) proposal that fear is evolutionarily protective because it signals potentially life-threatening situations to be avoided. Because many means of suicide are extremely painful, to engage in suicidal behavior, an individual must have a degree of fearlessness. Joiner posits that through repeated practice, an individual can overcome this fear by habituating to the frightening and physically painful aspects of self-harm and by convincing him- or herself that the pain associated with a chosen means of suicide is tolerable.

Joiner posits that the capacity for suicide is acquired through habituation (typically through a pattern of self-injury). Solomon and Corbit's (1974) model of opponent processing provides an understanding of how lethal actions can become a positive emotional valence. In opponent processing, an individual engaged in a repeat behavior will have an initial emotional response, which eventually becomes overtaken by an acquired opponent response. For example, the primary response to skydiving will likely be fear, but with repeated exposure, the opponent process of exhilaration will arise and become amplified. Eventually, this opponent process will overtake the initial response.

Van Orden and Joiner (2010) hypothesized that self-harm behaviors have a primary effect of fear and pain but acquire an opponent process of relief and analgesia. Through repeated practice, fear remains constant or diminishes, and as the opponent process becomes dominant, these behaviors come to be primarily associated with emotional relief. Opponent processing provides a framework to view prior attempts (one of the strongest predictors of eventual suicide) as rehearsals, leading to pain desensitization, cultivation of positive emotional valence surrounding suicidal behavior, and capability to overcome the naturally protective fears of pain and death.

In summary, Joiner's model provides elegance and intuitiveness, using only three proximal factors as the "danger zones" to predict suicidal behavior. Hypothetically, by evaluating for these factors, clinicians can screen for patients at high risk. The drawback is that in experiments, both perceived burdensomeness and thwarted belongingness have been associated with suicidal ideation but not behavior (Ma, Batterham, Calear, & Han, 2016). Furthermore, the concepts of acquired capability and opponent processing have been contradicted by research on military suicide (Griffith, 2012).

O'CONNOR'S INTEGRATED MOTIVATIONAL–VOLITIONAL MODEL OF SUICIDE

O'Connor's integrated motivational–volitional model of suicide uses Ajzen's theory of planned behavior to examine suicide as a volitional rather than impulsive action (O'Connor, Armitage, & Gray, 2006). This model, however, incorporates elements of the stress–diathesis model of suicidality in the premotivational phase. The suicidal process is considered along a timeline—starting with the biopsychosocial groundwork laid out by the stress–diathesis model and followed by the arrested flight model (Williams & Pollock, 2001) before making the transition from ideation to action. The emphasis of the integrated model is on the proximal predictor of suicide—suicidal *intention* rather than ideation—and the model explores the stages of suicidal ideation from background setting (premotivational phase) to ideation (motivational phase) through the transition from mere ideation to intention and ultimately suicidal behavior (volitional phase) (Figure 1.8).

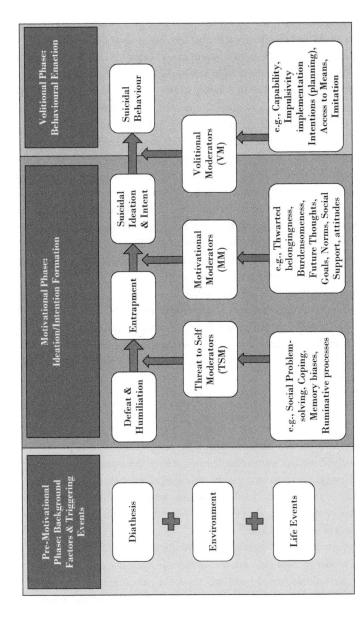

Figure 1.8 The integrated motivational–volitional model of suicide.
Source: OConnor (2011).

The *premotivational phase* provides the groundwork for suicidal ideation (Schotte & Clum, 1987). Combining nature and nurture, the premotivational phase explores the way that environmental factors or negative events can activate biological vulnerabilities. Personality traits such as perfectionism can provide vulnerability such that a stressful life event can push an individual to the motivational phase of suicidality. O'Connor (2011) showed that for adolescents with high levels of socially prescribed perfectionism, even low-level stress could lead to a dramatically increased probability of self-harm.

Once the groundwork is laid, suicidal ideation and intention can occur. The *motivational phase* is based on the arrested flight model (Williams & Pollock, 2001), in which feelings of defeat/humiliation lead to a feeling of entrapment. Once entrapped, suicidal ideation may arise as a possible solution to the seemingly hopeless situation. Feelings of defeat and humiliation can be compounded by "threat to self moderators," including overgeneralized memory and rumination, which can escalate feelings of defeat into entrapment. Once an individual feels entrapped, motivational moderators, including a paucity of positive future thinking, influence whether suicidal ideation progresses to intent. O'Connor considers all moderators to be targets for possible interventions.

Finally, the *volitional phase* provides the key transition from suicidal ideation to action, which is marked by volitional moderators, including access to means of suicide, knowing others who have engaged in suicide, and impulsivity. Interventions in this final phase are highly desirable, and studies are underway examining psychosocial interventions to prevent the transition from intention to action.

A prospective cohort study of the IMV model showed that its components could be somewhat predictive of future suicidal ideation (O'Connor, O'Carroll, Ryan, & Smyth, 2012; O'Connor, Rasmussen, & Hawton, 2009). Further research in other settings is needed to confirm these findings and to establish the model's predictability of behavior rather than ideation. The experimental evidence for specificity of the moderators of each step is also lacking.

SUMMARY

Understanding the suicidal process is essential for research and suicide prevention. The early psychoanalytic models were valuable because they influenced the view on suicide from that of a moral dilemma to a psychopathological and clinical phenomenon. The second-generation psychological models of suicide were backed with a modest degree of experimental evidence and were classified into four domains: affective, cognitive, diathesis–stress, and suicidal crisis.

The key concepts emerging from the affective theories, exemplified by the cry of pain/ arrested flight model by Williams, are the unbearable state of entrapment and Joiner's concepts of perceived burdensomeness and thwarted belongingness. The central concepts promulgated by the cognitive–behavioral theorists—Schotte and Clum's (1987) cognitive vulnerability model and Rudd's (2006) fluid vulnerability model—are impulsivity, cognitive rigidity, and maladaptive cognitive style.

Of the diathesis–stress models based on the concept of a biological trait vulnerability to stress, Beck's model is also based on cognitive–behavioral theories with the trait vulnerabilities of maladaptive cognitive style, personality, and impulsivity. On the other hand, Mann's model, in which the trait vulnerabilities are impulsive aggression and pessimism, modulated by low serotonin and low norepinephrine, respectively, emphasizes neurochemistry. The key feature of both models is separation of the long-term trait factors from dynamic precipitating stressors.

Finally, the suicidal crisis models of Fawcett, Hendin, and Galynker and Yaseen postulated the existence of a distinct clinical entity of the suicidal crisis syndrome, which culminates in suicidal behavior. The SCS model stands out in that SCS severity appears to predict imminent suicidal behavior.

Although these models have advanced the field of suicide research substantially, they also have limitations. The main flaw of these theories is that they are narrow in focus and insufficiently integrate the complex cognitive, affective, and trait vulnerability factors for suicide. Furthermore, these models do not address the evolution of the suicidal process over time, whereby stressful life events interact with trait vulnerabilities to form causal pathways making suicide possible. Finally, with the exception of the most recent SCS work by Galynker and Yaseen, no theory has been clinically useful in identifying patients at high risk for imminent or near-term suicide, which is essential if we are to slow the rise in suicide rates worldwide (Bertolote & Fleischmann, 2015).

O'Connor's third-generation integrated motivational–volitional theory of suicidal behavior attempts to overcome these limitations by considering the suicidal process in stages over time. The IMV model attempts to incorporate "disparate" static and dynamic factors into one comprehensive whole by including Beck's and Mann's stress–diathesis models in the premotivational phase of the IMV as the basis for Williams' entrapment-based psychological schema of the evolution of the suicidal process, which takes place during the motivational phase. The main limitations of the IMV are the lack of a framework for the multiplicity of suicidal behavior and for the diverse pathways subserving both impulsive and deliberate attempts, the lack of a clear definition of suicidal crisis, and its applicability to assessing actual risk of near-term suicidal behavior.

The significant progress in our theoretical understanding of suicidal process and suicide has not yet translated into our ability to identify imminent suicidal risk and to prevent suicide. There exists a need for a third-generation model that integrates the stress–diathesis vulnerability construct with both affective and cognitive aspects of the suicidal process, clearly differentiates the trait and imminent suicide risks, provides a satisfactory narrative connecting these two clinical concepts, and explains both impulsive and planned suicides. The comprehensive narrative crisis model, which meets these criteria, is described in Chapter 2.

2

The Comprehensive Narrative-Crisis Model of Suicide

With Jessica Briggs

INTRODUCTION

Trait Versus State Risk Factors

When assessing imminent suicide risk, the differences between trait and state markers are important. Although there is no universal definition, *trait* generally refers to stable characteristics of the individual, which may include genetic predisposition, temperament, and/or personality (Goldston, Reboussin, & Daniel, 2006). For example, some people may have persistently high levels of hopelessness and anxiety, regardless of life circumstances, whereas others may tend to remain hopeful and calm.

In contrast, *state* refers to characteristics that fluctuate with time. In the context of suicide risk assessment, state characteristics typically refer to mood, anxiety, and thought content/process, all of which may change over periods of time ranging from minutes to weeks.

Stressful life events can result both in state and trait changes in suicide risk. Victims of childhood emotional, physical, and/or sexual abuse often suffer severe episodic "state" anxiety and depression concurrent with the abuse. These same childhood adversities carry the risk of significant long-lasting increases in suicidal behavior in adults (Bruwer et al., 2014). It has been suggested that these changes have epigenetic mechanisms and are therefore trait risk factors, which may even be heritable (Labonte & Turecki, 2012).

The narrative-crisis model considers the immediate effects of childhood adversity to be state phenomena and the life-long consequences as trait vulnerability. Similarly, in regard to suicidal behavior, societal and religious values, typically established in childhood, are considered trait phenomena.

Overall, the narrative-crisis model of trait vulnerability for suicide comprises enduring characteristics that make an individual susceptible to suicide. This broad construct includes the cognitive dispositional vulnerability factors postulated by Beck's diathesis–stress model; the biological diathesis of low levels of serotonin/norepinephrine and impulsive aggression of Mann's model; the epigenetic factors related to childhood trauma; and societal, cultural, and religious norms.

Static Versus Dynamic Risk Factors

The newer construct of static versus dynamic risk factors for suicide resembles the older construct of state versus trait risk factors. Although both contrast long-term and short-term clinical phenomena, the trait–state dichotomy refers to personality and neurobiology, whereas the static–dynamic dichotomy pertains to demographic characteristics and elements of past psychiatric history that are associated with increased long-term suicide risk. According to this new model, the demographic static risk factors are age, sex, race, ethnicity, socioeconomic status, and geographic location. The most significant static risks are a history of psychiatric illness and of suicidal behavior by the patient, family member, or a close friend. Childhood trauma, abuse, neglect, and maladaptive parenting styles are static and trait risk factors for suicidal behavior.

The most common dynamic risk factors are socioeconomic and interpersonal stressors, including job loss, business failure, eviction, romantic rejection, and conflicts with family or friends. Substance abuse, exacerbation of a psychiatric illness, neglected friendships, abandoned hobbies, preparatory actions, and suicide attempts occur in response to these risk factors (Claassen, Harvilchuck-Laurenson, & Fawcett, 2014).

Static and trait factors for suicide are so distal to suicidal behavior that they have become enduring personal characteristics and are referred to in the narrative-crisis model as *trait vulnerability*. In contrast, the state and dynamic risk factors are transient phenomena that are proximal to suicidal behavior. Because state risk factors are acute characteristics, they are assessed as part of the suicidal crisis syndrome (SCS). Because dynamic risk factors are derived from stressful life events, which may form the foundation of the narrative identity, they are consequently discussed in the suicidal narrative part of the model.

OVERVIEW OF THE
NARRATIVE-CRISIS MODEL

The approach to imminent suicide risk evaluation is based on the comprehensive narrative-crisis model of suicide developed by Galynker and Yaseen. The narrative-crisis model is a third-generation model that expands and reconceptualizes the authors' earlier work that defined the boundaries of SCS and established its relevance to imminent risk (see the section titled "Suicide Crisis Syndrome and the Positive Feedback Model of Suicide" in Chapter 1).

The narrative-crisis model posits that suicide is a volitional process that develops over time. Individuals reach the suicidal crisis if they have trait vulnerability and if they experience their life narrative as a dead-end sequence of events, termed the *suicidal narrative*. The model has three components: trait vulnerability, the suicidal narrative, and the suicidal crisis syndrome.

Trait vulnerability includes all static risk factors, which are relatively stable over time and distal to acute suicidal behavior. It also incorporates innate temperament factors such as fearlessness and pessimism, early adverse experiences such as childhood trauma, and cultural and social factors such as societal acceptability of suicide as a solution to problems.

Suicidal narrative, the second component of the model, is derived from the theory of narrative identity, which postulates that individuals "form their identity by integrating their life experiences into an internalized evolving story of self which gives people the sense of wholeness and purpose in life" (McAdams, 2001, p. 100). The narrative-crisis model posits that suicidal individuals feel entrapped in their suicidal narratives or ideas of having a worthless past, intolerable present, or no future.

Suicidal crisis syndrome, the third component of the narrative-crisis model, is a distinct emotional state characterized by an unbearable mixture of anxiety, agitation, entrapment, and loss of cognitive control. The result is the suicidal act, brought on by an emotional urge to end the pain and circular ruminations.

The narrative-crisis model postulates that imminent suicide risk is primarily determined by the intensity of SCS, which can be measured by the Suicidal Crisis Inventory (SCI) scale. However, both trait vulnerability and a person's suicidal narrative contribute independently to imminent suicide risk. The overall imminent suicide risk is ultimately determined by all three components in the narrative-crisis model.

THE TRAIT VULNERABILITY COMPONENT

The trait vulnerability component of the narrative-crisis model draws from Beck's and Mann's well-developed and researched models of suicidal behavior that show discriminant validity for past suicidal behavior and long-term suicide risk.

Beck's diathesis describes dispositional vulnerability factors, which make one susceptible to SCS even under low levels of stress (Wenzel & Beck, 2008). He defined five main dispositional vulnerability factors: impulsivity, deficits in problem solving, overgeneral memory style, maladaptive cognitive style, and personality (Wenzel & Beck, 2008). Impulsivity and personality are biological temperament factors that are discussed within Mann's biological framework presented in Chapter 1. The other three—deficits in problem solving, overgeneral memory style, and maladaptive cognitive style—are cognitive abnormalities best considered within Beck's cognitive–behavioral approach.

Most of these have not been tested for predictive validity of near-term suicidal behavior or have only been predictive long term. It seems intuitive that the trait vulnerability factors moderate the intensity of SCS, but this relationship is yet to be tested experimentally (Figure 2.1).

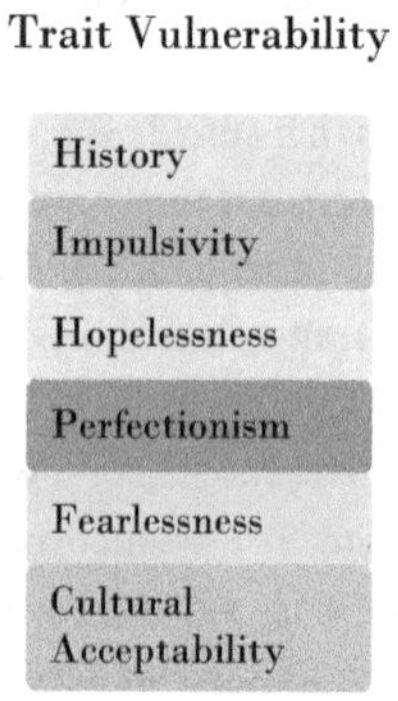

Trait Vulnerability

History

Impulsivity

Hopelessness

Perfectionism

Fearlessness

Cultural Acceptability

Figure 2.1 Trait vulnerability component.

THE SUICIDAL NARRATIVE COMPONENT

The suicidal narrative component of the narrative-crisis model describes the psychological processes of long-term trait vulnerability for suicide evolving into the feelings, thoughts, and behaviors that bring on the acute suicidal crisis and the associated high imminent suicide risk.

The SN construct focuses on the formation and power of the suicidal narrative identity as the prerequisite for SCS. The SN is also related to David Jobs' (2012) "drivers" approach to suicide risk, which posits that each suicidal person's story has to be examined for "drivers," or uniquely meaningful events or thought patterns that "drive" the suicidal process of each suicidal individual. The SN construct posits that all drivers have common elements, which form a characteristic life narrative arc applicable to most suicidal individuals. In fact, in the narrative-crisis model, it is the life narrative arc of suicidal individuals that is termed the "suicidal narrative." It evolves through the following phases:

- Phase 1: Unrealistic life goals
- Phase 2: Entitlement to happiness
- Phase 3: Failure to redirect to more realistic goals
- Phase 4: Humiliating personal or social defeat
- Phase 5: Perceived burdensomeness
- Phase 6: Thwarted belongingness
- Phase 7: Perception of no future

The popular psychological theory of narrative identity, which inspired the term "suicidal narrative," has received strong empirical support (McLean, Pasupathi, & Pals, 2007; Pals, 2006; Woike & Polo, 2001). It postulates that each person's identity is formed through the integration of life experiences into an internalized, evolving story of the self that provides a sense of wholeness and purpose (McAdams, 2001). The suicidal person's narrative evolves into one in which the past narrative of one's life leads to a present that is so intolerable that the future becomes unimaginable.

Although individual suicidal narratives are unique to particular individuals, many of the life plots and subplots that form suicidal narrative arcs are variations on only a few themes. The most prominent of these are the arrested flight model (Williams & Pollock, 2001), which emphasizes feelings of humiliation, defeat, and entrapment, and the interpersonal model, which highlights perceived burdensomeness and thwarted belongingness (Joiner et al., 2010).

The narrative-crisis model posits that although the specifics may vary, the SN applies to most suicides. Most elements of the SN included in the narrative-crisis model have been described in the literature and have been shown to have some association with suicidal behavior (Brown, Harris, & Hepworth, 1995; DeWall, Baumeister, & Vohs, 2008; Morrison & O'Connor, 2008; Yaseen, Chartrand et al., 2013). Work has begun to establish the cohesiveness of the SN construct and its predictive validity in determining imminent suicide risk (Figure 2.2).

THE SUICIDAL CRISIS COMPONENT

The narrative-crisis model postulates that suicidal behavior occurs when a person reaches a clinical state called the suicidal crisis (SC). The SC describes a fervorous negative affective state that combines cognitive and emotional dysregulation with an overwhelming sense of entrapment. The model further posits that the intensity of the SC is the most immediate indicator of imminent suicide risk. The SC component of the narrative-crisis is the direct extension of Galynker and Yaseen's model of suicidal behavior, which is based on their work on acute SCS and on their positive feedback model of suicide described in Chapter 1 (Galynker, Yaseen, Briggs, & Hayashi, 2015; Katz, Yaseen, Mojtabai, Cohen, & Galynker, 2011; Yaseen, Chartrand, et al., 2013; Yaseen, Fisher, Morales, & Galynker, 2012; Yaseen et al., 2012).

Building on the "suicidal crisis" and "psychic pain" constructs of Shneidman, Baumeister, Fawcett, Hendin, and others, Galynker and Yaseen designed and tested the SCI scale, which established the exact emotions and cognitions constituting SCS. Work is ongoing, but the most recent factor analysis of the SCI scores suggested that SCS consists of five intercorrelated negative affective states: entrapment, ruminative flooding, panic–dissociation, emotional pain, and fear of dying.

Galynker and Yaseen showed that in the emergency room setting, SCS intensity correlated with current and past suicidal ideation and behavior. Moreover, in high-risk psychiatric inpatients, it was also associated with future post-discharge suicidal behavior (Yaseen et al., 2014) and to date remains the only construct predictive of imminent suicidal behavior.

SCS, defined by the previously mentioned five affective factors, is a transient state condition, and in high-risk psychiatric inpatients hospitalized for suicidal risk, its intensity may change significantly from admission to discharge. Predictably, SCS

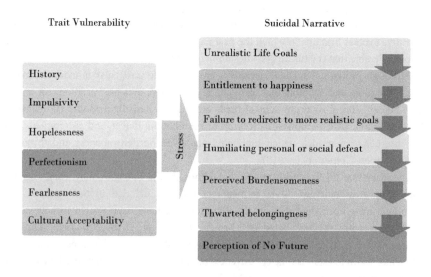

Figure 2.2 Trait vulnerability and suicidal narrative components.

magnitude at admission correlates with suicidal behavior proximal to the admission. SCS intensity prior to discharge is less reflective of the proximal pre-admission suicidal behavior but correlates strongly with the imminent suicidal behavior within 1 month after hospital discharge (Galynker et al., 2016). Thus, SCS appears to be a true and sensitive marker of the suicidal crisis. Further research is needed to determine whether the narrative-crisis model and the SCI scale can be used to track suicidal risk over time (Figure 2.3).

NARRATIVE-CRISIS MODEL FLEXIBILITY

Narrative-Driven Versus Crisis-Driven Suicidal Behaviors

The relative contribution of SN and SCS to overall suicide risk depends on the coherence and power of an individual suicidal narrative and on that individual's affective instability. Some narratives can be so compelling as to bring on suicidal behavior with minimal affective instability, resulting in meticulously planned suicides. Suicides of individuals with terminal illness or those facing torture and/or death in captivity are examples of such narrative-driven suicides (see Figure 2.2, bottom arrow).

Alternatively, a person with high affective lability could attempt and die by suicide after suffering a suicidal crisis even if his or her suicidal narrative is transient and reactive to a short-lived stressor. An example of such crisis-driven suicide is a response to business failure by somebody in a mixed manic state (see Figure 2.2, top arrow).

The narrative-crisis model is sufficiently flexible to explain varied suicidal behaviors from premeditated narrative-driven to impulsive crisis-driven. Although all suicidal narratives conclude in a dead end, the entry points into the narrative may differ depending on the nature of the life stressors.

For example, the suicidal narrative of an immigrant student from a country in which honor suicide is accepted culturally, who has a grade point average that is too low for a medical career, and who feels that he has disgraced his family is different from that of a high school student who is being ostracized for being "weird." The former may be described as a perfectionism–failure–burden narrative, whereas the latter is driven primarily by social defeat and thwarted belongingness. In both scenarios, individuals with trait vulnerability may believe that they have run out of options and develop an acute suicidal crisis.

SUMMARY

Suicidal Narrative: Clinical Guide to the Assessment of Imminent Suicide Risk is based on the comprehensive narrative-crisis model integrating most of the currently known long-term risk factors, the dynamic proximal risk factors conceptualized as a suicidal narrative, and the acute SCS. The trait component corresponds to traditional chronic risk factors and confers long-term chronic suicide risk. The seven-phase suicidal narrative provides a framework for the analysis of the psychological processes leading to the development of the suicidal crisis in those with long-term vulnerability for suicide. The crisis

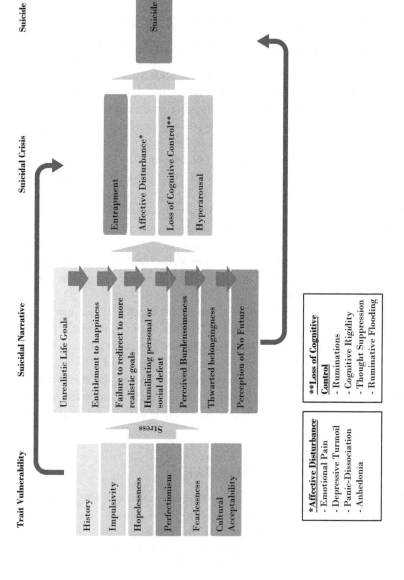

Trait Vulnerability

History
Impulsivity
Hopelessness
Perfectionism
Fearlessness
Cultural Acceptability

Suicidal Narrative

Unrealistic Life Goals
Entitlement to happiness
Failure to redirect to more realistic goals
Humiliating personal or social defeat
Perceived Burdensomeness
Thwarted belongingness
Perception of No Future

Suicidal Crisis

Entrapment
Affective Disturbance*
Loss of Cognitive Control**
Hyperarousal

Suicide

Suicide

Stress

*Affective Disturbance
- Emotional Pain
- Depressive Turmoil
- Panic-Dissociation
- Anhedonia

**Loss of Cognitive Control
- Ruminations
- Cognitive Rigidity
- Thought Suppression
- Ruminative Flooding

Figure 2.3 Narrative Crisis Model.

component, specifically SCS severity, is directly predictive of imminent suicidal behavior and confers a short-term suicide risk.

To date, some fairly solid experimental evidence supports the association of trait vulnerability with long-term suicide risk and of SCS intensity with the near-term risk for suicide. The validity of the suicidal narrative as well as the related integrated motivational–volitional and interpersonal models in predicting suicidal behavior is under active investigation. The narrative-crisis model provides a coherent and clear framework for comprehensive assessment of all aspects of suicidal behavior to ensure that no factor has been overlooked and at the same time uncovers useful targets for clinical intervention.

3

Trait Vulnerability Assessment

With Zhanna Gerlovina

DEMOGRAPHICS

Age, Race, and Ethnicity

Suicide rates and patterns differ according to age, race, and ethnic group. The suicide rate for men in the United States continues to be much higher than that for women, but this difference does vary across age groups. The highest differential between rates in men and women is for ages 10–24 years, with the ratio in that age group increasing from 3.7 in 1994 to 5.8 per 100,000 in 2012 (American Foundation for Suicide Prevention [AFSP], 2016; Curtin, Warner, & Hedegaard, 2016).

For the 35- to 64-year-old age group, which has the highest suicide risk, the gender ratio is somewhat lower at 3.34 per 100,000 (27.3 for men vs. 8.1 for women). This drop in risk ratio reflects relatively higher increases in suicide rates for women versus men from 1999 to 2010. During this time, the suicide rate for this age group increased by 27.3% for men and 31.5% for women. This shift is consistent with the overall trend among women, whose suicide rates increase with age (AFSP, 2016; Curtin et al., 2016).

It is worth noting that events precipitating suicide in children are different from those in the elderly, and events precipitating suicide in both these groups are different from those in adults. Parent–child conflicts are the most common precipitant for suicide in children, and hanging is the most frequent method (Soole, Kõlves, & De Leo, 2014). In the elderly, the major factor leading to suicide is depression, followed by physical disability. The majority of elderly suicide victims are not seen by a psychiatrist prior to their suicide (Snowden, Steinman, Frederick, & Wilson, 2009).

In terms of race and ethnicity, worldwide frequencies of suicidal behavior vary from country to country. According to the World Health Organization, the highest suicide rates are reported in Guyana, Surinam, Korea, Sri Lanka, India, the former Soviet Union, and Africa. Meanwhile, the lowest rates of suicide are reported in Arab countries. Guyana's annual suicide rate of 48 per 100,000 is the highest in the world, whereas the lowest is in Saudi Arabia, which has an annual rate of 0.4 per 100,000.

Within the United States, there are significant differences between individual states' suicide rates. States with the most suicides report rates that are two times higher than the national average and three times higher than the rates of states with the least suicides.

Currently, the highest suicide rates are in western states, including Wyoming (23.2), Alaska (23.1), and Montana (22.9). The lowest rates are in the East, including New York (8.0), New Jersey (8.2), and Maryland (8.9).

According to the Centers for Disease Control and Prevention, in 2010 the highest rates of suicide in the United States were observed in Caucasians (22.3) and in American Indians/Alaskan Natives (18.5), compared to relatively low rates in African Americans, Hispanics, and Asians/Pacific Islanders (6.8, 7.4, and 7.8, respectively). During the past decade, there has been a much sharper increase in suicide rates among Whites and American Indians/Alaskan Natives (40.4% and 65.5%, respectively) compared to Hispanics and African Americans (6.8% and 3.5%, respectively). As a result of these increases, the ratio of suicides in Caucasians versus African Americans increased from 2.5 to 3.3.

The overall suicide rate in the United States among children aged 5–11 years appears to have remained stable between 1993–1997 and 2008–2012 (from 1.18 to 1.09 per 1 million; incident rate ratio [IRR] = 0.96; 95% confidence interval [CI], 0.90–1.03). However, the overall rate does not reflect that during this time, in contrast with the adult statistics, suicide increased significantly in African American children (from 1.36 to 2.54 per 1 million; IRR = 1.27; 95% CI, 1.11–1.45) while decreasing significantly in Caucasian children (from 1.14 to 0.77 per 1 million; IRR = 0.86; 95% CI, 0.79–0.94).

Combining the previous demographic data on age, gender, and ethnicity creates clinically meaningful contrasts between higher and lower suicide risk groups. Although demographics alone are not predictive of imminent risk, they provide a valuable reference point.

Gender

The following is arguably the most quoted fact regarding the well-known gender discrepancy in suicide statistics: "Women attempt suicide three times as often as men, but men die by suicide three times as often as women" (AFSP, 2016). This statement generally holds true for the US and Western cultures as a whole; the pattern shifts dramatically in other areas of the world. In China, the most populous country in the world, women die by suicide more often than men (Zhang, Li, Tu, Xiao, & Jia, 2011). Nevertheless, many studies show that men generally use methods that are much more lethal in their suicide attempts, such as firearms and hanging. Given this trend, it makes sense that male suicide attempts tend to be more lethal than female attempts and that men are more likely to die from their attempts (Curtin et al., 2016).

Examining the data for the United States in more detail, the gender disparity in the lethality of suicide methods means that firearm decedents are more likely to be foreign born, elderly, non-Hispanic, Caucasian, married men. Decedents of hanging and suffocation also tend to be male and foreign born but never-married, young, and racial/ethnic minorities.

Regarding lower lethality methods such as jumping from heights and using sharp objects, decedents are more likely to be foreign born, older, non-Hispanic, African American, never-married women. Similarly, self-poisoned decedents are more likely to be unmarried females, middle-aged, and non-Hispanic Caucasian (Kleiman & Liu, 2013).

These gender differences may suggest disparities in the intentionality of suicidal behavior between men and women, with men being more determined to die even when using less lethal methods (Mergl et al., 2015).

Lesbian, Gay, Bisexual, and Transgender

Youth who report same-sex sexual orientation are at greater risk than their heterosexual peers for suicide attempts, and this risk persists even after controlling for other suicide risk factors (Russell & Joyner, 2001). This increase in suicide risk is mainly due to a negative familial response toward an adolescent's "coming out" process. Family rejection of an adolescent who is lesbian, gay, bisexual, or transgender (LGBT) can be associated with an eightfold increase in the likelihood of attempted suicide compared to that of adolescents who experience minimal or no family rejection (Cash & Bridge, 2009).

This increased risk of suicidal behavior in LGBT youth persists into adulthood. Gay and bisexual men are approximately four times more likely than heterosexual men to attempt suicide during their lifetime (King et al., 2008). In adult gay men, an increase in suicide risk is largely due to the perceived negative societal reaction. Men who experience three or more forms of anti-gay marginalization have twice the rate of suicide ideation compared to those with no marginalization (27.3% vs. 12.6%) and greater than four times the rate of suicide attempts (3.9% vs. 0.9%) (Ferlatte, Dulai, Hottes, Trussler, & Marchand, 2015).

HISTORY OF MENTAL ILLNESS
AND SUICIDE ATTEMPTS
History of Mental Illness

Having a diagnosis of a psychiatric disorder, with the exception of dementia, is also linked to an increase in suicide risk (Nordentoft, Mortensen, & Pedersen, 2012). According to findings in the United Kingdom (Windfuhr & Kapur, 2011), the risk of suicide for patients with psychiatric disorders is 5–15 times higher than that for patients without psychiatric disorders. The differences in suicide rates for each disorder are due to many factors, such as comorbidity, history of previous attempts, and gender differences.

Approximately 90% of individuals who die by suicide have a mental illness, although this varies globally (Chang, Gitlin, & Patel, 2011). The most common diagnoses are affective disorders (32–47%), schizophrenia (15–20%), alcohol dependence (8–17%), personality disorders (8–11%), and drug dependence (3–9%) (Varnik, 2012). Anxiety disorders are notably absent from this list; until very recently, they may have been underdiagnosed in suicidal patients because clinicians may have considered anxiety as too mild to contribute significantly to suicide risk. However, during approximately the past decade, it has become clear that anxiety and panic contribute significantly to suicide risk, especially short-term risk.

In an analysis of data from the ongoing National Epidemiologic Survey on Alcohol and Related Conditions (NESARC), inpatients with depression and panic attacks were independently associated with a twofold increase risk for suicide (Katz, Yaseen, Mojtabai, Cohen, & Galynker, 2011). In a prospective analysis of the same database, patients who had panic attacks with fear of dying were six times more likely to attempt suicide than those who did not have panic attacks (Yaseen, Chartrand et al., 2013). Retrospectively, other anxiety disorders were associated with approximately a threefold increased risk of lifetime history of suicide attempt (Thibodeau, Welch, Sareen,

& Asmundson, 2013). In developing countries, the percentage of mentally ill among suicide decedents is significantly lower (34% in India), presumably because many mentally ill individuals from the lower socioeconomic classes never see a psychiatrist (Varnik, 2012; Vishnuvardhan & Saddichha, 2012).

Approximately 25% of suicide decedents in the United Kingdom were in contact with mental health services prior to their suicide (Hoertel et al., 2015). In the United States, approximately 50% were in contact with some doctor during this time period. Similarly, suicide risk is thought to be greatly increased following discharge from inpatient mental health wards, although inpatient suicides have declined significantly during the past 20 years (see the next section).

Thus, it appears that many psychiatric disorders may increase suicide risk (Weissman, Klerman, Markowitz, & Ouellette, 1989). However, psychiatric disorders rarely occur in isolation and are too frequently comorbid to be a matter of chance (Kessler, Chiu, Demler, & Walters, 2005). This comorbidity can be explained through the manifestation and interaction of two genetic vulnerability factors known as internalizing and externalizing behaviors or disorders. These two transdiagnostic factors may explain the links between individual disorders and suicidal behavior.

The term internalizing behaviors originated in child psychiatry and refers to mood dysregulation caused by difficulties in managing negative emotions. In children, internalizing behaviors may manifest as withdrawn behavior, frequent worrying, self-denigrating comments, and low self-confidence, and they typically do not result in disruptive behaviors. The term externalizing behaviors refers to problems that are manifested in disruptive behavior and reflect a child's negative reactions to his or her environment. This may include aggression, delinquency, and hyperactivity. In general terms, internalizers tend to blame themselves for their problems, and externalizers tend to blame everyone around them.

In adults, the Axis I internalizing disorders include major depressive disorder, generalized anxiety disorder (GAD), dysthymia, panic disorder, seasonal affective disorder, and social phobias. Axis I externalizing disorders are primarily addiction disorders such as alcohol use disorder, drug use disorder, and pathological gambling. Internalizing Axis II disorders in adults comprise avoidant-dependent, histrionic, schizoid, and schizotypal personality disorders, whereas the externalizing personality disorder include antisocial, narcissistic, and borderline personality disorders (Cosgrove et al., 2011). Although distinctly different, both dimensions arise from a general psychopathology factor, which makes people vulnerable to both dimensions and increases the risk of suicidal behavior (Hoertel et al., 2015).

This mechanism of a general psychopathology risk factor, rather than (or in addition to) the alternative mechanism of distinct disorder-specific risk factors, may explain suicides, which occur after the worst symptoms of a disorder have improved or completely resolved. If the yet-to-be-defined generalized risk factor underlies most or even some suicidal behaviors, then treatments for specific symptoms typically associated with suicide risk may not eliminate it completely.

Many case histories describe suicides that took place after a person's depression has either improved or turned into euthymia. Sudden brightening of mood has been suggested anecdotally as a warning sign of imminent suicide. Similarly, patients with severe anxiety disorders or with psychotic disorders do not necessarily take their lives at the height of their anxiety or psychosis. Many suicides occur in individuals who in the eyes of a casual observer seemed normal and even happy.

In addition to the treatment of specific disorders and symptoms associated with increased suicide risk, interventions are needed for the underlying transdiagnostic or dimensional factor that increases suicide risk regardless of the *Diagnostic and Statistical Manual of Mental Disorders* (American Psychiatric Association, 2013) diagnostic structure. In other words, increased suicide risk could be considered a transdiagnostic syndrome and presents both an important research domain and a valuable treatment target.

History of Suicide Attempts

History of suicide attempts or of deliberate self-harm is one of the strongest risk factors for suicide (Sakinofsky, 2000). In industrialized nations, approximately half of all suicide decedents had at least one prior suicide attempt (Nordentoft et al., 1993). One in 100 suicide attempters go on to die by suicide in a subsequent attempt(s) within the first year (Hawton, Zahl, & Weatherall, 2003). Suicide death rates for previous attempters are on average 30 times higher than those for the general population. As many as 5% of suicide attempters will die by suicide within 9 years (Owens, Horrocks, & House, 2002).

The number of previous suicide attempts and advanced age further increase the risk of an upcoming fatal attempt, particularly in the elderly (300-fold increase in the age group older than 85 years compared to the general population without a history of attempts). Surprisingly, the ratio of men to women who die by suicide after previous attempts is close to equal. One possible explanation for this fact is that men are more lethal in their first attempt, and those who do not die are a self-selected group of men prone to using less lethal means of suicides (Nordentoft et al., 1993).

In those with a history of suicide attempts, the risk of death is highest in the first year after self-harm. The risk of dying by suicide within 1 year of a past attempt is similar to the risk of dying of suicide in the year after discharge from an inpatient psychiatric unit or after hospitalization for any reason (60-fold increase compared to the risk for those never hospitalized). Whereas a suicide attempt in the remote past could be classified as a trait vulnerability for suicide, a recent suicide attempt (up to 1 year in the past) represents a short-term risk factor. It appears that the stress of an acute episode of psychiatric illness, recent hospitalization, or suicide attempt sharply increases short-term suicide risk. For that reason, all of these factors are discussed in more detail in Chapter 4.

CHILDHOOD HISTORY
Childhood Trauma

A massive body of literature indicates that childhood maltreatment, particularly sexual abuse, is associated with increased suicide risk in adulthood. The link between childhood sexual abuse and adult suicide is strongest when the abuse was long-lasting, the perpetrator knew the victim, and there was force and/or penetration. Adults with a history of childhood sexual abuse may be 20 times more likely to engage in suicidal attempts compared to non-abused individuals and 70 times more likely to do so if the abuse involved penetration. It is clear that childhood sexual abuse, particularly physically invasive sexual abuse, increases the risk of suicide later in life (Santa Mina & Gallop, 1998). The link between childhood physical abuse and adult suicide risk is not as strong, but it is still significant.

Parenting Style (Parental Bonding)

Parental bonding is a construct, developed by Parker and colleagues (Parker, 1981, 1989; Parker, Tupling, & Brown, 1979), that classifies parenting style into four categories based on the level of care afforded to children and the level of control or overprotection exercised by the parents. Optimal parental bonding is described as a combination of high care and low overprotective behaviors, whereas poor parental styles involve the three other combinations. Neglectful parenting involves both low care and low control, whereas authoritarian ("helicopter") parents provide high care but also a high level of control. Parents who are emotionally distant and controlling exercise the parental bonding style of affectionless control. Research suggests that there exists a strong relationship between poor parental bonding and suicide (Adam, Keller, West, Larose, & Goszer, 1994; Gureje et al., 2010; McGarvey, Kryzhanovskaya, Koopman, Waite, & Canterbury, 1999; Miller, King, Shain, & Naylor, 1992).

All poor parental bonding, particularly low care, has a significant association with suicidal behavior. However, affectionless control, the combination of low care and overprotection, has a particularly strong association with suicidality. The data are less consistent with regard to overprotection alone because both parental gender and cultural factors appear to be pertinent (Goschin, Briggs, Blanco-Lutzen, Cohen, & Galynker, 2013). Affectionless control is a significant risk factor for both suicidal ideation and behavior in adolescents and adults. All of the studies on adolescents reviewed by Goschin et al. showed that affectionless control is a risk factor for suicidality, and studies using adult populations were nearly as uniform. This suggests that poor parenting style has long-term and possibly lifelong consequences.

The association between affectionless control and increased suicidality is noted more often in mothers than in fathers. This difference could be related to a historically dominant role of mothers relative to fathers in the family environment (McKinney, Donnelly, & Renk, 2008). This discrepancy also appears to be related to culture. In countries in which the mother is the primary figure in raising and educating children, the perceived maternal affectionless control is likely more important relative to the paternal bonding. Given the increasingly multicultural nature of societies, cultural characteristics are an increasingly important part of risk assessment.

It is unclear why affectionless control has a particularly strong association with suicidality. One hypothesis is that perceived overprotection can influence children's sense of their own identity and autonomy, which in turn can raise the risk of suicidal ideation. The literature shows that overcontrolling behaviors in mothers are associated with psychopathology in children and adolescents (Affrunti & Ginsburg, 2012) and that an overcontrolling style in both parents is associated with a variety of specific psychiatric disorders, including anxiety disorders (Spada et al., 2011), social phobia (Knappe,

Beesdo-Baum, Fehm, Lieb, & Wittchen, 2012), eating disorders (Lobera, Ríos, & Casals, 2011), and depression (Campos, Besser, & Blatt, 2010).

Attachment Style

Attachment theory, pioneered by Bowlby (1969, 1980), hypothesizes that early experiences with caretakers translate into internal representations of relationships that influence an individual's ability to navigate social situations (Crowell, Beauchaine, & Linehan, 2009). Research suggests a strong association between attachment styles and long-term (and possible short-term) risk of suicidal behavior (Levi-Belz, Gvion, Horesh, & Apter, 2013; Stepp et al., 2008). Griffin and Bartholomew's (1994) four-category model of "self" and "other" describes four attachment styles: secure, fearful, preoccupied, and dismissing. The attachment styles are defined by one's view of self and that of the other.

The secure attachment style is defined by a positive view of self and others (which translates behaviorally into low anxiety and low avoidance, correspondingly). Securely attached individuals have an internalized sense of self-worth and are comfortable with intimacy in close relationships. The three other attachment styles are known as insecure. The fearful attachment style is defined by a negative view of self and negative view of others. Fearful individuals are highly dependent on others for the validation of their self-worth; however, because of their negative expectations of others, they shun intimacy to avoid the pain of potential loss or rejection. The preoccupied attachment style is defined by negative view of self and positive view of others. Preoccupied individuals, like fearful individuals, have a deep-seated sense of unworthiness. However, their positive other model motivates them to validate their precarious self-worth through excessive closeness in personal relationships, leaving them vulnerable to extreme distress when their intimacy needs are not met. Finally, the dismissing attachment style is defined by a positive view of self and negative view of others. Dismissing individuals also avoid closeness with others because of negative expectations; however, they maintain their high sense of self-worth by defensively denying the value of close relationships and stressing the importance of independence.

It has been suggested that the likelihood of engaging in suicidal behavior could be related to how negative early attachment experiences are structured into internal adult working models of attachment (Adam, Lohrenz, Harper, & Streiner, 1982). Indeed, research has identified impaired parental attachment and bonding as one key risk factor for suicidal behavior later in life (Fergusson, Woodward, & Horwood, 2000).

It appears that early insecure attachment may operate as a general vulnerability factor, increasing the risk of poor work functioning and suicide attempts. Individuals with an insecure attachment style may exhibit impaired social and collaborative behaviors and thus lack the interpersonal skills required to be successful in a work environment (e.g., balancing teamwork with functioning independently, good communication skills, etc.). This may result in impaired self-esteem and depressed mood, thereby increasing suicide risk (Levi-Belz et al., 2013; Stepp et al., 2008).

However, depending on the patient population, there may be other mechanisms linking specific insecure attachment styles with suicidal behaviors. For example, in high-risk psychiatric inpatients, the relationship between the fearful attachment style and future suicidal behaviors is strong but indirect, and it is mediated entirely by entrapment (Clark, Li, & Cropsey, 2016). Clark et al. found that the secure attachment style had a protective effect on future suicidal behaviors, also fully mediated by entrapment, whereas dismissing and preoccupied attachment had no significant relationship with future behaviors.

TRAITS

Impulsivity

Beck's impulsivity vulnerability factor overlaps with the biological diathesis for suicidal behavior from Mann's stress–diathesis model (Mann et al., 2005). According to Mann, biological vulnerability is associated with genetically or epigenetically encoded low levels of norepinephrine and serotonin. The link between low levels of serotonin, past suicidal attempts, and completed suicides is supported by numerous well-designed studies (Mann, Waternaux, Haas, & Malone, 1999). These studies show that the aforementioned link is mediated by impulsivity, hopelessness, and depression, which in turn have been shown to be associated with past suicidality and may be related to long-term suicide risk.

Hopelessness and Pessimism

Although hopelessness is usually considered a state factor, it also has a strong trait component that remains stable over time. Some research suggests that trait hopelessness, also defined as pessimism of the future, may be a strong predictor for all indices of suicidal ideation and behavior (O'Connor, Smyth, Ferguson, Ryan, & Williams, 2013). In one classic long-term prospective study, hopelessness scores at baseline predicted more than 90% of all suicides in high-risk psychiatric inpatients during a 10-year follow-up period. Other studies showed that hopelessness was not predictive of suicidal behavior during short periods of time, suggesting that it is indeed a trait rather than an acute state condition (Goldston, Reboussin, & Daniel, 2006).

Perfectionism

Perfectionism was defined by Beck as a maladaptive cognitive style, and it refers to unrealistically high expectations that some individuals have for themselves, which set them up for failure. The concept of perfectionism is surprisingly complex and multifaceted, with research suggesting that many of its features are associated with suicidal behavior and ideation (reviewed by O'Connor, 2007). The aspects of perfectionism most consistently associated with suicidality are self-criticism, concern over mistakes, doubts over one's actions, and socially prescribed perfectionism, which is defined as the belief that others hold unrealistically high expectations for one's behavior and will only be satisfied if those expectations are met. Prospective studies of the predictive value of perfectionism for future suicidal behavior seem to suggest that this association exists. In short, perfectionism is a powerful motivating trait that forms the core of many suicidal narratives. It can be easily assessed both with psychometric scales and with direct questions, making it a useful target for imminent suicide risk assessment.

Trait Fearlessness and Pain Insensitivity

A capability for suicide is theorized to be a key ingredient in making it possible for someone to actually end his or her life (Joiner, 2005; Ohman & Mineka, 2001). With adequate support, this theory would provide a framework for why most people who have suicidal intent never attempt suicide. If true, the acquired capability for suicide would help explain the relatively high suicide rates in physicians (Cornette et al., 2009) and military personnel (Selby et al., 2010), which may be due to repeated exposure and habituation to death and dying.

Joiner's interpersonal model emphasizes the construct of acquired capability for suicide (see Chapter 2). However, it is important to note that this capacity could also be genetic. Some people are brave and fearless beginning in early childhood, whereas others are more timid and fearful. Research supports the notion that the former have externalizing personality traits, whereas the latter have internalizing ones. Psychopaths, for example, who are the most extreme externalizers, exhibit reduced anxiety and fear reactions—a phenomenon that has been shown to have a prominent genetic component.

Several studies reported that higher levels of fearlessness of death were associated with a higher number of suicide attempts (Anestis & Joiner, 2011). In the military, thwarted belongingness and perceived burdensomeness were associated with suicidal behavior only in those with high levels of fearlessness with regard to suicide. Clinically, however, the connection between capability for suicide and suicide intent or imminent suicidal behavior cannot be easily discerned.

Much more evident is the function of fear as a barrier to suicide, even when desire for suicide is palpable. For some patients, the fear of physical pain associated with most methods of suicide is visceral. This is usually expressed by the suicidal individual as some variation of "I am not afraid to die, but I am afraid of the pain." For others, the fear of pain is more vague and undifferentiated. In such cases, patients typically make statements such as "I will never do it; I do not have the courage." Such a statement could indicate fear of pain, of nothingness, of the unknown, or all of these.

CULTURAL ACCEPTABILITY

Cultural Attitudes and Immigration

Any person's suicide risk is significantly influenced by cultural attitudes. Historically, cultures that place a strong emphasis on personal honor tend to foster higher rates of suicide. For example, "honor suicides" (i.e., suicides in the face of defeat or capture) were common in Greek and Roman civilizations (Dublin, 1963). Japanese warriors who brought shame to their family voluntarily committed a ritualized form of suicide known as Seppuku to restore their honor. In Jodhpur, India, a wall by the fortress gate is full of 16th-century hand imprints left by women who fell to their death in response to the death of their husbands who died defending their city ("Sati Handprints," 2016). Thus, in many cultures, suicide has been (and, in some cases, still is) viewed as an appropriate response to certain types of perceived dishonor (Osterman & Brown, 2011).

In cultures in which family honor has historically been valued more than the wishes of the individual, people may feel unable to seek help for any distress caused by their cultural standards. In doing so, they would only amplify their shame, as well as impose additional dishonor on their families by revealing their distress. In such cultures, fear of reputational damage could create self-imposed barriers to seeking professional help, thus putting people at higher risk for suicide.

Finally, immigrant groups from "honor cultures" may exhibit high suicide rates under circumstances that would imply family dishonor in their native countries. A frequent scenario encountered in a psychiatric emergency room is a suicide attempt by an Asian student after failing to earn the grades needed for acceptance into a prestigious graduate program. In Asian families, failure to succeed can be a family disgrace (Chambers, 2010). College suicide attempts are not limited to Asian students, but this scenario highlights the pivotal role that culture can play in suicide risk.

Immigration Status

Interestingly, immigrants to the United States have lower suicide rates prior to their immigration compared to US-born citizens. However, suicide rates increase with acculturation and may exceed the rates of those who are born in the United States (Borges, Orozco, Rafful, Miller, & Breslau, 2011). Immigrants who migrated as children of Asian and African American ethnicity show higher lifetime prevalence of attempts than the US-born of the same ethnicity (Borges et al., 2011). The same is true for Middle Eastern immigrants (Nasseri & Moulton, 2009). Thus, when assessing imminent risk, clinicians must obtain a detailed cultural history. Paradoxically, despite high stress, recent immigration appears to be somewhat protective against suicidal behavior.

Moral, Philosophical, and Religious Objections

Religion generally disapproves of suicide, and having a religious affiliation is considered to be a protective factor with regard to suicide risk (Lawrence, Oquendo, & Stanley, 2015). Whereas for atheists, suicide may signify the end of life and escape from mental pain, for those with a religious affiliation, suicide is a sin and a violation of the divine code of behavior ("Catechism of the Catholic Church," n.d.; Holland, 1977; Roth, 2009). Thus, for many believers, religious affiliation is a protective factor against suicide.

Studies have confirmed the protective role of moral and/or religious objections to suicide against suicidal behavior (Galynker, Yaseen, Briggs, & Hayashi, 2015; Lawrence et al., 2015). Patients with depression and bipolar disorder (Dervic et al., 2011), as well as those without a specific psychiatric diagnosis, have been shown to have lower rates of suicidal behavior if they endorsed a religious affiliation. Conversely, lack of moral objections to suicide predicts higher rates of post-discharge suicidal behavior in high-risk psychiatric inpatients (Galynker et al., 2015).

The discussion of religious aspects of suicidal behavior would be woefully incomplete without addressing the topics of suicide terrorism and mass suicides, two rare but conspicuous circumstances, in which religious affiliation actually increases the risk of suicide. Scientific data on suicide terrorism are understandably lacking. The empirical data on suspected suicide terrorists suggest many discrepancies between suicide terrorists and other suicides (Townsend, 2007). This implies that such individuals are not truly suicidal and should not be viewed as a subgroup of the general suicidal population. Understanding suicide terrorism cannot be done outside of historical and cultural contexts, and it requires a multidisciplinary approach that includes not only psychological but also anthropological, economic, historical, and political factors.

The literature addressing mass suicides is even more sparse. Mass suicide is the simultaneous suicide of all members of a social group. The mass suicides of approximately the past 20 years are all related to the establishment of religious sects, which are defined as mystic, idiosyncratic, and often bizarre self-contained belief systems that may sometimes lead to the self-destruction of the sect under the guise of being an act of self-assertiveness (Mancinelli, Comparelli, Girardi, & Tatarelli, 2002). People who join cults are often psychiatrically ill with propensities toward dissociative states, histories of severe child abuse/neglect, tendencies to abuse controlled substances, debilitating situational stressors, and intolerable socioeconomic conditions. They are vulnerable to mass suicide when incited by the cult's charismatic leader. Two prominent cases of mass suicide are the 900 deaths in Jonestown and the 39 members of the Heaven's Gate group who committed suicide in order to reach an alien spacecraft following Comet Hale–Bopp (Lamberg, 1997).

Regional Affiliation

Even subtle differences in cultural attitudes result in significant differences in suicide rates. In the United States, western and southern states are sometimes classified as "honor states" due to their emphasis on self-sufficiency and negative view of federal entitlement programs. These states have higher suicide rates, particularly among Caucasians living in rural areas (Stark, Riordan, & O'Connor, 2011). Of note, in rural communities, suicides are more often associated with social isolation, and youth suicide rates are 2–10 times higher than the national average (Hirsch, 2006). Furthermore, levels of antidepressant prescriptions (an indicator of mental health help-seeking) are lower in honor states, despite levels of major depression being higher.

Suicide in the Family

Independent of familial history of mental illness, family history of suicide increases suicide risk, suggesting a social transmission effect. A familial history of mental illness increases suicide risk only in adults without a history of psychiatric illness, whereas a familial history of suicide increases suicide risk two- or threefold equally, irrespective of psychiatric illness history (Qin, Agerbo, & Mortensen, 2002). As such, familial history of suicide should be established in the assessment of acute suicide risk.

In adolescents, exposure to suicidal behavior of family or friends is associated with a threefold increase in future suicidal behaviors risk. In fact, exposure to a friend's or a family member's suicidal behavior significantly increased risk in adolescents (Nanayakkara, Misch, Chang, & Henry, 2013). Maternal suicidal behavior is more strongly associated with suicidal behavior in children compared to paternal suicidal behavior (Geulayov, Gunnell, Holmen, & Metcalfe, 2012). Children are more likely to be affected by parental suicidal behavior than are adolescents or adults, and the effects of maternal suicide on boys versus girls are the same. As in adults, there is no evidence of an interaction between exposure to a peer or family member suicide attempt and depression in children and adolescents.

Parental suicide weighs heavily on children throughout their lives, particularly when children approach the age at which their parent committed suicide. This is particularly pertinent for families with a genetic predisposition to a mental illness that causes deterioration later in life. As the suicide survivor's condition worsens, parallels with the deceased parent may become inevitable, thus increasing the sense of apprehension, hopelessness, and entrapment.

Suicide Clusters

A suicide cluster is defined as an excessive number of suicides occurring in close temporal and geographical proximity (Larkin & Beautrais, 2012). In the United States, it has been estimated that at least 2% of teenage suicides occur in temporal–spatial clusters. Clustering is thought to be two to four times more common among adolescents and young adults (aged 15–24 years) than among other age groups (Gould, Wallenstein, Kleinman, O'Carroll, & Mercy, 1990). Suicide clusters tend to occur in those who have contact with mental health services (McKenzie, 2005) or are in psychiatric hospitals (Haw, 1994), prisons (McKenzie & Keane, 2007), and schools (Brent et al., 1989).

We have a limited understanding of what triggers a suicide cluster and what causes it to continue and to eventually subside. A psychological explanation for this phenomenon is that suicide clusters occur when already vulnerable individuals, who are socially connected through shared characteristics, experience the suicide of a peer (Joiner, 1999). Other psychological processes, such as suggestion, identification, social learning, and susceptibility, are also implicated in the development of suicide clusters (Haw, Hawton, Niedzwiedz, & Platt, 2013). Most theories rely on the analogy of contagious illness, suggesting that clustering is a result of imitation of suicidal behavior. Novel channels of transmission for suicide contagion may include social networks (Mesoudi, 2009), media reporting (Niederkrotenthaler et al., 2010), and the Internet (Pirkis & Nordentoft, 2011).

The effect of the Internet on suicidal behavior is relatively new and requires careful investigation. Although the Internet facilitates help-seeking and support, it may also exert negative influences that discourage help-seeking. As many as 20% of adolescents with a history of suicide attempts state that social networking sites influenced their decision to self-harm (O'Connor, Rasmussen, & Hawton, 2014). The increase in suicide among Japanese adolescents and the emergence of Internet suicide pacts through suicide-related websites exemplifies this finding. The sites' visitors exhibit distinct existential suffering and focus their posts on the meaning of an individual's choice to die. In these instances, suicide clusters occur when individual suicides are sanctioned within a group of strangers too afraid to die (Naito, 2007).

In summary, cultural and religious factors play a significant role in moderating acute suicide risk. Aspects pertaining to personal and family honor, religious or moral prohibition, and moral acceptability of suicide are of particular importance. In the United States, attention should focus specifically on second-generation immigrants who may believe they have not met their parents' expectations and thus failed to repay them for the sacrifices made during immigration. In addition, exposure to suicide by family or friends, particularly to a mother's suicide, carries increased suicide risk. Cluster suicides are very real, and so are online suicide sites and groups. The still unresearched potential influence of social media on individual suicidal behavior is likely to be significant and should be explored in the course of suicide risk assessment.

Suicide Exposure and Practicing

In contrast to genetic trait fearlessness, the acquired capability for suicide is developed largely through environmental exposure to painful events, body injury, and/or violent deaths. Although this theory of gradual inoculation to the fear of the physical pain of death is intuitive, it is not well supported by research. Suicide rates in the military, for example, are not strongly related to the duration or type of combat exposure (Reger et al., 2011). Likewise, there does not seem to be a relationship between exposure to violence and suicide among policemen (Miller, 2006). It has been shown that surviving genocide, abuse, and loss of a family member to genocide are also not significantly associated with suicide (Rubanzana, Hedt-Gauthier, Ntaganira, & Freeman, 2014).

Suicidal behavior is an unambiguous and ominous sign of an imminent attempt. Although 50% of completed suicides occur on the first attempt (Schaffer et al., 2016), some of those may involve extensive preparation and remain undiscovered in the majority of cases. This preparatory behavior becomes known only in high-profile suicides or murder–suicides, as a result of considerable effort and resource expenditure. The clearest recent example of this is the German Wings copilot who crashed a plane into a mountain when the pilot left the cockpit to use the bathroom. The massive investigation that followed revealed that the copilot had been researching previous pilot suicides and that in the week preceding his murder–suicide, he practiced locking the cockpit door and initiating the accelerated descent that he ultimately used to bring down the plane.

The remaining 50% of unsuccessful initial suicide attempts differ greatly in their lethality. Statistically, the most common methods, in increasing order of lethality, are self-injurious cutting, drug overdose, poisoning, asphyxiation, drowning, hanging, jumping from heights, and firearms (Chang et al., 2011). Completed suicides are usually executed attempts by the same method used in the last attempt or attempts via a method of higher lethality. For example, a nonlethal overdose is followed by a lethal overdose with more pills or by jumping off the roof of a building. Failed attempts of high lethality are more likely to be followed by completed attempts compared to failed attempts of low lethality (Ajdacic-Gross, 2008).

In general, the lethality of the method used is significantly correlated with the intensity of the suicidal intent (Nishimura et al., 1999). Methods also differ regionally depending on their availability. In the United States, most people die by suicide using a firearm (AFSP, 2016). Overdose by pesticides, which are highly toxic and readily available in developing countries (Ajdacic-Gross, 2008), is most common worldwide. It is control of the means, rather than clinicians' improved ability to identify and treat suicidal patients, that is the most successful method of suicide rate reduction to date.

Case Examples

The first two parts of the imminent suicide risk assessment, the suicidal narrative and the suicidal crisis syndrome, intentionally do not contain any questions about suicide. The purpose of this omission is to avoid openly revealing the true purpose of the interview, making it difficult for those with high suicidal desire to hide the degree of their suicidal intent. The implicit risk/attitude/capability assessment uses the word "suicide" and asks general questions about suicide attitudes and exposure. Still, this module assesses suicide risk only indirectly, reducing the risk of the patient becoming defensive and giving misleading answers.

Interview Algorithm

1. Attitudes toward suicide
   a. Cultural
      i. General questions
         I am not sure about your exact cultural background, please tell me a little about your family.
         In your culture, how important is it to be loyal to your family?
         How far do people go in restoring family honor?
         What is your culture's attitude toward suicide?
         Is suicide sometimes the right thing to do?
         What is your personal opinion?
      ii. Suicide questions
         Do you think for some misdeeds suicide is the right solution?
         The only solution?
   b. Religious
      i. General questions
         Are you a religious person?
         How does your religion regard human life?
         How does it regard the human soul?
         Is there life after death?
         How does what you do in life affect what happens after death?
         Are you spiritual?
         Are we one with the universe?
      ii. Suicide questions
         Does suicide mean the end of one's immortal soul?
         Does it mean you will go to hell?
         Make you one with the universe?

2. Capability for suicide
   a. Trait fearlessness and pain insensitivity
      i. General questions
         Are you more fearless than most people?
         Are you less sensitive to pain than others?
         Are you afraid of death?
         Are you afraid of pain of death?
      ii. Suicide questions
         Would you be scared to kill yourself?
         Would you be afraid of the pain associated with suicide?
   b. Acquired capability: Exposure and practicing
      i. General questions
         Can you train yourself to be brave?
         To not be scared of death or pain?
         How?
         How do you think it should be done?
      ii. Suicide questions
         Have you tried to hurt yourself before? By what means?
         Have you attempted suicide? By what means?
         Did this make you less scared of suicide?
   c. Suicide in the military
      i. General questions
         How was military service for you?
         Did it provide purpose and self-respect?
         How is it to be a civilian?
         Was it a difficult transition?
         Do you feel like a burden?
         Do you feel a lack of understanding and respect?
         Do you feel alone?
      ii. Suicide questions
         Can it be so bad, it would not be worthwhile (possible) to continue?

3. Contagion
   a. Suicide of family and friends
      i. Suicide questions
         Has anybody among your family and friends died by suicide?
         What happened?
         Where were you?
         How did this affect you?
   b. Suicide clusters
      i. Suicide questions
         Has anybody among your friends died by suicide?
         What happened?
         Where were you at the time?
         How did this affect you?

Have any of your favorite celebrities died by suicide?

What happened?

Where were you at the time?

How did this affect you?

Do you know anybody who posted suicide messages on social media?

Have you gone on suicide sites? Chats?

What would friends do if they became suicidal?

Case 1: High Risk for Imminent Suicide

Randy, a 22-year-old college student, was brought to the emergency department after he staggered into a lecture hall and passed out on the floor. Six months prior, Randy was hospitalized after a suicide attempt via overdose. He was diagnosed with depression, treated with Wellbutrin, and discharged. He stopped Wellbutrin and did not follow up with his therapist.

1. Attitudes toward suicide
   a. Cultural
      i. General questions

      DR: Randy, please tell me a little about your family.

      RANDY: What do you want to know? They are stupid.

      DR: What do you mean?

      RANDY: They are wrapped up in their miserable lives, they have no idea what is going on.

      ii. Suicide questions

      DR: Let's say you were close to your parents. Could you do anything so shameful that the only way to redeem yourself would be suicide?

      RANDY: That's crazy. I can see many reasons why life may not be worth living, but failing to live up to parents' expectations is not one of them.

   b. Religious
      i. Suicide questions

      DR: Since you mentioned it, what would be such a reason?

      RANDY: The world is a miserable place.

      DR: Isn't suicide a morally wrong thing to do?

      RANDY: It's a choice. I see no intrinsic value to life.

2. Capability for suicide
   a. Trait fearlessness and pain insensitivity
      i. General questions

      DR: Are you a brave person?

      RANDY: I am not a coward.

      DR: Tell me something brave you have done.

      RANDY: I graduated from high school. I had to fight. I got beat up a lot.

      DR: Are you more or less sensitive to pain than others?

RANDY: See this? (Proceeds to show scars on forearms from cutting) I am not afraid of pain.

DR: Are you afraid of death?

RANDY: No.

    ii. Suicide questions

DR: Suicide can be a violent and painful, particularly when you are young and healthy.

RANDY: If you do it right you should not feel anything.

DR: Like how?

RANDY: With a gun

DR: Do you have a gun?

RANDY: I can get one if I need to.

  b. Acquired capability: Exposure and practicing

    i. General questions

DR: Have you seen a lot of violence in your life?

RANDY: No more than anybody else.

    ii. Suicide questions

DR: When you tried to kill yourself, what did you overdose on?

RANDY: Valium and vodka.

DR: Did you mean to die?

RANDY: Not sure. I kind of wanted to see what would happen.

DR: And?

RANDY: I wouldn't do that again. Too unreliable.

3. Contagion

  a. Suicide in family

    ii. Suicide questions

DR: Has anybody in your family committed suicide?

RANDY: My cousin shot himself when he was 18.

DR: Were you close with him?

RANDY: Pretty close.

DR: Did he kill himself on the first try?

RANDY: Yeah with a shotgun.

DR: Where were you at the time?

RANDY: Sleeping.

DR: How did this affect you?

RANDY: It seemed sudden. . . . He was not happy. It seemed like a solution.

  b. Suicide clusters

    ii. Suicide questions

DR: How long ago did your cousin kill himself?

RANDY: Six months now.

DR: Didn't you overdose at about the same time?

(Silence)

DR: Did you plan on it together?

RANDY: I don't want to talk about it.

DR: Did you research your overdose method?

RANDY: You don't need to research much. It's right out there.

Suicide Implicit Factors Assessment Table

Component	Risk Level				
	Minimal	Low	Moderate	High	Severe
Attitudes		X			
Moral religious prohibition/ permissiveness					X
Capability—trait					X
Capability— practicing					X
Family suicide					X
Suicide clusters					X
Total					X

Randy's risk for imminent suicide is very high. He does not value human life, has no moral or religious prohibitions, and has a philosophical position for justifying it. He is fearless and had a practice attempt. Finally, he had a suicide in the family, may have had a suicide pact with his cousin, and has access to a gun.

Case 2: Moderate Risk for Imminent Suicide

A 20-year-old Asian, Christian female with a previous suicide attempt by overdose was admitted to an inpatient unit. When asked about her mental state, she said she was fine other than she could not control her crying and screaming. During interviews, she would interrupt her answers with loud wailing.

1. Attitudes toward suicide
   a. Cultural
      i. General questions
         DR: I am not sure about your exact cultural background; please tell me a little about your culture.
         A: I am Korean, my parents are Korean.
         DR: I do not know much about Korean culture or about Korean values. How important is family honor in Korea?

A: Very important.

DR: What does a young person need to do to be honorable?

A: Study hard and get good grades.

DR: What if they try and can't? Can they live with that?

A: That would be shame on the family! They just need to study harder.

DR: In your culture, would one rather die than bring shame on the family?

A: Yes, sometimes, but I am a Christian—it's a sin. Your soul only goes to heaven if you are not a sinner.

    ii. Suicide questions

DR: If you were not Christian, would you think suicide the right solution?

A: Yes, if your family is ashamed of you (crying).

DR: The only solution?

A: I don't know.

  b. Religious

    i. General questions

DR: You said you are a Christian. What denomination are your parents, and you, as a matter of fact?

A: We go to the same church; it is Korean.

DR: For Christians, suicide is a sin, isn't it?

A: Yes.

DR: What happens to your soul when you die?

A: It goes to heaven if you are not a sinner.

    ii. Suicide questions

DR: And if you kill yourself?

A: Hell.

DR: You tried to kill yourself before . . .

A: I don't want to go to hell, I will never do that again, it was a mistake (wailing).

2. Capability for suicide

  a. Trait fearlessness and pain insensitivity

    i. General questions

DR: Are you a brave person?

A: No.

DR: Are you scared of pain?

A: No, pain makes me feel good sometimes.

DR: Are you scared of death?

A: Yes.

DR: Are you scared of the pain you would feel when you die?

A: Yes.

    ii. Suicide questions

DR: Would you be scared to kill yourself?

A: Yes.

DR: But you tried to overdose.

A: (Wailing) It was not serious . . .

DR: Was it painful?

A: When they pumped my stomach.

b. Acquired capability: Exposure and practicing

   i. Suicide questions

   DR: Now that you tried it once and it was not painful, would it be easier a second time?

   A: I am not going to. . . . I already told you—I am a Christian.

   DR: What about the last time? You took a whole bottle.

   A: I don't know what happened, I could not think straight.

3. Contagion

   a. Suicide in family

      i. Suicide questions

      DR: Has anybody in your family committed suicide?

      A: Yes, my grandfather jumped off a bridge

      DR: Where?

      A: Home in Korea. I was in the US.

   b. Suicide clusters

      i. Suicide questions

      DR: Has anybody among your friends recently died by suicide?

      A: No.

      DR: Do you know of anybody who did?

      A: Yes, Robin Williams. I think he hung himself.

      DR: Have you visited any suicide websites? Taken part in chats?

      A: No.

Suicide Implicit Factors Assessment Table

Component	Risk Level				
	Minimal	Low	Moderate	High	Severe
Attitudes				X	
Moral religious prohibitions/ permissiveness		X			
Capability—trait			X		
Capability— practicing				X	
Family suicide			X		
Suicide clusters	X				
Total			X		

A's risk for suicide is moderate. Her culture accepts honor suicide to avoid family disgrace, and she is aware of this. She is not intrinsically brave and is scared of pain, but she overcame that by finding a painless way to die. Her Christian faith still seems somewhat protective, the suicide in her family was remote, and she does not seem to care about the suicide of a public figure or want to be part of a "suicide community."

Case 3: Low Risk for Imminent Suicide

Mark is a 60-year-old married Jewish lawyer with a history of bipolar disorder who lost his practice while having a hypomanic episode. His depression was not improving despite the medications, and he was getting desperate. He felt like he had become useless and a burden to his family.

1. Attitudes toward suicide
   a. Cultural
      i. General questions
         DR: I know you are Jewish, what denomination are you?
         MARK: I am Orthodox.
         DR: How important is it in the Orthodox community to be loyal to your family?
         MARK: Our whole culture is about community, family, and tradition.
         DR: How does the community react to someone who brings shame on their family?
         MARK: We help the family, and we have rabbis who try to help the person too.
      ii. Suicide questions
         DR: What is your community's attitude toward suicide?
         MARK: Suicide means desertion of your family and religion.
         DR: Do you think for some misdeeds suicide is the right solution?
         MARK: It is never the right solution.
   b. Religious and moral attitudes
      i. General questions
         DR: Are you a religious person?
         MARK: Yes, I am very active in my synagogue.
         DR: How does Judaism regard the human soul?
         MARK: We have one.
         DR: And what happens to it when you die? Does it depend on how you live your life?
         MARK: It must. But we don't know.
      ii. Suicide questions
         DR: What if one dies by suicide?
         MARK: Nothing good—how can you do that to your family?

2. Capability for suicide
   a. Trait fearlessness and pain insensitivity
      i. General questions
         DR: Would you call yourself a brave person?

MARK: I guess so.

DR: Would you say that you are fearless?

MARK: I am not fearless, everybody has fears. I am average.

    ii. Suicide questions

DR: Would killing yourself be a scary act?

MARK: Of course it would.

3. Contagion
   a. Suicide in family
      i. Suicide questions

DR: Has anybody in your family died by suicide?

MARK: Yes, my mother. She was bipolar. She overdosed when she was depressed.

DR: That must have been awful. How old were you?

MARK: I was 40. I was at work. I got a call from her home attendant who found her dead when she came to work in the morning.

DR: How did this affect you?

MARK: I am scared that I will end up the same way.

DR: What has prevented you so far?

MARK: It's just the wrong thing to do. And my family.

   b. Suicide clusters
      i. Suicide questions

DR: Besides your mother, did anybody else you know attempt suicide?

MARK: Not personally. Just celebrities. Robin Williams.

DR: How did this affect you?

MARK: It was scary. They say he was depressed, but he was clearly bipolar. He was so manic when he was young.

DR: Do you know of any online suicide sites?

MARK: No.

Suicide Implicit Factors Assessment Table

Component	Risk Level				
	Minimal	Low	Moderate	High	Severe
Attitudes		X			
Moral religious prohibitions/ permissiveness		X			
Capability—trait	X				
Capability—practicing	X				
Family suicide				X	
Suicide clusters	X				
Total		X			

Although the acuity of Mark's suicidal state may be high, his capability for suicide is low. Mark has negative attitudes toward suicide both culturally and from a moral and religions perspective. However, his mother did kill herself, which elevates his suicide risk from minimal to low.

Test Case

Test Case 1

Lenny is a 60-year-old man, never married, with bipolar disorder. At age 57 years, he was hospitalized with a manic episode after being promoted at work and losing sleep due to stress. He subsequently lost his job and was depressed for 3 years with daily suicidal thoughts.

1. Attitudes toward suicide
   a. Cultural
      i. General questions
         DR: Tell me a little about your family.
         LENNY: My sister is a social worker, and my brother is a sound technician. My father is dead. My mother is in a nursing home with Alzheimer's disease.
         DR: Are you a close family?
         LENNY: No. I have not spoken to my brother in months. I talk to my sister once a week, but she does not want to talk to me right now because I am making her depressed. I am not even sure if they would miss me if I died.
         DR: I am sorry to hear that you feel alone in your family. When you have your thoughts about suicide, is your family holding you back?
         LENNY: No, just my fear of actually doing it.
      ii. Suicide questions
         DR: Do you think that there are situations when suicide is a legitimate option?
         LENNY: Yes, if the pain is unbearable
   b. Religious
      i. General questions
         DR: Are you religious?
         LENNY: I am Jewish, but I am not observant.
         DR: How does Judaism regard suicide?
         LENNY: I would imagine negatively.
         DR: What does this mean to you?
         LENNY: Not much.
         DR: Do you believe in God? In the human soul?
         LENNY: Maybe there is God—somebody had to create the Universe. I don't think there is an eternal soul or life after death.
      ii. Suicide questions
         DR: Should the fate of your eternal soul be a consideration when someone contemplates suicide?
         LENNY: For somebody like me? No.

2. Capability for suicide
   a. Trait fearlessness and pain insensitivity
      i. General questions
         DR: You said that it is the fear of actually doing it that would prevent you from killing yourself. Are you a brave person?
         LENNY: No.
         DR: Are you less sensitive to pain than other people?
         LENNY: About the same.
      ii. Suicide questions
         DR: A few minutes ago, you said that fear is holding you back. You mean that you would be scared to kill yourself?
         LENNY: Yes.
         DR: What is it you are afraid of? Pain?
         LENNY: Yes. The whole thing is so violent. Even "humane" lethal injection executions are violent—people die for hours. What if you miscalculate?
   b. Exposure and practicing
      i. General questions
         DR: Can you train yourself to not be scared of death?
         LENNY: Isn't that what military training is about?
      ii. Suicide questions
         DR: Do you think it is possible to train yourself not to be scared of suicide?
         LENNY: Maybe.

3. Contagion
   a. Suicide in family
      i. Suicide questions
         DR: Has anybody in your family died by suicide?
         LENNY: No.
   b. Suicide clusters
      i. Suicide questions
         DR: Have any of your friends died by suicide?
         LENNY: Yes. One of my friends. He hung himself.
         DR: How did this affect you?
         LENNY: It was very upsetting. I wished I were dead instead.
         DR: How long ago was that?
         LENNY: Two years.
         DR: Are you aware of any celebrities who died by suicide?
         LENNY: Robin Williams. He also hung himself. He was depressed.
         DR: Do you know of any suicide sites?
         LENNY: Yes, I went to some.
         DR: Did you post messages?
         LENNY: No, just read.

Suicide Implicit Factors Assessment Table

Component	Risk Level				
	Minimal	*Low*	*Moderate*	*High*	*Severe*
Attitudes					
Moral religious prohibitions/ permissiveness					
Capability—trait					
Capability— practicing					
Family or friend suicide					
Suicide clusters					
Total					

Lenny is alienated from his family and has no moral objections to suicide. He believes that suicide is justifiable if one is in too much pain. These two factors put him at high risk. He is fearful of pain and timid, decreasing his risk. However, he had a strong and personal reaction to his friend's suicide, increasing his risk. Overall, Lenny is at high risk for imminent suicide.

4

Stressful Life Events

With Shoshana Linzer, Adina Chesir, Tal Ginsburg, and Olivia Varas

INTRODUCTION

Stressful life events are some of the most critical factors precipitating suicidal behavior. They often occur during the week or month preceding suicide and are directly related. Up to 40% of suicide decedents experience a stressful event either on the day of a suicide attempt or on the day before. Commonly, the stressful life events leading up to the attempt are related to relationships with spouses or intimate partners (Heikkinen, Aro, & Lönnqvist, 1994). The links between stressful events and suicides are undeniable but not straightforward. Stress has many causes, including rejection, a humiliating business failure, or an incurable medical illness. The other most frequent reason found in psychological autopsies and in interviews with the survivors of high-lethality suicide attempts is mental illness (Lim, Lee, & Park, 2014).

Yet, taken as a whole, evidence supporting a direct casual and temporal relationship between life stressors, motives for suicide, and suicide attempts is not unequivocal. Although evidence for an association between negative life events and suicidal ideation and behavior is fairly consistent, there seems to be no direct relationship between stress severity and the lethality of suicidal ideation and behavior. Surprisingly, support for an inverse relationship between positive events and suicidal ideation and behavior is lacking. This may mean that so-called protective factors may not be as effective as hypothesized or may be strongly dependent on cultural factors (Liu & Miller, 2014).

For example, African American women are at high risk for suicidal ideation and suicide attempts, use emergency psychiatric services at higher rates than men and women of other ethnic groups, but have low suicide death rates. African American cultural variables may promote resilience and prevent fatal suicidal behavior among African American women, allowing them to generate and contemplate reasons for valuing life and protecting against life-threatening suicidal behavior (Flowers, Walker, Thompson, & Kaslow, 2014).

Regarding psychiatric illness, there is no apparent relationship between stressful life events and suicidal behavior for patients with major depressive disorder (MDD) without comorbid personality disorder, and there is only a weak correlation between suicide attempts and recent stressful events for depressed patients with borderline personality disorder (Oquendo et al., 2014). Another reason for lack of a strong association between sources of stress and suicide attempts may be that patients with mental illness lack the insight to identify the negative stressor as an exacerbation of their illness leading to suicide (Lim et al., 2014).

In addition, recently discharged military members explain suicide attempts as a means of alleviating emotional distress related to loss of respect, social isolation, and failure. However, both suicidal intent and the medical lethality of the attempt may be only weakly correlated with the corresponding measures of this distress (Bryan, Hernandez, Allison, & Clemans, 2012). Age may also play a role. Nearly 75% of US high school students who attempt suicide may do so for reasons other than death, such as revenge, sending a message, or regulating emotions. Whereas most suicidal adults understand that suicide is an act of killing oneself, the majority of adolescents may not be fully aware of this. Even in adolescents, however, stronger depressive symptoms and premeditation prior to the attempt are related to higher risk for suicide with death as a clear motive (Jacobson, Batejan, Kleinman, & Gould, 2013).

Still, most studies indicate that information on stressful life events is essential in the assessment of suicide motives, the most important of which are mental and physical illness, marital and relationship conflicts, parent–child conflicts, and economic hardship (Shiratori et al., 2014). Thus, examining these potential stressors related to imminent suicide risk is essential to our understanding of their impact on an individual's life. It is just as important, however, to understand the role of these stressors in the suicidal narrative.

WORK AND CAREER
Economic Hardship

Although a positive relationship between economic hardship and suicide rate is intuitive, it has been studied relatively little. Research shows that even in stable economic climates, suicide rates are higher in lower socioeconomic classes (Rehkopf & Buka, 2006). Low savings rates and lack of leisure time also correlate with higher suicide risk (Machado, Rasella, & Santos, 2015). Moreover, mental disorders mediate the relationship between family income and suicidality (Pan, Stewart, & Chang, 2013).

The relationship between lower socioeconomic status and suicidal behaviors is most evident during economic crises. For example, with a worsening economic climate, suicide rates in the United States started rising in 2005 after decades of decline. The most likely explanation for the reversal in trend lies in deteriorating economic conditions and the sharp rise in unemployment in 2007–2009. Indeed, during this time, there was a strong positive association between unemployment and suicide rates over time (Harper, Charters, Strumpf, Galea, & Nandi, 2015), specifically in middle age. Furthermore, for middle age there exists a temporal relationship between suicide and job loss (Chang, Stuckler, Yip, & Gunnell, 2013).

In the United States during the Great Recession, the association between unemployment and suicide appeared stronger with higher female labor force participation, suggesting that women working exacerbated the risk of male suicide associated with job loss. This surprising relationship was strongest for younger women in lower socioeconomic classes, in which unemployment for men may exact additional psychological pressure when women work. As a result, a low-income family with an unemployed man and an unemployed woman is at highest risk for adult male suicide. On the other hand, for older women, their unemployment may be positive for their entire family (Ying & Chang, 2009), lowering suicide risk for unemployed men in the family. Of note, American women had the highest increase in suicide rates, whereas in some European countries, the overall suicide rate for women continued to decline (Chang et al., 2013).

Business or Work Failure

Losing a job may serve in a suicidal narrative as failure to achieve a life goal, humiliating social defeat, or a feeling of burdensomeness. Shame and alienation combined with financial hardship and failure to find another job may result in intense entrapment and desperation (discussed further in Chapter 5). Thus, job loss could markedly increase suicide risk, contributing to different phases of the suicidal narrative.

Case 4

Paul was a 63-year-old lawyer with a history of bipolar disorder who died in the medical intensive care unit (MICU) of a large urban hospital after being admitted for overdosing on psychiatric medications. He overdosed impulsively after his wife left the apartment, saying that she was filing for divorce. Prior to this, he had not expressed suicidal intent to his wife, therapist, or psychopharmacologist. This was Paul's third marriage. He met his wife when he was 50 years old, and for him it was love at first sight. Despite fairly frequent fights about his wife's out-of-control spending, their marriage was generally happy. Yet after Paul was unexpectedly let go by his law firm during the Great Recession, their relationship started to deteriorate. At first, Paul was sure he would get a job at another law firm. After years of an unsuccessful job search, Paul retired and began living on a fixed income. Due to the stock market crash and some unwise investment decision, he soon became depressed. He told his therapist that each time he tried to tell his wife that they needed to budget their finances differently, she would threaten a divorce. He said that she made him feel like a failure. Paul was too ashamed to face his friends, so he stopped socializing and considered himself a failure, with no way out of the situation. Paul and his wife were scheduled to meet with his therapist 2 days after Paul took his life. Paul's case illustrates the relationship between business failure, economic hardship, and suicide. Because Paul had enough savings for him and his wife to live comfortably but not lavishly for the rest of their lives, his economic hardship was exacerbated by his wife's unrealistic expectations. However, given his predisposition to emotional dysregulation due to his bipolar disorder, he became acutely suicidal, resulting in a completed suicide.

Loss of Home

Homelessness is arguably the most visible sign of social and economic failure; thus, there is a direct and strong relationship between foreclosure rates and suicide rates. From 2005 through 2010, increased foreclosure rates explained 18% of the variance in the suicide rate, suggesting that the foreclosure crisis has likely contributed to increased suicides, specifically in middle-aged men, independent of other economic factors associated with the recession (Houle & Light, 2014). The Great Recession in Western Europe and North America was associated with at least 10,000 additional economic-related suicides. signifying that 1,800 of those were due to loss of home in foreclosure (Reeves, McKee, & Stuckler, 2014).

Critically, for imminent suicide risk assessment, 79% of suicides occurred before an actual housing loss, and 37% of decedents experienced acute eviction or foreclosure crises within 2 weeks of the suicide. Thus, impending foreclosure signifies a very high suicide risk for middle-aged men, requiring quick and preventive intervention (Fowler, Gladden, Vagi, Barnes, & Frazier, 2015). The overall increase in suicides due to foreclosure was five times higher than that due to eviction.

Particularly for those with mental illness, imminent eviction must be considered a significant risk factor for imminent suicide (Serby, Brody, Amin, & Yanowitch, 2006). The intervention must be quick and proactive because, as is the case with foreclosure, most people who are in danger of being evicted and become suicidal will kill themselves within a few days of being evicted.

In conclusion, eviction or foreclosure is often considered a traumatic rejection, a denial of basic human needs, and a shameful experience, particularly for those of middle-class background. Given the much higher suicide rates related to foreclosure compared to eviction, it is conceivable that higher socioeconomic status may contribute to psychological vulnerability to the loss of one's home.

Case 5[1]

Joan was a 58-year-old Caucasian woman with bipolar disorder. Although she had attempted suicide several times in recent years, her level of functioning and treatment adherence had improved considerably in the months before her death. When it became apparent that she would be evicted, plans were made for her to move into the home of friends. Her case manager and sister both spoke with her that evening and did not notice anything amiss. The next morning, she was found dead of a self-inflicted stab wound.

Case 6[2]

Jose was a 48-year-old married White man. Six weeks before his suicide, he was hospitalized with mixed mania, suicidal ideation, and compulsive gambling. He was nearly $250,000 in debt and facing eviction. He had petitioned to block the eviction and was optimistic that the judge would rule in his favor. On the day before his death, the court ruled that the landlord was entitled to evict him. He went missing and was found the next day dead from a drug overdose.

Both cases describe completed suicides related to eviction in the high-risk group of 45- to 64-year-olds. Characteristically, both took place prior to eviction and following a meeting with an official, which made the eviction inevitable. In Joan's case, the precipitating event was the meeting with the case manager, whereas in Jose's case it was the court decision.

[1] From Serby et al. (2006).
[2] From Serby et al. (2006).

RELATIONSHIP CONFLICT

Together with economic hardship or financial difficulties, intimate relationship conflict accounts for close to 80% of stressful life events preceding suicide (Kõlves, Värnik, Schneider, Fritze, & Allik, 2006). Intimate relationship conflict is a term used to describe serious and emotionally charged disagreements with a current or former intimate partner, typically involving divorce, breakups, infidelity, jealousy, or other problems (Ortega & Karch, 2010). In suicide notes, marital and intimate relationship conflict is the most frequent reason given (Ortega & Karch, 2010). In psychological autopsies, approximately one-third of suicides are either preceded by a serious relationship conflict in the past 2 weeks of life or precede the certainty of such conflict in the next 2 weeks. Furthermore, suicide attempt survivors frequently indicate that marital and intimate relationship conflict precipitated the attempt (Zhang & Ma, 2012).

Romantic Rejection

Among the many stresses inherent in relationships, romantic rejection leads most frequently to suicide attempts. Two-thirds of spouses who have survived their former partner's suicide perceive their recent separation (i.e., within 3 months of suicide) as the most critical event leading to suicide (Heikkinen, Aro, & Lönnqvist, 1992). In serious suicide attempts, the three most common precipitants are, in order, the end of a romantic relationship, other interpersonal intimate relationship difficulties, and economic hardship (Beautrais, Joyce, & Mulder, 1997). The numbers are similar for those in the military: Half of Air Force decedents experience a failure in spousal or intimate relationships, one-third of which typically occur within the month prior to suicide (Reger et al., 2011).

Case 7

Gus was a 27-year-old genetics graduate student at a major university who overdosed 2 weeks after his girlfriend ended the relationship. His girlfriend Mary was a chemistry graduate student 2 years his senior. After several months, Mary felt that she was being used and that Gus was too ambitious and self-absorbed. She believed that she was getting nothing out of the relationship. She suggested that they have a closure dinner, which turned into a prolonged fight. Gus called several times to apologize and asked to meet again. Mary accepted the apology but said that she needed a break. Gus continued to text her, but Mary stopped answering. A week later, she received a call from Gus's PhD adviser saying that he was found dead in his lab. An e-mail with a heading "This is how I killed myself" arrived almost simultaneously.

Gus's is a typical case of suicide of a young person because of romantic rejection. He killed himself a week after his girlfriend stopped answering his texts, which was a message of irrevocable rejection. In response, although he clearly understood that he was about to die, Gus's last e-mail about how he had died was meant to connect him to her for the last time by providing the details of his death. Perfectionism, failure to disengage, thwarted belongingness, and other elements of the suicidal narrative are clearly discernable.

Intimate Relationship Conflict

Despite findings that married individuals are at lower risk for suicide compared to unmarried individuals (Smith, Mercy, & Conn, 1988), relationship quality appears to supersede marriage integrity. Marital dissolution and dissatisfaction have been associated with suicide risk (Prigerson, Maciejewski, & Rosenheck, 1999; Stack & Wasserman, 1993). Married or not, those who die by suicide are likely to have experienced recent intimate relationship conflict (Cheng, Chen, Chen, & Jenkins, 2000; Phillips et al., 2002). More than half of these stressful events occur in the final 24 hours before suicide (Marttunen, Aro, & Lonnqvist, 1993). In general, marriage appears to be a protective factor against suicide, particularly for men (Goldsmith, Pellmar, Kleinman, & Bunney, 2002), whereas for women, suicidal behavior does not depend on marital status. Compared to married or cohabitating men, divorced and separated men are up to six times more likely to die by suicide. This is possibly due to the vulnerability associated with interpersonal stressors during the separation phase (Cantor & Slater, 1995). In fact, recent separation may confer more than a fourfold greater suicide risk over current married, cohabiting, widowed, or single status, especially in men between the ages of 15 and 24 years (Wyder, Ward, & De Leo, 2009).

Nearly half (46%) of all the suicide deaths among females occur between the ages of 15 and 44 years, during reproductive age when relationship issues are of primary importance. In this age group, suicide is the fourth leading cause of death for women, ranking higher than death due to homicide, HIV, cerebrovascular disease, and diabetes (Centers for Disease Control and Prevention [CDC], 2014). After mental health-related causes, the most frequent precipitants for women are problems with a current or former intimate partner (36%), and 28% of women disclosed their intent to die by suicide to another person with enough time for someone to have intervened (CDC, 2014). Women who experience higher rates of domestic violence, current physical or sexual abuse, or who have a history of childhood abuse are at increased risk for attempts under these circumstances (Baca-Garcia, Perez-Rodriguez, Man, & Oquendo, 2008).

Women report experience of domestic and intimate partner violence somewhat more often than men, but the difference is not dramatic. Domestic violence tends to occur most often in families with lower educational status and during times of economic adversity. Furthermore, repetitive violence has been linked to more serious consequences compared to single violent events. However, recent population studies indicate that the association between reports of domestic violence and suicide attempts exists among both women and men, although it is more well established for women. Moreover, the association between suicide attempts and intimate partner violence appears stronger for men. It is possible that men with suicidal ideation go on to attempt suicide (Hawton & Van Heeringen, 2009) or that men are often reluctant to seek help for domestic violence due to the shame and humiliation of appearing weak (Galdas, Cheater, & Marshall, 2005). Thus, when assessing suicide risk, evaluation of intimate partner violence should not exclude either sex. Overall, the risk for suicide attempt in families with domestic violence compared to those without is six times higher for women and eight times higher for men (Dufort, Stenbacka, & Gumpert, 2015).

Case 8

Josh was a 60-year-old married accountant. He had a long history of bipolar II disorder with fairly predictable seasonal cycling. With age, his hypomanic episodes had become shorter, and his depressive episodes grew longer; thus, by age 61 years, he was depressed 10 months of the year and hypomanic for 1 month, with only 1 month of euthymia. As his disease progressed, he had an increasingly difficult time keeping his clients, and his relationship with his wife grew more strained. She had always been the main breadwinner in the family and was very critical of Josh, including when they were with friends. At home, she was hostile and disdainful, verbally abusive, and cast herself as both a saint and a victim for putting up with such a loser and wasting her life on him. These fights made Josh feel like a failure, and he often thought of suicide during his depressive episodes. During hypomanic periods, he was fairly successful in getting new clients but was also overspending and having affairs. Josh's last depression was particularly severe, and after missing several deadlines at work, he lost his only major client. When he told his wife, she was furious; she slapped him, threw his books at him, and told him to get out of the house because she was filing for divorce. Josh begged to stay, but his wife physically pushed him out of the door. He banged on the door several times, but she did not open it. He went to the roof of their apartment building, sent her a text stating "I am jumping off, you will be better off without me," and then jumped to his death.

As in Gus's case, Josh's suicide also followed rejection, but it was primarily the result of ongoing domestic emotional abuse and the onset of physical abuse. His shame in telling others—their children, his friends, and relatives—about his failure and the feeling of entrapment are almost palpable.

Parents in Conflict with Children

Conflict with children is a less frequent stressful life event and suicide trigger than romantic rejection and economic hardship, but it can still be a significant contributor to suicidal behavior. Just as the meaning and the emotional significance of parent–child conflicts strongly depend on culture, religion, and ethnicity, so does the association between these factors and suicidal behavior. Some studies indicate that such conflicts are most damaging in Asian cultures that value close family ties, and they are of lesser importance in countries that value individualism and independence, such as the United States. Even from a sociocultural standpoint, the Asian view of the self is more dependent on correlations with others than it is in Western countries, and this is likely to affect the suicide narrative (Tanaka, Sakamoto, Ono, Fujihara, & Kitamura, 1998). In this respect, acute life stresses evoked by family conflicts and job and financial security issues should not be viewed as isolated stressors but, rather, can be grouped as negative relationships with others. These relationships play more important roles for suicide in Asian than in Western countries (Chen, Wu, Yousuf, & Yip, 2012). Thus, it is not surprising that in Japan, for example, conflicts with children, after depression and physical illness, are most strongly associated with long-term suicide risk, on par with severe economic hardship and ahead of romantic rejection and loneliness (Shiratori et al., 2014).

Case 9

Lin was a 58-year-old Chinese woman with a long history of schizophrenia who was admitted to an inpatient unit. Lin immigrated to the United States with her husband and two boys in her early 30s when she was already ill but fairly functional; at the time, she was able to take care of her household and also help out at her brother-in-law's grocery store. However, when Lin was in her mid-40s, she had several violent psychotic episodes requiring hospitalization. The patient's husband and sons, who described their mother as dysfunctional, were clearly tired of taking care of her, and there was much angry talk between them at the family meeting. The patient did not participate and just sat in her chair staring at the floor. The husband asked to place Lin in a nursing facility, but she had worked off the books and had no insurance. The social worker told them to apply for disability, and Lin was discharged home. Three hours later, she jumped to her death off the roof of her building.

Lin had many risk factors for suicide. She had a trait vulnerability of severe mental illness and cultural acceptability of suicide conferring chronic suicide risk. Her agitation, ruminations, and affective disturbance were part of severe suicidal crisis syndrome (SCS), indicating imminent risk, but it was primarily during her last admission that her life narrative took the shape of the suicidal narrative. Her family behavior made it painfully obvious that she was a burden and that she had lost the respect of the entire family. Moreover, her medical team placed all control of her life into her family's hands, creating a dead end. Thus, according to the narrative crisis model, Lin was at a very high risk of suicide. Tragically, Lin's culture added the final risk factor. Lin's language barrier made her isolated from her treatment team, which could not perform an objective mental status examination. If it had, team members might have realized that placement in a nursing facility by her family was rejection according to her culture.

Children in Conflict with Parents

Suicides in pre-teenager children are relatively rare. However, they do occur, with parent–child conflicts being their most frequent precipitants. In identifying children at high risk for suicide, it is important to assess for the presence of such conflicts and to understand the incremental risk contribution due to other sociodemographic variables. According to a recent review, a neglectful and yet controlling parenting style known as "affectionless control" is likely to contribute to the role that parent–child conflicts play in suicide risk in children, adolescents, and adults (Goschin, Briggs, Blanco-Luten, Cohen, & Galynker, 2014).

During the past two decades in the United States, the suicide rate for children 10–14 years old tripled from 0.5 to 1.5/100,000. However, when ethnic and racial differences are considered, during this time there has been a dramatic increase in suicide incidence for Black children and a decrease in suicide incidence among White children (Curtin, Warner, & Hedegaard, 2016). The reasons for this divergent trend are not yet clear, but this needs to be kept in mind during risk assessment (Bridge et al., 2015).

With regard to parental styles, some parenting features appear to be protective for suicide risk, whereas others increase it. Maternal and paternal warmth in childhood and maternal control in adolescence have protective influences on suicide risk. Surprisingly, authoritative parenting is protective as well. On the other hand, rejecting–neglecting parenting strongly increases the risk for suicide attempts. Seven other factors increase suicide risk in prepubescent children: attention deficit hyperactivity disorder, female sex, smoking, binge drinking, absenteeism/truancy, migration background, and parental separation (Donath, Graessel, Baier, Bleich, & Hillemacher, 2014; Goschin et al., 2014).

The relative importance of trait suicidality and stressful life events in the etiology of suicide in children appears to differ from that in adolescents and adults. Whereas 90% of suicide decedents in this age group had a psychiatric diagnosis (Chang, Gitlin, & Patel, 2011), for suicide decedents younger than age 12 years, only 25% met the criteria for a psychiatric diagnosis and 30% had depressive symptoms at the time of death. In contrast, 60% of the parents of these suicide victims reported that the child experienced some kind of stressful conflict prior to death, whereas only 12% of the parents of accident victims reported such conflicts (Freuchen, Kjelsberg, Lundervold, & Groholt, 2012).

In retrospect, the stressful conflicts preceding child suicides were considered unimportant or even trivial at the time (Groholt, Ekeberg, Wichstrom, & Haldorsen, 1998), but were likely to involve shame (Lester, 1997; Orth et al., 2010). The parents' descriptions revealed behaviors of which children typically are ashamed, such as being caught stealing, having done something wrong, having been humiliated, and having experienced hurtful comments. In general, shame is a difficult feeling to deal with, and in combination with the personality traits of vulnerability and impulsiveness, it may prove dangerous. From this perspective, suicide may represent a child's attempt to resolve a shameful situation perceived as unbearable (Freuchen et al., 2012).

With regard to adolescents, as discussed in Chapter 3, those who die by suicide are more likely to have a family history of suicide and/or significant psychopathology (Shaffer, Gould, & Hicks, 1994). Not surprisingly, childhood abuse, a history of parental separation or loss of a parent (by death or divorce), as well as physical and/or sexual violence in the family are also associated with suicidality (Schilling, Aseltine, Glanovsky, James, & Jacobs, 2009). Adolescents with suicidal behaviors are more likely to be living in non-intact families (Afifi et al., 2008; Brent & Mann, 2005; Zayas, Bright, Álvarez-Sánchez, & Cabassa, 2009) and in an atmosphere of problematic communication, poor attachment, and high levels of conflict (Afifi et al., 2008; Bridge, 2008; Gould, 1996; Libby, Orton, & Valuck, 2009; Martin, 2005; Qin, Mortensen, & Pedersen, 2009). In depressed adolescents, poor family function and family conflict are predictive of suicide attempts within 1 year after initial assessment (Bridge, 2008). Independent of parental conflict, adolescents aged 11–17 years who frequently moved during childhood were more likely to make suicide attempts during adolescence (Qin et al., 2009). There is a dose–response relationship between the number of moves and risk of attempted suicide: Youth who had moved 3–5 times were 2.3 times more likely to have attempted suicide compared to those who had never changed residences, whereas those who had moved more than 10 times were 3.3 times more likely to attempt suicide, controlling for birth order, birthplace, and paternal and maternal factors. The same is true of suicide completers (Cash & Bridge, 2009).

The new concept of emerging adulthood has been created to describe those between ages 18 and 25 years who are still not independent of their families. In *The New York Times* column titled "How Adulthood Happens," David Brooks (2015) discusses a widespread phenomenon of young people not reaching maturity until their 30s. Correspondingly, the most common proximal risk factor for completed suicide for subjects younger than 30 years was not financial distress but, rather, conflict with family members, partners, or friends (Foster, 2011). In this age group for both men and women, a negative relationship with either or both parents or conflicts between parents are significantly associated with suicide risk (Consoli et al., 2013).

Case 10

The mother of an 11-year-old boy came home and found that her son, Scott, had hanged himself with her scarf from their second-floor stair balcony. Scott had behavioral and academic problems in the past, and his suicide followed an incident at school for which he was sent home for hitting another student in his class. The school principal told his parents that if Scott became violent one more time, he would be expelled and have to attend a school for children with behavioral problems. When they were driving home following the conference, Scott's parents told him that if he got kicked out of school, they would send him to boarding school and never visit. Scott had been threatened with boarding school before and did not appear scared. The mother later remembered that approximately 1 year ago, Scott and his sister play-acted hanging after watching a Western movie on TV in which men were hanged.

Scott's suicide illustrates most major points about suicides by small children. It took place as a result of a major conflict with his parents involving shame, although the stressful life events preceding the suicide were only a continuation of his life as usual. As is often the case, his parents did not realize the danger or actual suicide risk.

Ongoing Childhood and Adolescent Abuse and Neglect

Results from dozens of studies generally suggest that childhood sexual, physical, and emotional abuse and neglect are associated with childhood and adolescent suicide attempts. This relationship holds true for children from different cultures and ethnicities, from families with or without mental illness, and with different peer relationships. All four aforementioned types of childhood abuse or neglect are associated with adolescent suicidal ideation and suicide attempts, and their effects are additive. However, there is evidence that sexual abuse and emotional abuse may be relatively more important in explaining suicidal behavior compared to physical abuse or neglect (Miller, Esposito-Smythers, Weismoore, & Renshaw, 2013).

The strongest and clearest evidence exists between sexual abuse and childhood and adolescent suicide attempts. This link is significant regardless of the child or adolescent age and grade level (Waldrop et al., 2007), sex (Esposito & Clum, 2002a), IQ (Fergusson, Woodward, & Horwood, 2000), and race or ethnicity (Brown, Cohen, Johnson, & Smailes, 1999; Thompson et al., 2012). However, although the previously mentioned associations are generally true, most may be stronger for boys than for girls, in whom they are present only if comorbid with hopelessness and depression (Bagley, Bolitho, & Bertrand, 1995).

The strong relationship between sexual abuse and suicide attempts in adolescents appear to be remarkably independent from family structure, pathology, and peer relationships. The link remains robust for any family structure regardless of parental separation, parental role changes, mother's level of education, family socioeconomic status, parental violence or imprisonment, adolescent's attachment, parenting style or family functioning (Fergusson, Horwood, & Lynskey, 1996; Fergusson et al., 2000), parents' psychiatric symptoms and substance abuse (Johnson et al., 2002), parental suicide, or general feelings of social connectedness (Rew, Thomas, Horner, Resnick, & Beuhring, 2001).

Of note, the associations between childhood sexual abuse and adolescent suicide appear to be invariant to categorical psychiatric diagnosis and persist whether or not an adolescent has been diagnosed with major depressive disorder, conduct disorder, adjustment disorder, and social phobia (Glowinski et al., 2001). Individual symptom dimensions such as depressive symptoms (Fergusson, Beautrais, & Horwood, 2003; Rew et al., 2001), hopelessness (Martin, Bergen, Richardson, Roeger, & Allison, 2004; Rew et al., 2001), dissociative symptoms (Kisiel & Lyons, 2001), personality factors (Fergusson et al., 2000), and previous suicide attempts (Johnson et al., 2002) also do not appear to affect the link between childhood sexual abuse and suicidal behavior.

Results from studies of physical abuse also reveal a clear association with suicide attempts in adolescents, regardless of whether they live at home or are psychiatric inpatients, delinquent youth, homeless youth, or runaways. Similar to sexual abuse, the associations of childhood physical abuse with adolescent suicide attempts do not depend on youth gender, youth age, race/ethnicity, family socioeconomic status, or caregiver education level (Brown et al., 1999; Esposito & Clum 2002b; Johnson et al., 2002; Rew et al., 2001;Thompson et al., 2012). The link between physical abuse and suicide attempts in adolescents persists regardless of their psychological distress in childhood and early adolescence; depression severity; disruptive and risky behavior; comorbid internalizing and externalizing symptoms; diagnoses of major depressive disorder, conduct disorder, adjustment disorder, or social phobia; and prior suicide attempts (Fergusson et al., 2003; Glowinski et al., 2001; Johnson et al., 2002; Rew et al., 2001).

As with sexual abuse, the association between physical abuse and youth suicidal behavior is not related to family factors such as history of suicide within the family, family alcohol and drug problems, maternal care, parent attachment, family composition, and parent psychiatric symptoms (Johnson et al., 2002; Rew et al., 2001). Nor is it related to peer variables such as social connectedness, suicide of a friend, and attachment to friends (Rew et al., 2001).

Emotional abuse, but not neglect, appears to be associated with suicidality, regardless of youth demographics and mental health problems, and family variables (Thompson et al., 2012). The influence of family and peer relationship variables on this link is unknown.

Physical abuse and sexual abuse often take place simultaneously; when they do, it is sexual rather than physical abuse that is associated with suicide attempts, regardless of family socioeconomic status, youth dissociative symptoms, negative life events, parental violence, mental health symptoms, separation, imprisonment, education, attachment, and changes in caregiver (Brent et al., 1993; Fergusson et al., 2000; Kisiel & Lyons, 2001). Somewhat unexpectedly, when all four forms of abuse co-occur, adolescent suicide attempts are primarily associated with sexual and emotional abuse (Locke & Newcomb, 2005); suicide has no link to physical abuse and neglect.

Childhood maltreatment affects boys and girls differently, and the differences are most pronounced for sexual abuse (Bagley, Bolitho, & Bertrand, 1995), for which the risk of a suicide attempt is 15 times greater for male victims of sexual abuse than for female victims (Martin et al., 2004). Physically abused boys may also be at higher risk for suicide attempts compared to physically abused girls (Rosenberg et al., 2005).

Regardless of the victim's gender, sexual abuse experiences that involve contact (i.e., touching and intercourse) with the perpetrator are more likely to lead to a suicide attempt compared to noncontact sexual abuse (i.e., verbal sexual harassment). Suicide attempt risk is higher with a later age of onset of sexual abuse, when the perpetrator is an acquaintance rather than a parent or caregiver, and when a parent denies the abuse occurrence and expresses anger for the abuse incident toward the child rather than the perpetrator (Plunkett et al., 2001).

In summary, childhood maltreatment, particularly sexual and emotional abuse, is associated with increased risk of suicide attempts in childhood, adolescence, and adulthood. The risk is much higher for males than for females and also when abuse involves physical contact and is perpetrated repeatedly within the family. Because most suicide attempts are preceded by a stressful life event within 1 month, when assessing risk for imminent suicide, it is important to establish whether the abuse is recent or ongoing.

Bullying

Bullying is unwanted, aggressive behavior among school-aged children that involves a real or perceived power imbalance. The behavior must be repeated or must have the potential to be repeated over time. Both kids who are bullied and kids who bully others may have serious, lasting problems (for more information, see https://www.stopbullying.gov). It has been reported that both perpetrators and victims of bullying are at an increased risk of suicidal behaviors (Dilillo et al., 2015). Students who are bullied, threatened, or injured by someone with a weapon, physically hurt by their partner, or have ever been forced to have sex are twice as likely as students who have not experienced victimization to attempt suicide (Van Geel, Vedder, & Tanilon, 2014).

The relationship between bullying and suicide risk is gender dependent and affects the victims and the perpetrators differently. Female victim-perpetrators and female victims have the highest risk for suicide attempts (Cook, Williams, Guerra, Kim, & Sadek, 2010). Bullying is rarely the only factor contributing to suicidal behavior. Suicide in youth usually arises from a complex interplay of various biological, psychological, and social factors, of which bullying is only one.

Late adolescent victims of bullying are less likely to seek help from school administration and mental health professionals if they are suicidal compared to victims who are not suicidal; for bullied adolescents, there seems to be an inverse relationship between the severity of suicidal ideation and help-seeking. Even more remarkably, targets of bullying with the most severe suicidal ideation tend to not seek help from peers and family members, who are the most frequent source of help for adolescents. Thus, for known victims of bullying, an abrupt and unexplained end to complaints about bullying or a sudden denial of previous distress may be a sign of increased risk for imminent suicide.

Bullying is not limited to children and adolescents, and it is surprisingly common in the workplace. Among 642 completed work-related suicides from 2000 to 2007, 55% had an association with work stressors, identified as business difficulties, work injury, or conflicts with supervisors/colleagues (including workplace bullying). Thus, bullying in the workplace should be assessed whenever difficulties at work are identified as stressors (Routley & Ozanne-Smith, 2012).

Case 11

Sergei, a 17-year-old high school senior, was admitted to the emergency department (ED) after he tried to stab himself in his chest with a knife in a suicide attempt after being raped at his school. Once he was stabilized, he was admitted to an acute psychiatric unit on constant observation for suicidal ideation. Sergei was a student at an exclusive boarding high school for boys. He did not like the school from the very beginning and begged his parents to take him home. Sergei was also overweight and awkward, and he was quickly given the nickname "the Oligarch Fag," which was used by everybody behind his back but not to his face. He completed 9th grade without making any friends but was not bullied or abused. At the beginning of 10th grade, however, he was jumped in the bathroom and his watch was stolen. Sergei complained to the principal's office, the dorms were searched, and the watch was found in a night table of one of the popular kids. The delinquent student was expelled from school, and from that moment on, Sergei's life became a living hell. His classmates beat him up at least one night a week, always putting a pillowcase over his head so he could not recognize the perpetrators. He was threatened that if he squealed one more time, he would be dead. The beatings continued until one night Sergei was dragged to the gym, gagged, and raped with a plastic beer bottle. He was left bleeding on the floor, where he was found by one of the cleaning staff.

Case 12

Yana, the 16-year-old daughter of Greek immigrants, was brought to the ED after her mother found her lying on her bed, unresponsive, with two empty bottles of her psychotropic medications by her side. There was no note. Yana was attending one of the small, elite private schools in New York on a scholarship and had trouble fitting in with the rest of the students. The parents told the treatment team that Yana's only friend in her class was the other scholarship student, who was from Iran. Both girls were often teased for being overweight and wearing the wrong clothes and makeup. Yana begged her parents to transfer her to another school, but her parents were adamant that she should continue because of the high quality of the education and the high admission rates into Ivy League colleges. Yana had never threatened suicide before, and recently she had complained less about the school, which made the family think that the situation may have improved. However, during the physical exam, the team saw multiple scarred cuts on her forearms and thighs. Yana was admitted to the MICU with hypotension and bradycardia and was stabilized. When she woke up, she told the medical team that the girls were cruel, worse than in the movies; that they made her feel like she was trash; and that her parents did not listen. On the day of the attempt, her only friend told her that she needed some space because Yana was just "too weird." Yana said she gave up on talking to her parents because it was useless.

Sergei's case is a result of ongoing relentless bullying and heinous physical one-time sexual abuse, tacitly condoned by the school. Yana's case illustrates most aspects of bullying: a power imbalance between her wealthy classmates and the two second-generation immigrants from lower-income families, no help-seeking, and fewer complaints to the family before the attempt because of the breakdown in communication and trust. Also, fairly characteristically, the suicide was precipitated not by bullying but, rather, by a friend's rejection, suggesting that Yana's psychopathology may have involved some borderline and avoidant-dependent traits. In both cases, the parents' neglectful and controlling parenting exemplifies the affectionless control parenting style associated with suicide attempts.

SERIOUS MEDICAL ILLNESS
Recent Diagnosis

Being diagnosed with a serious medical illness may bring on reassessment of one's life narrative. If the reconfigured life narrative involves significant narrowing of life's remaining options and perception of a looming end, a suicidal crisis may ensue. Although some degree of increased suicide risk is present in all age groups, the increases in imminent versus long-term suicide risk are different for adolescents and young adults than for older adults.

Patients who have recently received a cancer diagnosis are at increased risk for imminent suicide in the first year after being diagnosed, with the highest increase occurring in the first week. Elderly patients, who may have a better understanding of the diagnosis and may have had friends or relatives die of cancer, are at particularly high risk. In contrast, younger patients who lack such experiences and who may be in denial of its meaning do not experience as prominent an increase in risk (Fang et al., 2012).

Of note, people with serious hereditary disorders, such as Huntington's disease, who choose to learn about their diagnosis and do so by consulting trained specialists are at no higher risk for imminent suicide than healthy individuals. Even after learning that they will develop a terminal neurological disorder in the future, such persons almost never have catastrophic reactions to learning about their fate and express satisfaction regarding their decision to be tested. Training medical staff in how to deliver appropriate support to these individuals in a timely manner is critical (Dufrasne, Roy, Galvez, & Rosenblatt, 2011).

Finally, people with psychiatric illness who are told of their diagnosis of a life-threatening medical illness are at much higher risk of attempting suicide than those do not have a psychiatric disorder. Of note, suicide risk in physically ill people varies substantially by the presence of psychiatric comorbidity, particularly the relative timing of onset of the two types of illness. Unexpectedly, the risk of suicide attempt is even higher in those who have developed a psychiatric disorder, primarily depression, soon after learning of their medical diagnosis. This means that patients who develop a major depressive or psychotic episode after being informed of a serious medical illness have increased suicide risk. Thus, closer collaboration between general and mental health services should be an essential component of suicide prevention strategies (Qin, Hawton, Mortensen, & Webb, 2014).

Case 13

Alonso was a 25-year-old man who was admitted to an intensive rehabilitation unit. At the time of his diagnosis, he was working and engaged to be married the following spring. His biopsy results showed that the disease had already metastasized. Alonso was told the biopsy results and researched his treatment options and his dismal life expectancy on the Internet. He told his oncology team that with such a poor prognosis, he "might as well kill myself, because what is the point?" Psychiatry consultation was called to assess Alonso's suicide risk. When the psychiatrist came to see him, Alonso denied suicidal ideation. During the interview, he was anxious but upbeat. He told the psychiatrist that after speaking to his fiancée and his family, he felt much better. His fiancée told him she loved him no matter what and that the wedding was still on and they had to finalize their guest list. His parents told him that he needed to take care of himself and not to worry and that they would help financially, if needed.

Alonso's case is a good example of how adaptive denial may help young people diagnosed with terminal illness and also how a family can reduce the risk. With their actions and words, Alonso's girlfriend and his family quickly reminded Alonso that he is part of the family and that he is anything but a burden to them. Instead of feeling trapped by his diagnosis of terminal illness, Alonso was being asked to help make wedding choices with many options. This approach eliminates or weakens phases 5–7 of the suicidal narrative and makes suicidal crisis less likely.

Prolonged and Debilitating Illness

The association of medical illness with suicide is not limited to instances of recent diagnosis. Having a prolonged, terminal illness also increases suicide risk. One-third of persons who died by suicide and left a suicide note gave health-related reasons for taking their lives, and two-thirds of those had underlying chronic medical conditions (Cheung, Merry, & Sundram, 2015a). Surprisingly, in only a small minority were their illnesses possibly terminal (Cheung Merry & Sundram, 2015b), and it appears that type of illness may be more directly related to suicide than how life threatening the illness may actually be. Psychological autopsies show that of medical illnesses, cancer, prostatic disorder, and chronic obstructive pulmonary disorder (COPD) may be associated with completed suicide, whereas ischemic heart disease, cerebrovascular disease, peptic ulcer, and diabetes mellitus may not (Quan, Arboleda-Flórez, Fick, Stuart, & Love, 2002). The elevated risk of suicide increases progressively with the number of comorbid illnesses. Among the commonly reported diagnoses, cancer, stroke, and a group of illnesses comprising dementia, hemiplegia, and encephalopathy have a particularly strong incremental effect on risk for suicide (Jia, Wang, Xu, Dai, & Qin, 2014).

It also appears that functional impairment due to illness, rather than illness severity per se, is associated with increased risk for suicide. Studies have shown that lung cancer, gastrointestinal cancer, breast cancer, genital cancer, bladder cancer, lymph node cancer, epilepsy, cerebrovascular diseases, cataracts, heart diseases, COPD, gastrointestinal disease, liver disease, arthritis, osteoporosis, prostate disorders, male genital disorders, and spinal fracture conferred higher risks for completed suicide even 3 years after the initial diagnosis (Erlangsen, Stenager, & Conwell, 2015). Thus, evaluations of imminent suicide risk in the medically ill should include detailed assessments of their functional status. Furthermore, treatments aimed at reducing suicide risk in seriously medically ill individuals must also aim to improve these individuals' level of functioning and their satisfaction with it (Tanriverdi, Cuhadar, & Ciftci, 2014).

Health care and the ability of the health care system to address the functional needs of medically ill persons differ between countries, as does suicide risk due to medical illness. Countries with superior health care, such as the United Kingdom, have lower incremental risks of suicide due to medical illness. In the United Kingdom, of the physical illnesses, modest increases in risk of self-harm are associated with epilepsy (risk ratio = 2.9), asthma (1.8), migraine (1.8), psoriasis (1.6), diabetes mellitus (1.6), eczema (1.4), and inflammatory polyarthropathies (1.4). On the other hand, compared to the general population, lower risks for suicide are associated with cancers (risk ratio = 0.95), congenital heart disease (0.9), ulcerative colitis (0.8), sickle cell anemia (0.7), and Down's syndrome (0.1) (Singhal, Ross, Seminog, Hawton, & Goldacre, 2014).

Case 14

Sheridan, an 80-year-old retired businessman, was brought to the ED by ambulance after he told his wife of 55 years that he had just taken an entire bottle of propranolol. For 14 years since his retirement, he had been teaching a business class in a local community college as a volunteer. He had chronic congestive heart failure, which had increasingly limited his mobility, and he was considering ending his volunteer work after the spring semester. Sheridan told the team that the MICU scared him and that he was no longer suicidal. He believed he was strong enough and was discharged home with no physical therapy or psychiatric follow-up. A few months later, he was admitted with another overdose. The patient was very articulate in that he did not want to live anymore because his disability prevented him from doing anything he enjoyed; he had nothing good to look forward to. His wife said that she tried many times to dissuade him but was not successful and that she doubted that the medical team would be either. His wife said that she did not believe in psychiatry and was doubtful that medications would succeed where she had failed.

Sheridan's case illustrates how functional disability due to chronic and debilitating medical illness may reach a threshold when it suddenly narrows one's options in life, creating a sense of entrapment with no good solutions and sharply increasing imminent suicide risk. Physical therapy, antidepressant treatment for Sheridan's depression, and couples' therapy focused on improving commutation between partners and helping Sheridan's wife be more supportive in words and deeds of her husband's teaching could be life-saving for Sheridan.

Acute and Chronic Pain

Chronic pain, affecting one-third of the US population annually (Elman, Borsook, & Volkow, 2013), could be the most feared manifestation of any illness. Similar to mental pain, physical pain or its anticipation is associated with increased risk of suicide.

Independent of psychiatric and medical comorbidities, suicide attempt rates in chronic pain patients are two or three times higher than those in the general population (Tang & Crane, 2006). The greatest increase in suicide risk occurs in the context of chronic back pain (9-fold risk of completed suicide) (Penttinen, 1995), followed by severe headaches (6.5-fold), non-arthritic chronic pain (6.2-fold), and other generalized pain conditions such as fibromyalgia and irritable bowel syndrome (4-fold) (Spiegel, Schoenfeld, & Naliboff, 2007). Approximately 20% of poisoning deaths in pain patients are misidentified as accidental overdoses (Cheatle, 2011), so the actual suicide rates are probably 20% higher.

Case 15

Betty, a 55-year-old woman with a history of back trauma and multiple past surgeries, was admitted to the spine service with severe back pain. An infected rod was removed, and a psychiatric consult was called to assess the patient's suicidal risk. Betty's postsurgical pain was 10/10, and she was told that the insertion of a new rod was not feasible. Betty was a thin, ill-appearing woman lying in an orthopedic bed equipped with complicated-looking hardware. She was in visible discomfort. Her husband, at her bedside, was very distraught and told the consultant that Betty was at the end of her rope and that he could understand why. He said that the painkillers were not working, the staff was inattentive to his wife's needs, and that something needed to change—quickly. The consultant tried to reassure the husband, who seemed to then feel better. The consultant diagnosed Betty with adjustment disorder and prescribed a stat dose of a benzodiazepine. That same evening, the patient had a respiratory arrest and was intubated. An empty bottle of oxydone was found in her night table. The husband said that he brought it into the hospital because he could not watch his wife suffer.

This case describes a suicide attempt by a woman with chronic pain, brought on by the new acute pain post-surgery and a sense of entrapment and desperation due to both ineffective analgesic treatment and no clear path to relief in the future. Her husband unknowingly, or possibly even knowingly, helped his wife's overdose by bringing her the pills. He even indirectly alerted the team to a possible suicide attempt by telling them that she was "at the end of her rope." In cases such as Betty's, rooms should be routinely searched for "contraband" painkillers, and imminent suicide risk should be assessed forcefully.

SERIOUS MENTAL ILLNESS
Recent Diagnosis

As discussed in Chapter 3, carrying a diagnosis of a psychiatric disorder, except dementia, is linked to increased risk of suicide (Nordentoft, Pedersen, & Mortensen, 2012). The suicide rates are different for different disorders. Whereas the type of psychiatric disorder, the comorbidities, and the demographics confer trait vulnerability to suicide and are more related to the long-term suicide risk, the timing of the diagnosis is significantly related to suicide risk in the near term.

For many psychiatric disorders, including depression, substance use disorders, and schizophrenia, the risk of dying by suicide is particularly high within the first 90 days after initial diagnosis. During this time period, patients newly diagnosed with schizophrenia are 20 times more likely to die by suicide than those without a psychiatric diagnosis. The risk of completed suicide within 3 months after being diagnosed is 10 times higher for major depression and substance use disorders. The elevated risk for suicide attempts persists during the first year following a diagnosis of major depression and anxiety disorders but not schizophrenia. Thus, clinicians should be aware of the heightened risk of suicide and suicidal behavior within the first 3 months after initial diagnosis (Randall et al., 2014).

Some of the elevated short-term suicide risk in newly diagnosed individuals may be due to having just been hospitalized in an inpatient unit (discussed further in Chapter 5). However, high rates of suicide in the first 3 months after diagnosis are more related to self-awareness of mental illness and its implications for the future. Adolescents with psychotic symptoms who are aware of their mental illness and who do not seek help are 20 times more likely to be suicidal than those without psychotic symptoms who do seek help; for psychotic adolescents who do seek help, risk is 10 times higher. This suggests that insight into mental illness may increase risk for suicide (Kitagawa et al., 2014) and that lack of awareness or denial may actually be a very adaptive coping mechanism. Indeed, it appears that mentally ill who do not use denial as a coping mechanism may be at higher risk for suicide, indicating that self-deception may be a coping response to stressful life events in general (Pompili et al., 2011).

Case 16

John, a 19-year-old man, was brought to the ED by his parents because he started putting newspapers over his windows out of fear that the drug dealers in his neighborhood were watching him. He had not washed himself in weeks and was malodorous. His parents said that he was always a quiet kid and mostly kept to himself, spending a lot of time online. He liked to follow stories about organized crime. He parents said that recently he had become even more withdrawn and only left his room to use the bathroom. In the ED, John sat quietly in his chair, avoiding eye contact and staring at the floor. He was clearly psychotic, and the ED team told the parents that their son might have schizophrenia. The parents said they believed that John was stressed from spending so much time on the Internet and needed to rest more. They refused to hospitalize him but promised to watch him carefully for signs of worsening mental illness and to limit his time on the computer and have him read more books. John was discharged, but 2 weeks later he was brought, unconscious, to the ED by emergency medical services after he attempted to hang himself in his room. He later died in the MICU. His parents said that after his first ED visit, he stopped sleeping and obsessively read postings about schizophrenia on the Internet.

John's story is a classic case of suicide by a patient newly diagnosed with schizophrenia. His parents' lack of insight and denial of the diagnosis demonstrate a frequent contributing factor to increased risk conferred by recent diagnosis. Parents' naive assurances of safety are also fairly common in such cases.

Recent Hospitalization

Psychiatric hospitalization is an intensive treatment modality reserved for the most seriously mentally ill, for whom outpatient care is insufficient. In the United States, inpatient psychiatric hospitalization is covered by health insurance only if patients present danger to themselves or others. The unspoken assumption is that inpatient psychiatric hospitalization could be life-saving. However, the first psychiatric hospitalization, in particular, is a significant stressful life event that labels an individual as mentally ill and exposes him or her to others with severe mental illness (Cohen, 1994).

Paradoxically, but not unexpectedly, high-risk suicidal patients are at the highest risk for imminent suicide when either just admitted to a psychiatric unit for protection from self-harm or just discharged from an inpatient psychiatric hospital stay (Lawrence, Holman, Jablensky, & Fuller, 1999; Mortensen & Juel, 1993). According to a review of completed suicides in Denmark during a period of 16 years from 1981 to 1997, the odds ratio for completing suicide during the first week after discharge from an inpatient unit is approximately 250:1 for women and 105:1 for men, compared to those who have not been hospitalized (Qin & Nordentoft, 2005). In a Swedish study, one-third of drowning suicide decedents were discharged from an inpatient facility in the preceding week (Ahlm, Lindqvist, Saveman, & Björnstig, 2015). The reversed gender ratio, compared to a higher ratio of completed suicides for men versus women overall, is probably due to suicidal men not being hospitalized in the first place; men tend to use more lethal methods, increasing their likelihood of completing their initial attempt (Sue, Sue, Sue, & Sue, 2013). This explanation is consistent with a well-known statistic that 10 times as many women as men attempt suicide, whereas 3 times as many men as women die by suicide (Chang et al., 2011).

The increased risk of death from suicide following a psychiatric admission, compared to that of the general population (see later for data on the US military), decreases with time but remains elevated for at least 1 year. Not surprisingly, past history of self-harm and symptoms of depression present prior to hospital admission increase the risk of post-discharge suicide, as do, to a lesser degree, unplanned discharge and recent social difficulties (for review and meta-analysis, see Large, Sharma, Cannon, Ryan, & Nielssen, 2011). Post-discharge suicide risk depends somewhat on the day of the week the patient is discharged. Suicide and nonfatal suicide attempts have a 6–10% excess occurrence on Mondays and Tuesdays and are 5–13% less likely to occur on Saturdays (Miller et al., 2012).

Approximately 3% of patients categorized as being at high risk can be expected to commit suicide within 1 year of discharge from psychiatric hospitalization. In a Danish study, 60% of patients who went on to die by suicide were characterized at the time of their discharge as low risk for suicide using administratively approved scales (Qin & Nordentoft, 2005). Thus, as discussed in the Introduction, the post-discharge suicide risk assessment methods based on long-term risk factors are of little or no value in assessing short-term risk following an inpatient psychiatric hospitalization.

Historically, the military has had lower suicide rates than the general population. However, due to a recent steady increase, the suicide rate in the military is 71.6 suicides per 100,000 people yearly compared to 14.2 per 100,000 in the general population. Among the US military, personnel released from a psychiatric hospitalization are five times more likely to die from suicide than those who were not hospitalized (Luxton, June, & Comtois, 2013). The risk of dying from suicide within the first 30 days after a psychiatric hospitalization is 8.2 times higher than the risk after the first year post-discharge from hospitalization (Luxton et al., 2013). Thus, in the first weeks after discharge from an acute psychiatric facility, military personnel need even closer psychiatric follow-up than civilians (Luxton et al., 2013).

Of note, recent hospitalization in a general hospital ward may also increase short-term suicide risk. In the United Kingdom, two-thirds of individuals who die by suicide have hospital records within 1 year of the suicide, and the majority are discharged from general, rather than psychiatric, facilities (Dougall et al., 2014). Although this high ratio is likely an artifact of a 30:1 ratio of general to psychiatric admissions, it is clear that there exists an association between general hospital discharge and subsequent completed suicide. Diagnosis of psychiatric comorbidity at admission appears to be related to the time interval between hospital discharge and suicide: Those with psychiatric diagnoses are much more likely to die by suicide within 3 months after discharge compared to those without psychiatric diagnoses (Dougall et al., 2014).

Finally, among people receiving treatment for drug dependence, discharge from hospitalization marks the start of a period of heightened vulnerability to drug-related death. It is not possible to determine which of these are suicides and which are unintentional overdoses (Merrall et al., 2010).

Although the data are still new and need to be replicated in other hospital settings, currently, the best predictor of post-discharge suicidal behavior in high-risk psychiatric inpatients is the severity of SCS at the time of hospital discharge (Galynker et al., 2016; Yaseen et al., 2014). High scorers on the Suicide Crisis Inventory are 15 times more likely to attempt suicide within 6 weeks after discharge than those who do not meet the high score threshold (Galynker et al., 2016).

High-risk psychiatric inpatients exhibiting no signs of SCS are also at a high risk for post-discharge suicidal behavior (Yaseen et al., 2014). Indeed, high-risk psychiatric inpatients not infrequently report and also demonstrate this incongruous quick resolution of their intense emotional pain. Although it is difficult to imagine a patient who has just survived a serious suicide attempt not to have any residual symptoms or signs of SCS, there are at least two possible reasons for this unexpected phenomenon: (1) Patients with dramatic improvement of SCS hide their suicidal intent and (2) such patients are unable to identify their emotions due to their poor emotional differentiation skills.

Regardless of whether such patients hide their suicidal plans or are so out of touch with their emotions that they are not aware of their intent to die, they are at high risk for imminent suicide and are likely to make an attentive clinician intensely uncomfortable. Instead of relief at their patient's rapid improvement, such clinicians often experience an eerie mixture of anxiety, discomfort, mistrust, and apprehension regarding the candor of their patient's self-report. However, because on the surface these are often the "model patients," they give their doctors no overt reason to question the honesty of their self-report. Moreover, they strictly follow treatment plans, take their medications on time, and become leaders when participating in therapeutic activities. Such patients often express vocal remorse about their recent suicidal behavior and promise to comply with all recommended treatments upon discharge. And yet, these assurances often sound hollow.

Clinicians are often aware of their negative and seemingly irrational emotional responses and try to suppress them because, on paper and in the emergency medical records, these patients deny suicidal ideation. Such denials force clinicians' hand in documenting these patients' low suicide risk and clearing them to be discharged from the hospital. However, the clinicians' responses are often correct, and some of these patients are the ones who die by suicide within weeks and sometimes within hours after being documented as having low suicide risk. The use of clinicians' emotional responses for imminent risk assessment is discussed in Chapter 7.

Case 17

Sean was a 60-year-old single man who admitted to an inpatient psychiatric unit following a serious suicide attempt by hanging while in his apartment alone. Sean had recently lost his business, leaving him without income. He could not find a job, and after several weeks he became depressed and started drinking. Before hanging himself, he drank an entire bottle of bourbon. After admission, the team contacted Sean's best friend, who came to the unit and offered to help Sean financially until he could find a job. The patient suddenly brightened up and requested discharge so he could start looking for a job. He called his suicide a sucker's mistake and said that he would accept his friend's offer and try again. He attended groups enthusiastically and requested to go to Alcoholics Anonymous meetings.

There was something unnatural about his turnaround, and the staff felt apprehensive discharging him. They questioned the patient repeatedly about his future suicidal intent and about his plans. Sean described elaborate future plans and repeatedly denied suicidal intent. On the day of discharge, the patient was cheerful and motivated to use his second chance on life well. He had an appointment scheduled for the following day with his new outpatient therapist. Sean's friend took him home and safely brought Sean to his apartment. However, as soon as the friend left, Sean leaped off his 17th-floor balcony to his death.

Sean's case starkly illustrates imminent suicide by a high-risk patient following discharge from an inpatient psychiatric unit. The case also illustrates difficult challenges faced by inpatient psychiatrists when discharging patients at high risk for imminent suicide who vehemently deny their suicide intent. Sean's failed attempt by hanging confers a very high risk for future successful suicide (see Attempt Lethality). Clinicians' anxious emotional responses to Sean are typical of those to patients at ultra high risk (see Chapter 7). This case illustrates that the combination of a high-lethality failed recent attempt and a strong negative emotional response on the part of the staff, even in the presence of explicit denial of suicidal intent, indicates high risk for imminent suicide warranting extraordinary attempts at establishing the patient's real intent and setting up close follow-up mechanisms.

Recent Suicide Attempts

One of the strongest risk factors for suicide is a history of suicide attempts or of previous deliberate self-harm (Sakinofsky, 2000). The distinction between the two is that *suicide attempt* implies knowing the intent to die, whereas *deliberate self-harm* is purely behavioral and includes intentional self-poisoning or self-injury, irrespective of motivation (Hawton, Zahl, & Weatherall, 2003). Because in most studies the intent to die cannot be established with certainty, a purely behavioral definition of deliberate self-harm, rather than suicide attempt, may be more accurate for describing past self-injurious behavior.

Regardless of definition, longitudinal studies of past self-injurious behavior as a risk factor for future suicide attempts and completed suicide show very similar results. In developed countries, a history of deliberate self-harm or suicide attempt is found in approximately half of all suicides (range, 40–60%) (Nordentoft et al., 1993). Approximately 0.7–1% of suicide attempters go on to die by suicide in a subsequent attempt(s) within the first year (Hawton et al., 2003). Suicide death rates in previous attempters are on average 30 times higher than those in the general population.

The number of previous suicide attempts and advanced age further increase the risk of an upcoming fatal suicide attempt. The distribution of risk by age is particularly striking, ranging from 15 times in the 45- to 55-year-old age group to 300 times in the older than 85 years age group compared to the general population without a history of suicide attempts. Those with histories of past suicide attempt in other age groups have suicide rates 30–50 times higher than that of the general population. Although this is a very high rate, it is an order of magnitude lower than that in the elderly (Hawton et al., 2003; Nordentoft et al., 1993).

The ratio of men to women who die by suicide after previous attempts is lower than that for all suicides. In contrast to the 3:1 men-to-women ratio, some studies show only a 2:1 ratio, whereas in others, equal numbers of men and women die by subsequent suicide attempt. Considering that men tend to use more lethal means of suicide, one possible explanation for this discrepancy is that those who do not die in their first attempt are a self-selected group of men less prone to using lethal means of suicides (Qin & Nordentoft, 2005).

In those with histories of suicide attempt and nonsuicidal self-injury, the risk of death is highest in the first year after self-harm; in the United Kingdom, this risk is 66 times the annual risk of suicide in the general population. This risk is similar to the risk of dying by suicide in the first year after discharge from an inpatient psychiatric unit, to which many patients are admitted after a suicide attempt (discussed previously). Although risk of suicide is highest in the first year following self-harm, there remains a significant risk 5 and even 10 years later. As many as 20% of those who have attempted suicide will make another attempt within the first year, and as many as 5% will die by suicide within 9 years (Owens, Horrocks, & House, 2002). Thus, it may be that self-harm confers an increased risk for suicide over a lifetime.

The incremental increase in risk due to previous suicide attempts appears to be higher in the West than in the developing world and in developed Asian countries. For example, compared to 30–47% in the West (Gunnell & Frankel, 1994), only 8% or 9% of patients in rural Sri Lanka and only 17% of patients in urban areas of this country report previous episodes of self-harm (Mohamed et al., 2010). In India, only 13% of those who died by suicide had previously self-harmed (Gururaj, Isaac, Subbakrishna, & Ranjani, 2004); whereas a figure of 25% was reported in a large study from China. Suicide attempts and the suicide rate in previous attempters in Taiwan were also lower (Weng, Chang, Yeh, Wang, & Chen, 2016) than those in the West (Phillips et al., 2002).

One possible explanations for the comparatively lower levels of repeat self-harm in rural Asia compared to the West may be that the high fatality rates associated with the first episode of deliberate self-harm mean that high-risk patients are removed from the pool of patients at risk of repetition. Another explanation is the longer lengths of hospital stay in Asian hospitals (average of 3 or 4 days), in part due to the greater toxicity of the substances taken in episodes of self-poisoning. In these cases, decisions to observe patients on the medical ward may contribute to the reduced risk of repeated and more serious suicide attempts; patients are relatively protected from a reattempt while in hospital, which is critical considering that the risk of repeat self-harm is greatest in the days immediately following an original attempt. In contrast, in the West, many patients who present to hospital following self-harm are not admitted (Gunnell, Brooks, & Peters, 1996) and may be returned within hours to their community and the preexisting circumstances that surrounded their original attempt.

Interestingly, immigrants to the United States, who are a self-selected group, have lower suicide rates prior to their immigration than those of Americans. However, suicide rates increase with acculturation after several years and may exceed the rates of those who are American-born (Borges, Orozco, Rafful, Miller, & Breslau, 2011). Immigrants who migrated as children of Asian and Black ethnicity show higher lifetime prevalence of attempts than the US-born of the same ethnicity (Borges et al., 2011). The same is true for Middle Eastern immigrants (Nasseri & Moulton, 2009). Thus, when assessing imminent risk, clinicians must obtain a detailed cultural history, including that of immigration and acculturation.

Case 18

Prameet, a 24-year-old Indian Hindu man, was admitted to an inpatient unit after he confessed to his Internet girlfriend, an American-born Indian woman, that he had overdosed on Tylenol because he felt rejected by her. The emergency room assessment established that he had bought two bottles of Tylenol to kill himself but took only 10 pills. Prameet immigrated with his parents when he was 3 years old and did well in high school until the 11th grade, when he started failing his classes despite studying days and nights.

He had been depressed since then, except for two brief periods of time when he was taking antidepressants. In the hospital, his diagnosis of depression was confirmed, and treatment with venlafaxine was initiated. He was discharged when his mood improved, and he committed to safety. Two months later, after his girlfriend defriended him on Facebook, Prameet was readmitted after taking all the pills from one of the two bottles of Tylenol he bought before his prior admission.

Prameet's case describes escalating deliberate self-injury in an immigrant from Asia, and it illustrates how a history of deliberate self-harm may increase the risk for future deliberate self-harm. The vignette is also an example of increased suicide risk in child immigrants.

Attempt Lethality

Although history of a failed suicide attempt is one of the most serious long-term risk factors for eventual suicide, this risk differs based on the previous attempt's method and lethality. The connection between the lethality of the past attempt and suicide risk is twofold: The more lethal the means of the previous attempt, the higher the lifetime risk for the next attempt, and the next attempt will use either the same or more lethal means of suicide as the previous attempt.

In the United States, firearms are both the most lethal and the most frequently used means of suicide (CDC, 2015a). More than 50% of all American suicide decedents die by firearms, 25% by hanging and asphyxiation, and 20% by poisoning. Suffocation has a lethality rate similar to that of firearms, typically 69–84% (Miller, Azrael, & Barber, 2012). Recently in the United States, across all racial/ethnic groups and Census regions, increases of suicide by hanging have been outpacing those of other means.

In the industrialized West, where firearms are not as available to the general public, the most frequent means of suicide are hanging and suffocation, followed by poisoning. In the East, the most widespread method of suicide is pesticide ingestion (Krug, Dahlberg, Mercy, Zwi, & Lozano, 2002). Because Asia is the most populous continent, in numerical terms, more people in the world die by pesticide ingestion than by any other means (Gunnel, Eddleston, Phillips, & Konradsen, 2007). In the United States, poisoning includes primarily drug overdose and nondrug chemical ingestion, such as bleach (CDC, 2016).

Death rates of repeat suicide attempt differ depending on the method of the previous failed attempt. Compared to poisoning, those with a failed hanging suicide attempt are six times more likely to die by suicide, with the majority of suicides occurring in the first year after the initial attempt. The likelihood of completed suicide following a failed attempt by drowning is fourfold. Failed attempts by jumping off heights and using firearms are three times more likely to be followed by suicide deaths (Runeson, Tidemalm, Dahlin, Lichtenstein, & Langstrom, 2010).

In all cases except cutting, more than 50% of suicide decedents die by the same means they used in their unsuccessful previous attempt (Runeson et al., 2010). This persistence is most pronounced among those who used hanging in their initial attempt, of whom 93% of men and 92% of women later died from suicide by the same method. High proportions also used the same method for the final successful attempt after previous attempts by drowning, use of a firearm (men), or by jumping from a height.

In summary, although previous suicide attempt is one of the strongest single predictors for future suicide, there are differences in the subsequent suicide death rates depending on the method of the previous failed attempt. Pertinent to assessment of imminent suicide risk, the majority of suicide deaths occur within 1 year after an initial failed attempt, and up to one-third of all completed suicides may occur within 1 week after the previous attempt.

Case 19

Joe was a successful sculptor who was very attractive and known as a womanizer. However, Joe was quite unhappy and lonely because nobody ever met his criteria for an ideal partner. Finally, when Joe was 40 years old, he met Irena. Irena was a 40-year-old painter. She was very beautiful, smart, and successful. She was also childless. They had a passionate romance, and Irena got pregnant. Joe married Irena, and they had a daughter. One day, Joe looked through his wife's e-mails and discovered that she was having an affair with her manager. Joe was crushed. The love of his life was lying to him, and he was not sure whether he was his daughter's father. Joe begged Irena to end the affair. She initially refused, saying that her manager was vindictive and stopping their affair would end her career.

Devastated, Joe implored her. Finally, Irena promised to stop seeing the manager. Things were quiet for about a month, but then Joe looked through Irena's phone bill and discovered that she continued to exchange multiple texts daily with her manager. The next day, while driving, Joe confronted her again. Angry, Irena had a fit in the car and told him that she never loved him and that she married him only to have a baby, and now that she had a child, she wanted a divorce. They stopped at a gas station. Irena said she was calling a lawyer and went inside. Joe took out a rope from the trunk of the car and tried to hang himself from a branch of a tree next to the gas station. Irene came outside just as he was jumping. The tree branch broke, and Joe fell to the ground.

A rope burn was visible on his neck. Scared, Irena brought him to the emergency room, and he was hospitalized on the psychiatric ward. While Joe was in the hospital, Irena came daily and apologized, saying that what she said was in anger because he was so possessive. At the family meeting, Irena told the team she wanted to start couples therapy. Joe was mistrustful but too ashamed to reveal Irena's betrayal to his friends and felt lonelier than ever. Instead of sharing his pain, he hired a private investigator, who discovered that Irena still spent time in her manager's apartment, had met with a lawyer, and was planning a divorce. Joe hung himself using nylon cord on a cabinet handle in his apartment. The handle did not break.

This case is illustrative of high risk associated with failed previous attempt by hanging in men. Characteristically, the successful suicide followed the failed attempt within weeks. Joe's suicide crisis was precipitated by romantic betrayal and rejection. Joe's narrative identity became a perfect fit for a suicidal narrative: setting an unrealistic goal for his personal life, finding it and then failing to achieve it with Irena, followed by a humiliating defeat, failure to disengage, alienation, and entrapment.

Exacerbation and Acute Episodes

Most of the data on the relationship between exacerbations/acute episodes of mental illness and suicidal behavior derive from large-scale epidemiological studies (Kessler, Chiu, Demler, & Walters, 2005). It is well known that as many as 90% of suicide attempters meet criteria for one or more disorders in the *Diagnostic and Statistical Manual of Mental Disorders* (DSM; American Psychiatric Association, 2013) during the 12 months preceding the suicidal act (Kessler et al., 2005), with depressive disorders being the most common diagnosis (Mościcki, 2001). Vigilance for mood disorders and routine screening for the signs of acute suicidal crisis are therefore warranted.

In general, for relapsing–remitting psychiatric disorders, such as depression, time spent in high-risk major depressive episodes or mixed states is likely to be a dominant factor determining overall risk for suicidal behavior. The incidences of attempts during major depressive episodes and during partial remission are 21 and 4 times higher than in full remission, respectively (Isometsa, 2014).

Among patients with bipolar disorder (BD), the risk of suicide attempts is different for different phases of the illness; the highest (38-fold) risk involves mixed and depressive mixed phases, whereas the second highest (18-fold) risk occurs during major depressive episodes (Fiedorowicz et al., 2009; Valtonen, Suominen, & Haukka, 2008). In patients with BD, 86% of all suicide attempts occur during major depressive episodes and mixed states (Valtonen et al., 2008). Thus, time spent in high-risk illness phases carries the highest risk for near-term suicide attempts.

The previously discussed findings demonstrate that risk of both completed suicide (Nordentoft, Mortensen, & Pedersen, 2011) and attempted suicide (Valtonen et al., 2008) may be slightly higher in BD than in MDD (Novick, Swartz, & Frank, 2010). Both are also higher in BD II than in BD I. This paradoxical association of higher suicide risk with the less severe form of the disorder may be accounted for by differences in the duration of depressive and mixed episodes relative to the overall illness duration, which is higher for BD II. Spending more time in depressed or in the mixed illness phases may well explain why BD II is often associated with more frequent suicidal behavior than is BD I.

On a clinical level, the reasons for peaking suicidal behavior during acute episodes in the chronically mentally ill may be complex, including the changes of one's mental state and the inability to recognize one's emotions. Even patients who have already experienced several episodes of their illness, and who were suicidal previously, may not have the insight to appreciate the onset and escalation of SCS. Their caregivers and significant others, even if they have already lived through their loved ones' previous illness exacerbations, may still not recognize subtle early signs of the new episode and thus may not appreciate the increasing risk for imminent suicidal behavior.

Moreover, patients with schizophrenia or related illnesses having an exacerbation of their psychotic symptoms rarely express worsening suicidal ideation. In schizophrenia, the signs of worsening psychosis often obscure signs of depression, anxiety, or even panic attacks. Even patients who experience severe distress due to worsening psychotic symptoms and depressive mood exhibit only minimal or no increase in their help-seeking behaviors, which may not even be recognized as a change in the patient's mental condition (Yamaguchi et al., 2015).

Finally, of all the psychotic conditions (schizophrenia included), the highest risk for suicide and even infanticide is brought on by psychosis within 4 weeks after delivery. Excluding acute postpartum exacerbations of known schizophrenia, puerperal, bipolar disorder, and schizoaffective disorder, the risk of completed suicide and of high-lethality suicide attempt within weeks of delivery in this population was reported to be as high as 10% (Kapfhammer & Lange, 2012). Overwhelmingly, the suicides were committed when patients were both depressed and suffering from delusions. Although the majority occurred during the mood episode, which had started imminently after delivery, others took place weeks after a seemingly good symptomatic remission.

Case 20

Walt, a divorced musician with a history of bipolar II disorder, hung himself in his bathroom after dinner with friends one evening. Walt was a successful pianist and teacher in his early 60s who started having difficulty playing after he was diagnosed with Parkinson's disease. Walt had several episodes of depression in the past and was even hospitalized, but he always recovered. After his death, his children discovered that their father's business calendar was empty, and the executor of the estate discovered that Walt's finances were in disarray. His medicine cabinet had bottles of psychotropic medications.

Walt took his life during one of his many depressive episodes. As many depressed working people do, he found ways to keep his illness out of the public domain. Using his very public (in musical circles) hypomanic persona, he was able to keep his illness secret, even from his children. As often happens, he killed himself in the middle of a depressive episode.

Medication Changes

Initiation of a new psychopharmacological treatment regimen is a relatively perilous time for a patient, and during this time he or she requires closer monitoring by a prescribing psychiatrist. Even with ultimately successful treatment, during the first days and weeks of taking a new drug, the patient encounters new side effects, such as antipsychotic-induced akathisia and antidepressant- or stimulant-related insomnia, which may exacerbate the initial condition. In addition, he or she almost always continues to experience the residual target symptoms of depression, anxiety, or psychosis. Finally, during treatment initiation, troublesome transient mood symptoms, such as increased anxiety in the early stages of selective serotonin reuptake inhibitor (SSRI) treatment for depression (or anxiety), may often temporarily worsen the overall clinical picture and increase near-term suicide risk.

In response to concerns about this suicide danger zone with treatment initiation, in 2007 the US Food and Drug Administration (FDA) ordered that all antidepressant medications carry an expanded black box warning incorporating information about an increased risk of suicidality in young adults aged 18–24 years, as well as children and adolescents (FDA, 2007; Friedman & Leon, 2007). The FDA justified its decision by identifying a possible activation syndrome (AS), which at times emerges during the antidepressant therapy process as a possible suicidal ideation and behavior precursor. AS is composed of the following 10 symptoms: anxiety, agitation, panic attack, insomnia, irritability, hostility, aggressiveness, impulsivity, akathisia (psychomotor restlessness), and hypomania/mania.

The AS anxiety, panic attacks, and, to some degree, akathisia overlap with the SCS entrapment, panic–dissociation, and fear of death. Hypomania/mania overlap with SCS affective disturbance and anabolic–androgenic steroid-induced mood swings and affective instability. Finally, impulsivity and aggressiveness correspond to the narrative crisis model's trait suicidality as well as the stress–diathesis model's suicide diathesis and the O'Connor's premotivational stage. In other words, AS empirically overlaps somewhat with SCS, but this hypothesis needs to be tested experimentally.

AS can also be interpreted as symptoms of dysphoric mania/hypomania and is phenomenologically similar to the syndrome of depressive mixed state (DMX) or mixed depression (Benazzi, 2007; Benazzi & Akiskal, 2001). DMX is observed predominantly in patients with bipolar depression, particularly those with BP II (Akiskal & Benazzi, 2005; Takeshima & Oka, 2013), and could be one of the strongest risk factors for suicidality (Valtonen et al., 2009). In line with the phenomenological similarities between AS and DMX, Akiskal and Benazzi (2006) and Rihmer and Akiskal (2006) argued that AS could be understood as antidepressant-induced DMX. In this context, it can be inferred that antidepressant treatment-emergent AS can be understood as antidepressant-induced DMX, which could substantially increase risk of near-term suicide. Consequently, the FDA recommended to consider changing the therapeutic regimen, including discontinuing the antidepressants if these symptoms are severe, abrupt in onset, or were not part of the patient's presenting symptoms (Culpepper, Davidson, Dietrich, Goodman, & Schwenk, 2004; FDA, 2007).

When patients a priori known to be at higher risk for developing treatment-emergent manic symptoms are excluded, antidepressant initiation is associated with increased rates of suicide attempts within 120 days only in children, whereas the rate is decreased in adult males (Olfson & Marcus, 2008).

Discontinuation of prescription psychotropic medication may be even more troublesome than initiation because almost all, if not all, prescription psychoactive drugs have been associated with significant withdrawal syndromes. These syndromes have been well described for benzodiazepines (Voshaar, Couvée, Van Balkom, Mulder, & Zitman, 2006), antidepressants (Warner, Bobo, Warner, Reid, & Rachal, 2006), first- and second-generation antipsychotics (Viguera, Baldessarini, Hegarty, van Kammen, & Tohen, 1997), and mood stabilizers (Howland, 2010), and they are often concomitant with the relapse of the initial target symptoms for which they were intended—anxiety, depression, psychosis, and affective dysregulation. To a lesser degree, these considerations apply to instances of stopping and restarting medication due to nonadherence to treatment.

As a consequence, suicidal risk and behaviors, which are core features of depression, anxiety, panic, and psychosis, wax and wane in intensity at the times of treatment initiation and adjustment, often reflecting not only the mood fluctuations intrinsic to a particular illness but also drug initiation and discontinuation phenomena. Thus, in assessing near-term suicide risk specifically, it is always important to assess and understand possible fluctuations of mood, agitation, insomnia, and cognitive disturbances due to possible initiation and withdrawal symptoms associated with licit and illicit drugs. Once such symptoms are identified, maintaining careful surveillance and vigorous treatment are equally essential (Zisook et al., 2009).

Some discontinuation signs and symptoms are class specific and some are drug specific. Patients report significantly fewer discontinuation symptoms with escitalopram compared to paroxetine and venlafaxine XR. The discontinuation profiles for these drugs remain the same regardless of whether they have been used for the target symptoms of anxiety, panic, or depression. For each antidepressant, no differences in discontinuation symptoms were observed between the three indications, and surprisingly, there seemed to be no evidence of increased symptom incidence with increased length of treatment (Baldwin, Montgomery, Nil, & Lader, 2007). Thus, discontinuation profiles differ between antidepressants of the same class and are broadly similar in different disorders.

Discontinuation syndromes also differ between different people who may experience similar symptoms with different drugs in the same class. A woman who had developed a discontinuation syndrome with paroxetine tapered from 10 to 5 mg/day may present the same syndrome when she occasionally misses her 75 mg q 12 h venlafaxine doses. The symptoms—comprising agitation, numbness, pricking sensations, sweating, difficulty concentrating, weakness, derealization, and perceived xerophthalmia—immediately subside upon drug dose reinstitution of either drug (Montgomery, 2008).

Unlike the case with SSRIs and selective norepinephrine reuptake inhibitors, the severity of benzodiazepine withdrawal symptoms does depend on treatment duration and is more severe in patients who have taken a benzodiazepine for more than 5 years. Benzodiazepines are commonly prescribed in primary care for anxiety disorders and insomnia. The withdrawal can be so severe that even a relatively slow drug dose taper over 4 weeks on a scheduled 25% dose reduction per week may be associated with repeated high-lethality suicide attempts and completed suicide (Murphy & Tyrer, 1991). Withdrawal symptoms are most marked in those with personality disorders, predominantly dependent ones (Murphy & Tyrer, 1991).

Benzodiazepines are prescription drugs that are frequently sold on the street. As with all street drugs, their misuse is associated with severe symptoms of intoxication and withdrawal. Although both intoxication and withdrawal symptoms may be quite obvious in the ED setting, subclinical symptoms of withdrawal may not be readily observable and patients may not be able to differentiate them from their non-drug-related anxiety, agitation, or depression. With the strong suicidal diatheses and a suitable suicidal narrative, both intoxication and withdrawal symptoms would contribute to the intensity of the acute suicidal crisis. Hence, an inquiry into possible changes in licit or illicit drug use should be an important part of the imminent risk assessment.

Case 21

Marge was a 53-year-old lawyer who was brought to the ED by her husband for paranoid thinking and irrational behavior. His wife thought that her partners at work were trying to fire her from the company. Convinced that they hacked her home computer to collect incriminating evidence, Marge started staying up at night watching the computer screen for suspicious activity. Marge's husband believed that there was no truth to her suspicions. Marge was an ambitious and anxious woman who was highly regarded and respected at work. She had few interests outside her work and family. Three months ago, after she lost an important client resulting in lower income for her and the other partners, Marge was diagnosed with major depression and was started on an SSRI. On medical screening examination in the ED, Marge was guarded but cooperative and well related. Her affect was anxious but appropriate, and her thinking was organized. When her delusions were challenged during the interview, she conceded that she had no evidence for them and that she may just be stressed from increasing pressure at work. Marge was given a stat dose of risperidone, and her anxiety and paranoia decreased. She was diagnosed with bipolar mod disorder II depressive episode, kept overnight, and discharged on a small dose of risperidone and lithium; the SSRI was continued. Marge's family was supportive and involved in treatment. Marge gained weight, and 2 weeks after discharge her husband and daughter asked the outpatient psychiatrist to stop risperidone because Marge seemed to have improved and they had read online that antipsychotics should not be used for maintenance treatment. Marge was still very anxious, had a difficult time sleeping and concentrating, but was now saying that she had overreacted and that her partners were fine. Risperidone was stopped, and Marge became more anxious and agitated. She stopped sleeping altogether but was refusing risperidone because of the weight gain. There was no reason to admit her to the hospital because she was not suicidal and the family kept a close watch over her. The psychiatrist prescribed clonazepam and the patient, with her family, left the office. Despite the clonazepam, Marge did not sleep at all. She went to work early but never made it because she jumped to her death in front of a subway train.

Marge's case is an illustration of a preventable suicide brought on in part by diagnostic uncertainty and misguided medication management. Marge had an undiagnosed bipolar II disorder and was living in a state of productive hypomania. The first time she became depressed, she was misdiagnosed with unipolar depression rather than bipolar depression and treated with an SSRI without a mood stabilizer. This treatment resulted in a gradual emergence of a mixed manic episode with psychotic features, which included insomnia and premonition of social defeat, alienation, and entrapment. Marge's mixed manic episode was also misdiagnosed as depression with psychotic features. As a result, her SSRI treatment, which had created the mixed state in the first place, was continued and resulted in continuing worsening of her mania and psychosis. Both of the latter symptoms were partially treated with risperidone and, to a lesser degree, lithium. When, tragically, the risperidone was stopped due to the family's request, the psychosis quickly returned. Because the psychotic content of the mixed episode had the typical themes of humiliating defeat (revoked partnership) and the dead-end life narrative (failed career), in the context of insomnia and agitation, this delusional entrapment in a delusional reality quickly evolved into a severe SCS, culminating in suicide.

RECENT SUBSTANCE MISUSE

Drug and Alcohol Use Disorder

Although the relationship is not straightforward, suicide has been linked to the use of alcohol and drugs. It is further complicated by recent changes in the nomenclature of alcohol-related disorders from DSM-IV to DSM-5.

DSM-IV described two distinct disorders, alcohol abuse and alcohol dependence, with specific criteria for each. DSM-5 integrates the two DSM-IV disorders into one called alcohol use disorder (AUD) with mild, moderate, and severe subclassifications. The number of criteria met determines the AUD severity.

According to psychological autopsies and other research studies worldwide, AUD and other substance use disorders are the second most common group of mental disorders among suicide decedents (Conner et al., 2014). AUD on its own is a risk factor for suicide attempts and completion (Kessler, Borges, & Walters, 1999). Compared to nonsuicidal individuals with AUD, those with AUD who attempt or die by suicide are more likely to have comorbid depressive disorder, drug use disorder, aggressive behaviors, and medical illness or complaints. Suicidal persons with AUD have lower social support and more interpersonal stressful life events such as unemployment or other indications of economic adversity (Conner, Beautrais, & Conwell, 2003). Just like the two other commonly assessed risk factors, mental illness and previous history of attempts, AUD is associated with long-term suicide risk. Whether and how AUD confers risk for near-term suicide or suicide attempts is unclear. Much clearer is the association between imminent suicide risk and acute alcohol intoxication.

Acute Alcohol Intoxication and Recent Drug Use

Acute use of alcohol (AUA), describing alcohol intoxication, is related to but distinct from AUD. Although AUA is not a DSM diagnosis, it is a significant risk factor for suicidal behavior and is independent of drinking patterns or AUD (Borges & Loera, 2010). Acts of suicide among individuals with a history of AUD can occur either while intoxicated or outside periods of acute intoxication (Simon et al., 2002; Wojnar et al., 2008), and the phenomenology of suicides while intoxicated and while sober may be quite different.

A remarkable 37% of suicides and 40% of suicide attempts are preceded by AUA (Cherpitel, Borges, & Wilcox, 2004). Many studies have consistently demonstrated that AUA confers a 5- to 10-fold increase in risk of suicide. There are also data indicating that risk for suicidal behavior is increased at high drinking levels (Borges et al., 1996) and that use of firearms and hanging, the two most deadly methods of suicide, are associated with high drinking levels (Conner et al., 2014). This underscores the importance of alcohol dose in the link between AUA and suicidal behavior. Most important, although the SAD PERSONS scale as a whole is not predictive of suicidal behavior short term, recent increase in alcohol use is one of the SAD PERSONS scale items that does indicate increased near-term suicide risk within 6 months.

Consequently, to best inform prevention and intervention efforts concerning the association between AUA and suicidal behavior, it is important to understand its specifics. According to some studies (Bagge et al., 2013), one-third of participants drink before the attempt, and most who use alcohol (73%) do not do so to facilitate the attempt. The others, however, deliberately use alcohol prior to suicidal behavior in order to remove psychological barriers to suicide through increasing courage, numbing fears, and anesthetizing the pain of dying. Thus, suicide attempters may use alcohol as an additional drug to make death more likely (e.g., "I mixed alcohol with pills"). It may be that approximately one-fourth of suicide attempters with AUA fit this pattern (Hawton, Fagg, & McKeown, 1989), suggesting it is common.

Paradoxically, the minority who deliberately use alcohol to facilitate suicide are more similar to suicide attempters who do not drink prior to their attempt at all than to those who drink for other reasons. The latter, on the other hand, differ from non-intoxicated attempters in that they are more impulsive and have lower suicide intent.

Thus, alcohol-involved suicide attempts are heterogeneous (Bagge et al., 2013). The attempters who become intoxicated without specific intent to reduce pain of suicide appear to be more impulsive; for these individuals, suicide risk may decrease when they sober up. On the other hand, suicide attempters who drink for attempt facilitation will continue to be high risk even upon a decrease in blood alcohol level.

There may be other mechanisms by which AUA increases suicidal thoughts and behavior. These mechanisms may include, but are not limited to, alcohol-related psychological distress, disinhibition, depressed mood and anxiety, aggressiveness, impulsivity, and cognitive constriction (Bagge & Sher, 2008; Hufford, 2001). Through these and other mechanisms, AUA may also evoke or exacerbate acute interpersonal conflicts, thereby escalating stress levels and stress-reactive suicidal behavior (Conner et al., 2014). It is also possible that suicidal acts preceded by AUA are a distinct phenotype of suicidal behavior (Fudalej et al., 2009).

The data on the relationship between suicide attempt lethality and alcohol use are conflicting. Some reports indicate that alcohol use is associated with more lethal means of suicide (Sublette et al., 2009), whereas others find no such association and suggest that cannabis use may be related to more lethal means, such as jumping from heights (Lundholm, Thiblin, Runeson, Leifman, & Fugelstad, 2014). The highest blood alcohol levels at the moment of suicide were recorded with rare suicides by explosive device, with the average blood alcohol concentration of 1.71 g/kg. This especially drastic method of suicide (distinct from suicide bombing, which is a murder–suicide) was frequent in Croatia during the period after the Croatian Independence War (1991–1995), possibly as a consequence of a high incidence of war-related post-traumatic stress disorder (Čoklo et al., 2008).

Finally, the use of alcohol in suicide decedents prior to their deaths differs widely by ethnicity. Autopsy blood alcohol levels are consistently the highest for American Indians and Alaskan Natives and the lowest for Asian Americans and Pacific Islanders (Caetano et al., 2013). The frequencies of legal intoxication (i.e., blood alcohol concentration at or above the legal limit of 0.08 g/dl) follow the same pattern, ranging from 37% in American Indians and Alaskan Natives to 23% in Asian Americans. Hispanics had the second highest frequency with 29% (CDC, 2005b).

Case 22

Wendy was a 28-year-old woman diagnosed with bipolar disorder. She was hospitalized during a manic episode and treated with a second-generation antipsychotic that brought on an episode of treatment-resistant depression. She was discharged in her parents' care and was treated with increasingly complicated combinations of medications but did not improve. Despite all the treatment efforts, Wendy's depression kept getting worse, and after several months she told her family that she could no longer take the pain and that she would kill herself. The parents put her on a pharmaceutical trial waiting list that was several months long. Wendy was getting desperate and started drinking to control her emotional pain. Her comments to her psychiatrist were becoming hopeless and despondent. She came to several appointments intoxicated. The psychiatrist alerted Wendy's parents to her acute suicidality and instructed them to stay with her and to remove liquor from the house. Finally, Wendy was interviewed for the trial, but she did not meet the criteria. She made up a story and asked one of her friends to come over and sneak two bottles of vodka into the house, which he did. As soon as he left, Wendy drank one bottle. The parents noticed that Wendy was drunk, searched her room, and found both bottles. The parents made an appointment with Wendy's psychiatrist for the next day. However, they never made it to the appointment because the next morning they found her dead in her room with a plastic bag around her head.

This case shows an increase in alcohol use proximal to a suicide attempt, where Wendy's AUA was likely an attempt to self-medicate refractory depression, emotional pain, and anxiety. Given that Wendy suffocated herself hours after an impulsive episode of acute intoxication, her AUA was not a conscious attempt to minimize pain of death with alcohol. This is the case for 75% of suicide decedents who drink before their suicide. On the other hand, anxiety and depression from alcohol withdrawal (discussed next) may have also contributed to her death.

Drug or Alcohol Withdrawal

Whereas alcohol and drug intoxication may contribute to acute suicide risk due to disinhibition or intentional use to diminish fear of death or numb its pain, the negative affective states of anhedonia, depression, anxiety, and panic intrinsic to drug and alcohol withdrawal may increase risk for suicide by intensifying the syndrome of the acute suicidal crisis. As demonstrated by Galynker and Yaseen in patients with depression, panic attacks in general are associated with past attempts (Katz, Yaseen, Mojtabai, Cohen, & Galynker, 2011), and those with panic attacks with fear of death are seven times more likely to attempt suicide in the future (Yaseen et al., 2013). Thus, the turmoil of negative mood symptoms, including depression, anxiety, panic, and affective instability, which is a distinguishing feature of many drug withdrawal symptoms, turns periods of alcohol and drug withdrawal into times of high suicide risk.

The ethanol withdrawal syndrome specifically may be observed in the ethanol-dependent patient within 8 hours of the last drink, with blood alcohol concentrations in excess of 200 mg%, and it can be life threatening. Symptoms consist of tremor, nausea and vomiting, increased blood pressure and heart rate, paroxysmal sweats, depression, and anxiety. Thus, alcohol withdrawal in these patients may be a time of heightened vulnerability to suicide and must be assessed carefully, particularly prior to discharge from the ED (Terra, Figueira, & Barros, 2004).

Unlike alcohol and benzodiazepine withdrawal, opiate withdrawal per se is not as life threatening. However, during both acute and protracted opiate withdrawal, patients experience severe anxiety and dysphoria, which could exacerbate and increase the intensity of the underlying suicidal crisis that may have led to opiate misuse to begin with.

Thus, opiate misuse can be dangerous to a person's life both through an overdose and through withdrawal syndrome. In some patients, opiate withdrawal may cause panic, presumably through possible opiate noradrenergic interaction. Clonidine decreases opiate withdrawal-related anxiety (Gold, Pottash, Sweeney, & Kleber, 1980), but one uncontrolled case series showed its association with lower self-injurious behavior (Philipsen, Schmahl, & Lieb, 2004).

Cocaine withdrawal was initially described using a triphasic model (Kleber & Gawin, 1986). However, subsequent studies have failed to support the phasic nature of cocaine withdrawal. After cessation of cocaine use, rather than being phasic, cocaine withdrawal symptoms tend to decrease linearly, reaching their maximum in the first 24 hours and decreasing rapidly 48 hours after the last dose. The withdrawal symptoms consist of a "crash" along with a number of other symptoms, including paranoia, depression, anhedonia, anxiety, mood swings, irritability, and insomnia (Walsh, Stoops, Moody, Lin, & Bigelow, 2009). Some cocaine users also feel like they are losing their mind. All of the the previously mentioned symptoms are part of the acute suicidal crisis, making the first 48 hours of cocaine withdrawal a high-risk time period for suicide.

Cannabis withdrawal syndrome has been described only recently and consists of two factors—one characterized by weakness, hypersomnia, and psychomotor retardation and the other by anxiety, restlessness, depression, and insomnia. Both are associated with significant distress to the patient and with depression. Thus, cannabis withdrawal, like alcohol and heroin withdrawal, can increase the intensity of the acute suicidal crisis (Hasin et al., 2008).

Last, although barbiturate abuse peaked in the second half of the 20th century, it can still be encountered clinically. Someone who is addicted to barbiturates will begin to feel acute withdrawal symptoms within 8–16 hours after the last dose. Symptoms can be very severe, particularly in the beginning of withdrawal, and they include anxiety, insomnia, weakness, dizziness, nausea, sweating, and anxiety. There may be tremors, seizures, hallucinations, and psychosis, and users may become hostile and violent. Without proper treatment, hyperthermia, circulatory failure, and death may result.

Case 23

James was a 19-year-old high school senior with antisocial and borderline personality disorder as well as alcohol and substance use disorder. His drugs of choice were antihistamines, which made him hallucinate, and benzodiazepines, which caused euphoria and sedation. On the day of his suicide, James was staggering and falling asleep in classes and was brought to the local ED at 9 a.m. Although his urine toxicology was positive for barbiturates and marijuana, James denied drug use. As a routine, he was asked about his suicidality, which he adamantly denied. His parents were not available, and after hours in the ED he was given his cell phone to pass time. When his father arrived at 6 p.m., he noticed that James was texting furiously. James barely acknowledged his father and refused to talk to him. The father told the ED staff that this behavior was uncharacteristic for James. Prior to being discharged from the ED, James denied suicidal intent and was released to his father. On the way home, James continued to use his cell phone nonstop.

When they got to their house, James ignored his mother and his sister and went to his room, closing the door. Fifteen minutes later, the family heard a gunshot. James was found lying dead on his bed. He left a digital suicide note addressed to his girlfriend, who had just broken up with him, and to his parents. The note accused them of not caring about his life.

Although James had character pathology and substance use disorder, his suicide took place in the context of acute barbiturate withdrawal manifested by his increased hostility and anxiety. Given that his behavior was described as out of character, the withdrawal had likely intensified his negative affect and contributed to his suicide.

5

Suicidal Narrative

THE SEVEN PHASES OF THE SUICIDAL NARRATIVE

Suicide may be conceptualized as the ultimate phase of alienation from the world when all connections to everything a person loves in it—people, achievements, aspirations, or possessions—become irreversibly lost in one final action. This level of alienation is perceived by a suicidal person as a literal "end" from which there is no way out. Patients describe it variously as running out of options, having no good solutions, being in a tunnel with no light ahead, being backed into a corner, or being stuck in a dark department store after hours.

According to the narrative crisis model proposed in this Guide, people with trait vulnerability for suicidal behavior develop a fatalistic perception of their future. When stressors accumulate, these individuals increasingly see their lives as moving toward "a dead end" with no possibility of an acceptable or livable outcome. This perception of having no future and no power to effect change is unbearable and gives rise to the Suicide Crisis Syndrome. Establishing the extent to which the suicidal person's state of mind corresponds to this process is critical to the assessment of imminent suicide risk as well as to the development of corresponding interventions. To underscore the story-like process that characterizes the mind's progression toward the Suicide Crisis Syndrome, we've termed it the *suicidal narrative*

As mentioned in Chapter 2, the suicidal narrative echoes the concept of life narrative from a psychological theory of narrative identity (McAdams, 2001). Currently, the similarities between the suicidal narrative and the narrative identity are semantic and conceptual. Because both are new concepts, this hypothetical relationship has not been tested experimentally and may warrant future studies.

According to McAdams (2001), narrative identity is a person's internalized and evolving life story, integrating the reconstructed past, the present, and the imagined future to provide life with some degree of unity and purpose. Research into the relationship between life narratives and psychological adaptation shows that narrators who find redemptive meanings in suffering and adversity, and who construct life stories that feature themes of personal agency and exploration, tend to enjoy higher levels of mental health, well-being, and maturity (McLean, Pasupathi, & Pals, 2007; Pals, 2006). Conversely, those who cannot find positive meaning in adverse experiences and for whom the future becomes unimaginable may find themselves entrapped with no alternate solutions, placing them at increased suicide risk. This is a testable hypothesis, and future research will need to examine the relationship between narrative identity, the construct of suicidal narrative, and suicidal ideation and behavior.

The content and structure of the suicidal narrative are based on information gleaned from research studies on static risk factors underlying the second-generation *suicide risk models*, which have revealed pervasive themes in how acutely suicidal individuals perceive the evolution of their suicidality in response to stressful life events. Very common among these themes are perfectionism (O'Connor, 2007), setting up unrealistic life goals (O'Connor, Smyth, & Williams, 2015), failure to meet these unattainable life goals (Zhang & Lester, 2008), failure to redirect to more realistic goals (O'Connor, 2007), humiliating personal or social defeats (Siddaway et al., 2015), perception of being a burden to others (Joiner, Pettit, Walker, & Voelz, 2002), and alienation (Joiner, Brown, & Wingate, 2005).

As introduced in Chapter 2, the suicidal narrative component of the narrative crisis theory of suicidal behavior organizes these themes into seven phases that follow a coherent life story of progressive failure and alienation leading to a dead end, when the future becomes impossible:

- Phase 1: Unrealistic life goals
- Phase 2: Entitlement to happiness
- Phase 3: Failure to redirect to more realistic goals
- Phase 4: Humiliating personal or social defeat
- Phase 5: Perceived burdensomeness
- Phase 6: Thwarted belongingness
- Phase 7: Perception of no future

Although the body of experimental evidence linking the individual themes of the suicidal narrative to suicide is substantial, to date there are few data on how their exact sequence, overlap, and evolution over time interact to form causal pathways making suicide possible. Moreover, the available data are conflicting. Some reports suggest that defeat and entrapment are distinct constructs, each associated with increased risk for suicidal ideation and behavior, whereas one study suggests that defeat and entrapment are closely related and form a single construct (Taylor, Wood, Gooding, Johnson, & Tarrier, 2009). In addition, there are no data to explain whether someone who has a tendency to set unrealistic life goals and has also suffered a humiliating career setback is at higher risk for suicide than someone who has had a similar career setback but does not have such tendencies.

The individual stressors that induce these themes and contribute to the formation of the suicidal narrative may differ between individuals. As discussed later, some of these stressors, such as not being invited to a party, receiving a B on a college exam, or being scolded by a parent, may appear insignificant or even trivial to an outsider. Other stressors, such as overwhelming financial loss, death of a spouse, or divorce, are significant and tragic by any standard. Still, the vast majority of people eventually overcome even catastrophic losses, viewing them as an inevitable part of life. Although one can hypothesize that people with trait vulnerability for suicide are more likely than others to become suicidal when facing relatively trivial life stressors, little is known about what exactly in the interaction of stressful life events and trait vulnerabilities leads to suicide.

Ongoing research aims to establish whether a perception of one's life as a sequence of the suicide narrative phases increases one's risk of developing the suicidal crisis syndrome and of dying by suicide in the near future. One of the aims of these studies is to design a clinical scale to evaluate the intensity of the suicidal narrative and its relationship to suicide risk. In the interim, assessing the suicidal individual's life stories according to suicidal narrative phases, or constructing a suicidal narrative, is a useful way to establish whether perception of life story is evolving or has already evolved toward the suicide crisis.

Although all suicidal narratives share a common last phase, the dead end, the relative importance of the other phases varies among people. Many suicidal narratives are dominated by unrealistic expectations of success either in work or in personal life, and they are driven by unfulfilled narcissism. Many college student suicides, failed business-related suicides, and some suicides related to romantic rejection fall into this category. Life goals of those who killed themselves due to relentless bullying may be quite realistic, and their suicidal narrative is driven primarily by humiliation, alienation, and burdensomeness. Narratives of the seriously mentally ill could be quite short and appear irrational, and they may be primarily driven by the last phase's sense of no future, leading to a highly intense suicide crisis syndrome.

Although the suicidal process typically follows the arc of the suicidal narrative, even when all the phases can be identified, only one or two phases may dominate. The series of real-life suicide cases presented in this chapter are grouped according to the suicidal narrative phases that were most dominant in the causative mental process leading to the suicidal crisis and that made the suicide (or a high-lethality suicide attempt) possible.

PHASE 1: UNREALISTIC LIFE GOALS

Life is a pursuit of happiness, but happiness is often achieved by pursuing goals. Some life goals are unique and individualistic, but many are shared by a vast majority of people in most cultures. Most of us set life goals to be employed and independent, to create and maintain a happy home, to have a family, or to acquire material possessions ranging from smartphones to automobiles and homes. Very few of us, however, fulfill *all* hopes we have, and those who do so quickly expand their horizons to goals that were previously unimaginable. The most common goals are tangible and related to achievements and relationships; other less quantifiable goals pertain to emotions such as happiness, contentment, curiosity, or agency.

The first phase of the suicidal narrative, setting up unrealistic life goals, originates in trait perfectionism. Individuals with trait perfectionism tend to set lofty life goals, particularly if they carry a belief that others hold unrealistically high expectations of their behavior and will only be satisfied if these expectations are met (socially prescribed perfectionism or social perfectionism). As mentioned in Chapter 3 on trait vulnerability to suicidal behaviors, cross-sectional and population studies support the association of social perfectionism with both suicidal ideation and behavior (O'Connor & Forgan, 2007). Perfectionism is a powerful motivating trait that can be easily assessed during an interview, often by direct question, "Do you think or do others think that you are a perfectionist?" with a proper follow-up.

Setting up life goals appropriate to one's strengths, weaknesses, and available resources is an exceedingly complicated task. Assessing the suicidal patient's life goals in relation to his or her talents, flaws, personality features, and social aspects of the person's background will give an astute clinician invaluable clinical material for understanding the first phase of the suicidal narrative and for helping its assembly. Life goals taken for granted by an individual can be perceived as realistic by someone else and completely unachievable for others. As a simple example, a goal of having a family, owning a home, and having an income at the level of national average would be taken for granted by a young person from a middle-class background with traits of social perfectionism; this would be a realistic goal for a child of a first-generation immigrant, and it would be unreachable for a high school dropout with a drug problem and an impoverished family.

Although unrealistic life goals often relate to money and status, they are invariably symbolic of larger social expectations of behavior, such as their social roles as providers, parents, children, leaders, or community members. For example, several Indian farmers recently killed themselves after a drought because they would fail to deliver on the microloans they had taken.

The following are two case examples in which unrealistic life goals contributed to the suicidal narrative of failure, leading to the dead end of the acute suicidal crisis.

Case 24

Kimiko is a 21-year-old Japanese woman who was brought up in Japan as the only daughter in a wealthy family who owned a financial business. She was a bright girl, and her parents had shown off her talents to their friends since her early childhood. Kimiko was raised with the expectation that she would attend a prestigious university and succeed her father as head of the family business. She was privately tutored and had little free time and thus very few friends. As a teenager, she attended a private school in Massachusetts where she was the only Asian student. She did not get along with her classmates but was by far the best student in her grade and quickly became teachers' favorite.

Kimiko was a hard worker and was meticulous in her assignments. She had developed very close relationships with teachers who all told her, as did her parents, that she had unlimited potential and a spectacular future. This made Kimiko feel proud and special. However, she continued to have very few friends and spent most of her time reading and dreaming about joining her father's company at age 21 years as a highly paid executive. In the last year of high school, she started having panic attacks, which were treated with a selective serotonin reuptake inhibitor (SSRI) and an "as needed" benzodiazepine.

Kimiko graduated first in her class and was accepted at Princeton University. There, she had very few friends and again tried to distinguish herself with professors. Princeton was a large school, however, and her professors were busy. Kimiko felt lost and insignificant. Her grades were good but so were those of other students, and people no longer lauded her "unlimited potential." She got B pluses and A minuses on her midterms, which made her feel embarrassed. She could not bring herself to reveal her grades to her parents. She felt trapped and, not knowing how to face her parents, took all of the prescription medications prescribed for her panic disorder. After the overdose, she got scared and went to the emergency department, where she was treated; she survived.

Kimiko's suicidal narrative arc is a story of unrealistic expectations set for her by her parents, her single-minded pursuit of goals at the expense of age-appropriate social and emotional development, and abrupt and catastrophic humiliating personal defeat after getting B's in college, all of which led to her perception of her life narrative heading for a dead end. In her case, the dead end was "I will not be the CEO of my father's company."

Her narrative is dominated by an unrealistic life goal set up for her by her parents. Becoming a company CEO by merit is a setup for failure, even if one's father is the owner.

Kimiko's parents fueled her single-minded drive for a success so narrow that her failure was inevitable. Kimiko's Millon Clinical Multiaxial Inventory personality testing scores were high on narcissistic, dependent, avoidant, and schizotypal traits, as well as on anxiety and depression. At the time of her suicide attempt, she was convinced that she had failed her family, that she was unworthy of her parents, and that she was not smart enough to ever achieve what was rightly expected of her. After Kimiko was released from the hospital, she was treated with an SSRI for her depression and anxiety, as well as with an intensive crisis intervention in individual and family psychotherapy, helping Kimiko accept alternative measures of success.

Case 25

Stella was a 33-year-old woman who overdosed on Tylenol the day before her planned move into an independent living facility after 10 years in a psychiatric residence. Stella grew up in a middle-class family as a shy and reclusive girl with very few friends, but she studied hard and was a B student. She had one brother with attention deficit hyperactivity disorder and a sister with a drug abuse problem who dropped out of high school. Her father killed himself when Stella was 10 years old, and since his death, her mother relied heavily on Stella for emotional support and for housework help to the extent that Stella assumed a parent role to her mother (paternalized child). Her mother was unaware of the parental burden she was placing on Stella; Stella was always simply "the good kid."

However, in the last year of high school, Stella's grades started dropping. She could not concentrate and started having fears that classmates were laughing at her behind her back for being awkward and overweight. She stopped going to school, stopped eating, her hygiene worsened, and finally she locked herself in her bedroom and refused to leave because she said the TV started sending her coded threatening messages. Stella was hospitalized in an inpatient psychiatric unit and was diagnosed with schizophrenia. She was treated with neuroleptics and had several more hospitalizations before she was stabilized on clozaril and placed in a psychiatric residence, where she lived until her eventual suicide.

The residence staff members liked Stella and, just like her mother, called her "a good kid." Over time, she became a "star patient" who attended all the group meetings and activities, knew the residence rules better than some of the staff, and even helped the staff members with taking care of sicker patients, assuming the same role she had in her own family. Her treatment goals included job training and eventual transition to independent living. However, several times throughout the years as she approached transition, she required hospitalization for acute psychosis.

After a staff change, Stella's new psychiatrist decided that she was too high functioning for the residence, and as Stella was being prepared for discharge and a transition to independent living, the psychiatrist added a first-generation antipsychotic. To everybody's surprise and relief, Stella did not become psychotic, and a discharge day was scheduled for the following Monday. On Friday, the residence held a goodbye party for Stella. At the party, she seemed upbeat and cheerful, and she thanked everybody for all they had done for her.

Stella overdosed on two bottles of Tylenol on Friday evening. She wrote a suicide note explaining that she was killing herself because she knew she would get sick again and would let everybody down. After taking Tylenol, she got scared of what staff would think when they found her dead and told a health aide about her overdose. She was taken to a local hospital and placed in the intensive care unit. She told the visiting residence staff that she was so happy not to have died so that she could have another chance at transitioning to a residence. However, the next day she died of liver failure.

The first phase of Stella's suicidal narrative was written when she assumed the role of caretaker for her mother. Stella had a family history of serious mental illness and also suffered childhood trauma from her father's suicide, which increased her trait risk for suicide and for developing a major Axis I disorder. After her father's death, when Stella assumed a caretaker role for her mother, she also internalized her mother's unrealistic expectations of her as a perfect caretaker. The stress of these expectations most likely contributed to her developing schizoaffective disorder. During her 10 years in residence, Stella stepped into the role of perfect caretaker and was fulfilled by it. Graduation to independent living was a setup for certain failure; she would have nobody to take care of, she was destined to lose her sense of belongingness to the residence, and she felt like a burden to the new doctor. Even her opportunity of escape into psychosis was taken from her by the addition of the second antipsychotic.

Consequently, Stella's life fell into the suicide narrative of an unfulfillable expectation of being a perfect caretaker, followed by a 10-year experience of acting like one in a psychiatric setting, and ending in a suicide due to fear of humiliation, the expected defeat of letting down her substitute family, in addition to losing her connection with them. This fear was the dead end that led to the suicide crisis and suicide.

Two additional points in Stella's case are worth noting. First, unlike Kimiko's life goals, which had a concrete performance aspect and could be measured in grades, Stella's goals were entirely emotional. Concrete performance-oriented suicidal narratives like that of Kimiko are easier to detect and monitor clinically. Purely emotional life aims are much more difficult to identify, track, and monitor.

Second, although losing a supportive structure could be catastrophic for seriously mentally ill and psychotic patients such as Stella, patients may lack the cognitive skills to communicate their distress and fears appropriately. Such cases are further complicated by alexithymia, which prevents patients such as Stella from recognizing their own emotional distress. As a result, the danger of such transitions may be underestimated by staff, who have limited resources and are typically under pressure to discharge patients who are doing well. Many suicides of seriously mentally ill patients at the time of a reduction in level of care fall into this category.

PHASE 2: ENTITLEMENT TO HAPPINESS

Suicide is an irreversible act that ends a person's life and, with it, puts an end to all expectations that person may have had for his or her future. All of us have future expectations that start developing early in our childhood. As we grow older, future expectations are encouraged and often actively cultivated by our parents and other parental figures—grandparents, teachers, college professors, and mentors. Our life partners, friends, and acquaintances actively support our future expectations. Finally, society, industry, and the media bombard us with messages of success and happiness, creating the expectation that once we succeed in our goals, happiness and fulfillment will follow. Sometimes, our expectations are not met and we are left to come to terms with reality.

Hopelessness has been identified as one of the strongest predictors of suicide (Beck, Kovacs, & Weissman, 1975; Fawcett et al., 1990). However, hopelessness is only predictive of suicide long term, over a period of 10–20 years, and is not a predictor of imminent suicide (Simon, 2006) or even of a suicide within 12 months after the assessment. One possible reason is that although hopelessness is often experienced acutely in the present, and is thus viewed as a state condition, it is largely a temperament and a trait (Mann, Waternaux, Haas, & Malone, 1999). Moreover, hopelessness and pessimism are also cultural phenomena and may carry adaptive advantages in some cultures (e.g., Russia) but be maladaptive in others (e.g., the United States) (Kassinove & Sukhodolsky, 1995). Thus, hopelessness may not necessarily be related to short-term risk for suicide.

The ability or inability to think positively about the future is a state rather than a trait phenomenon, which may be more directly related to short-term suicide risk. Positive future thinking is defined as anticipation of positive experiences in the future, and it can be assessed experimentally via the future thinking task (MacLeod, Pankhania, Lee, & Mitchell, 1997), during which participants are asked to generate as many future events or experiences as possible that they are looking forward to. Most of these questions can also be asked during a clinical interview. Future positive experiences are divided into the following categories (O'Connor et al., 2015): Social/interpersonal expectancies involve at least one other person (e.g., marriage); the category of financial and home describes any aspect of financial or material gain or home improvement (e.g., making money, saving, buying a car, and decorating the house); achievement relates to the anticipation of an accomplishment (not including money), such as an accomplishment at work, promotion, and fame; leisure/pleasure refers to fun or pleasure (e.g., vacation); health of others describes expectations of health for friends and family; intrapersonal positive thinking involves the individual and no one else; and the last category is "other." Although all of these are related to suicide risk and are often intercorrelated (e.g., those who expect to achieve in one category tend to also expect an achievement in others), the primary expectation most directly connected with the risk of suicide ideation/suicide attempt in the next several months is "intrapersonal thinking" (i.e., expectation of happiness). Thus, short-term suicide risk seems to be intimately connected with a patient's expectations of his or her own fulfilling inner state, such as a state of exhilaration or that of inner calm and peace.

The relationship between expectations of happiness and suicide risk is not straightforward. Some reports suggest that low levels of positive future thinking are associated with suicidality, and this association is independent of depression and some other possible confounds (O'Connor, Connery, & Cheyne, 2000). In other words, high levels of intrapersonal positive future thinking appear to be protective from suicide. This finding is intuitive and could also be clinically important because creating positive future thinking would provide intuitive and easily understood treatment targets for clinicians. In the single short-term suicide risk study Morrison and O'Connor (2008) found that low levels of positive future thinking were better predictors of suicidal ideation (no data on attempts) than global hopelessness 2 or 3 months following a suicide attempt.

On the other hand, a 15-month study showed the opposite finding (O'Connor et al., 2015), and the likelihood of a repeat suicide attempt was elevated among those who reported more intrapersonal positive future thinking at baseline. These findings are crucial because they show that high levels of positive future thinking are not always protective. On the face of it, this may seem counterintuitive, given the generally accepted view that high levels of positive thinking buffer against distress in the face of life stressors (O'Connor, O'Connor, O'Connor, Smallwood, & Miles, 2004). However, if a person's expectation of future happiness is so high that it is unrealistic, this positive future thinking becomes an unreachable life goal of the kind described in the previous section.

A good way to probe the entitlement to happiness is to ask if the patient expects to be happy in life and how much unhappiness is reasonable to expect and tolerate. If the answer to "How are you feeling today?" is "I have never felt this bad in my life," it should bring on a probing "Did you think that you should be feeling happier than you are now?" or "How did you expect to feel at this point in your life?" The answer "I thought if I do all that is asked of me, I would be happy" should serve as a red flag that the person being interviewed felt entitled to happiness that is now starting to slip out of reach.

Entitlement to happiness appears to be a prominent phase in suicidal narratives among young people, or "millennials," who have come of age in the first two decades of the third millennium. In the United States, Japan, and the countries of the European Union, many millennials continued their education and remained dependent on their parents well into their young adult years. This historically new social behavior created a whole generation of highly educated young people entering an oversaturated job market with few jobs available requiring a high level of education, thus frustrating their future expectancies of success and happiness (Knowlton & Hagopian, 2013) and creating fertile ground for suicidal narratives based on thwarted entitlement to happiness.

A new life stage of "emergent adulthood" was defined to describe young people aged 18–25 years who, although adult in biological age, continue to live lives of adolescents. The term "moratorium" was coined to describe the decade between ages 20 and 30 years when millennials typically postpone making both career and personal commitments, taking time to enjoy themselves and find occupations that will bring them future happiness (Knowlton & Hagopian, 2013). At the end of the "moratorium," some of these 30-year-olds do not have the emotional maturity needed to make age-appropriate decisions necessary for full financial independence. This often requires accepting jobs they believe they are overqualified for with salaries well below those they believe they are entitled to, given their level of education. Many millennials believe that they have been cheated out of the bright future promised to them by society and by their parents. This generational conflict is a frequent stressor, which often precipitates the suicidal crisis.

The following are several case examples of the early phases of the suicidal narrative anchored in unrealistic positive future expectancies and in the entitlement to happiness.

Case 26

Angelia, a 27-year-old woman with a history of heroin and cocaine use disorder and an externalizing personality disorder, nearly died of a heroin overdose after her mother told her she was cutting off her financial support. Angelia's mother was a writer and an untreated alcoholic who drank daily and had frequent blackouts. When she was pregnant with Angelia, she divorced Angelia's father to marry a well-known artist 30 years her senior, who was also an alcoholic. Angelia's mother and stepfather fought frequently, and the split occasionally for short periods of time. Her mother's parenting style was unpredictable, alternating from hands-off to smothering and overbearing. Angelia dealt with her mother's erratic parenting and lack of boundaries primarily by trying to avoid her and by lying when necessary.

Having only episodic oversight, Angelia started using drugs in ninth grade but was able to hide it from her mother until her mid-20s, when she started using her mother's credit cards to support her heroin habit. Despite the drug use, she was a fairly good student, showed some promise as a writer, and was accepted into a good private university where she became an English major. Her college grades, however, were mediocre. When her parents suggested during her junior year that she should consider an alternative career, Angelia flatly said that only writing could make her happy and that if her mother would not help her pursue her passion, she would never speak to her again. Angelia's mother continued her financial support.

Because of Angelia's heroin and cocaine addiction, it took her 6 years to complete college. During this time, she was supported primarily by her parents, but she also made some money via tutoring and occasional freelance writing. During these years, she became dependent on prescription opiates and Adderall. Her drugs were prescribed by several doctors, but because none were illegal, she was able to keep her parents in the dark about the extent of her drug misuse for several years. However, after she developed a stimulant-induced psychotic episode and was hospitalized, her parents finally appreciated the severity of the problem. Angelia's addiction treatment was not successful. She skillfully used confidentiality and HIPAA laws to manipulate her parents to continue supporting her drug habit and her so-called writing career. She was hospitalized three times for low-lethality suicide attempts. After her mother canceled all her credit cards, Angelia made a high-lethality attempt with the intent to die.

Angelia was not a perfectionist. Her modest life goals consisted of becoming an intellectual like her parents and stepfather. She grew up expecting a bright and happy future. However, like some millennials, she felt entitled and expected it to arrive without much effort. Her suicidal narrative was anchored in her entitlement to happiness. Her family supported her entitlement because they set high goals for Angelia; in a way, the first phase of her narrative was written by proxy (as is often the case with helicopter parenting).

With substance abuse history on her mother's side of the family, Angelia discovered early on that using drugs was the easiest way to relieve her dysphoria and maintain the illusion of a happy future. The later phases of her suicidal narrative were related to her drug use, but it was the entitlement to happiness that laid the foundation of her future setbacks, alienation, and eventual suicide attempt.

Case 27

David was a 29-year-old man who died by hanging after his parents refused to fund his cannabis-growing enterprise following the legalization of marijuana in Colorado. David grew up in New Jersey, one of two children in a middle-class family. His family had no significant psychiatric history, his parents were happily married, and he had a happy childhood. On the surface, he was a well-adjusted student who was able to get A's and B's effortlessly. He was a recreational marijuana user, smoking weed weekly with his many friends.

David went to college without an idea for a major. He expected that he would get A's and B's without studying, but the courses were difficult and he flunked his midterms. He was embarrassed to tell his parents the truth, so he told them that everything was fine. In reality, he stopped going to classes and spent all day in his dorm smoking weed and binge-watching TV. When his parents found out, they suggested that David take a semester off. David searched for a job but could not find anything he liked. Instead of working, he stayed at home and tried to become a professional poker player. He was initially successful but soon quit, saying that the game involved luck and no skill.

It took David 6 years to graduate from college. He changed majors several times and ended up majoring in English. His parents paid his tuition and living expenses. David had several short-lived part-time jobs, which he lost due to his inability to handle feedback. After graduation, he got an assistant job at a start-up company but was let go after 3 months. He moved back in with his parents and lived there for several years rent-free. He worked occasionally, but he used his income as spending money. His parents eventually retired, sold their house, and rented a small apartment. They began living on a fixed income. For David's 30th birthday, they gave him $30,000 and told him that from that point on he would have to be independent.

David moved to Florida, where his friend was starting a business. He rented an inexpensive apartment and invested most of his money in a friend's Facebook-based dating app. Eventually, the start-up folded. David parents bailed him out "for the last time," telling him to get a job. He did so, only to be fired. When David's parents told him they could not afford to support him anymore, David threatened to kill himself. His parents gave him the money, taken from their individual retirement accounts.

David ran out of money and asked for his parents' support several more times. They would initially refuse but would cave to his threats of suicide. They consulted a psychiatrist on how to give their son financial independence and whether his suicide threats were real.

Just like Angelia, David grew up expecting a happy future but had neither the talent nor the work ethic to back future expectancies of success and happiness. The suicidal narrative of his life trajectory was rooted in his entitlement to happiness. His goals were quite achievable when he was in college, but they became increasingly unrealistic as he aged. With time, his lack of age-appropriate life experiences made it increasingly difficult for him to keep up with his peers. His parents repeatedly let him know that he was burdensome to them. A quick business success remained the only viable option until, in his mind, that door was shut by his parents' refusal to support his cannabis business. In summary, David's suicidal narrative had all the usual phases, but it was driven by his entitlement to happiness.

PHASE 3: FAILURE TO REDIRECT TO MORE REALISTIC GOALS

Striving for goals is a universal human experience. People work to attain goals with expectations of self-fulfillment, happiness, and other positive emotions. When goals cannot be attained, humiliation, anxiety, depression, and other negative emotions result. People's goals change throughout their life cycle. As people mature, inevitably some unattainable goals need to be discarded (Carver & Scheier, 1998). With age, the number of unattainable goals that need to be re-evaluated grows. Goal losses accumulating with age can be disheartening, but older adults have the highest life satisfaction (Stone, Schwartz, Broderick, & Deaton, 2010) as a result of the many realistic goals they have accomplished after discarding unattainable ones (Morrison & O'Connor, 2008). In the aforementioned cases, if Kimiko and David were able to appreciate that their life goals were unattainable, their life stories may not have followed the arc of a suicidal narrative.

When goal accomplishment is thwarted, the brain activates psychological processes of goal regulation, which differ by individual. These processes result in response patterns used to abandon commitment to a goal that has become unachievable (Wrosch, Scheier, Miller, Schulz, & Carver, 2003). From an evolutionary perspective, continuing the quest for an unachievable goal could result in exhaustion of cognitive, behavioral, or emotional resources (Wrosch et al., 2003). When goal attainment is unlikely, disengagement helps avoid feelings of failure (associated with suicide risk) (Nesse, 2000) and allows redirection of efforts toward more realistic goals in a process called goal re-engagement (Heckhausen, Wrosch, & Schulz, 2010). The latter adaptive process is associated with lower suicide risk.

Disengaging from unattainable goals is only adaptive when there are alternative meaningful goals available (Wrosch et al., 2003). Availability of goals varies by age (Wrosch et al., 2003). Older populations that possess limited options (Heckhausen et al., 2010) may be forced to abandon difficult-to-attain goals without re-engagement with new goals. Disengagement without re-engagement in older populations is associated with emptiness, thoughts of meaninglessness, and feeling irrelevant (Wrosch et al., 2003). Consequently, depression, hopelessness, and increased suicide risk may result (Carver & Scheier, 1998).

In industrialized societies, redirection post-retirement is essential for well-being. Failure to disengage from decades-old career goals to new goals may bring tragic consequences, particularly for men (Andreassen, Griffiths, Sinha, Hetland, & Pallesen, 2016). With the slow disappearance of the glass ceiling and emerging equal opportunities in the workplace, women approaching retirement are increasingly experiencing the same problem. It is not surprising that recent data from the Centers for Disease Control and Prevention (2014) show that the highest increases in suicide rates are among women in their 50s and 60s, followed by men of the same age group.

Recent increases in suicide rates for professionals of both genders in the later years of their careers suggest that without new worthwhile goals to engage in, goal redirection may not be adaptive. In these cases, retiring without having a groundwork for new meaningful activities may be more harmful than continuing work, even when work goals become unrealistic. Working to identify goals and redirect one's engagement in them may be the most adaptive pre-retirement strategy (Leinonen, Martikainen, Laaksonen, & Lahelma, 2013).

In contrast to older populations, young people have numerous choices for goal redirection. For them, low levels of goal re-engagement are strongly associated with higher levels of depressive psychopathology and suicide (Wrosch et al., 2003). Those who continue pursuing unachievable goals may do so because of "painful engagement" with those goals (MacLeod & Conway, 2007)—a dysphoric state defined by the perception of being painfully trapped in thwarted goal pursuit. Some instances of painful engagement are invaluable in teaching young people to recognize attainable goals.

Extended the pursuit of a high-risk career path that promises stardom against the odds, such as acting, music, or professional sports, is a common example of painful engagement. Most, realizing that their chances are low, disengage from unachievable goals of stardom and re-engage in pursuit of a lower-risk, more realistic goal with higher chances for success. Those who do not disengage may become entrapped in increasingly painful experiences of repeated failure, which bring on depression and increased suicide risk.

Another common setting for "painful engagement," both literally and figuratively, is a once-promising romantic relationship gone wrong. The pain the couple experiences may feel unbearable. Often, the more intense the initial attraction that brought the couple together, the more difficult it is to accept that the goal of mutual happiness has become unattainable. The following case examples illustrate situations in which individuals were aware that their goals had become unattainable but were unable to quit and find alternatives.

Case 28

Irena was a 32-year-old divorced woman of Polish descent who worked as a social worker. She had one 7-year-old son. She had recently divorced her husband of 7 years. Nothing was particularly wrong with her marriage, but Irena wanted something more. She met another social worker, Mark, at a meeting and fell in love. For her, it was love at first sight, but being Catholic, she considered infidelity a sin. Mark was the director of a department at a large hospital and had recently separated from his wife. He was Armenian, which Irena found exciting and exotic. Irena knew Mark was attracted to her too.

Once she made it known she was available, Irena and Mark started an affair. They were both madly in love and could not get enough of each other. Mark was everything Irena wanted—smart, ambitious, attractive, and sensitive. Their tastes were the same, their conversations were great, and their sex was fantastic. Irena thought she found a perfect man with whom to spend the rest of her life.

After approximately 10 weeks of bliss, Mark suddenly changed. Without warning, he told Irena that he needed space. Irena tried to give him space, but because she was afraid that he might leave her, she kept a close watch on him and kept finding different reasons to call or text him. That irritated Mark, who kept telling her he loved her, that he had no intention of leaving her, and that he just needed breathing room. Irena tried to give him space, but she could not.

Their fights were upsetting to Irena but also to Mark, who started pulling away. Irena resented him for ruining their perfect relationship. They had many talks and attempted to bring back the blissful first weeks of their relationship but could not. Mark wanted to break up. Irena told him that she could not live without him and if they just tried harder—if he tried to appreciate her love for him—they would be happy again. But the clock could not be reversed.

This continued for months. All Irena's girlfriends were telling her that she needed to stop seeing Mark and look for somebody else. They were telling her that she was young, beautiful, had a wonderful personality, and that Mark just did not appreciate her. They found him shallow and selfish. Irena agreed that this may have been the case, but she could not stop seeing him.

There were many breakups and reconciliations initiated by Irena. Mark thought Irena was "unstable" and could not see himself living with her long term. But he was also attracted to her and could not resist seeing her when she reached out. Passionate sex would ensue followed by fighting and another breakup. Despite everything, Irena was not willing to let him go. One night after yet another breakup, Mark stopped answering her frantic text messages. Irena could not bear his silence. She left work and waited for him at his hospital. Mark appeared, laughing and flirting with another woman. Devastated, Irena went home and jumped to her death from her 21st-floor balcony. Her son was at home in his room.

Irena's case is a typical example of a romantic "painful engagement." What makes it typical is the realization that the relationship is doomed and the inability to end it. This cognitive–emotional dissonance results in a rollercoaster of break-ups and reconciliations, which are prompted by extremes of attraction and despair and rationalized by cognitive schemes of "working on the relationship." In the end, Irena's inability to disengage from a doomed relationship was at the core of her suicidal narrative.

Case 29

Professor Andrew was a promising Assistant Professor of Geology in one of the larger Midwestern universities. He joined the faculty when he was in his 30s, which was later than most of his colleagues. Once he joined, he published often, was popular among students, and was quickly promoted from instructor to associate professor. However, when he was an associate professor, he had an affair with a student that resulted in a sexual harassment complaint, followed by a meeting with a dean. The dean was discreet but firm. Because he liked Andrew, he would keep the allegations quiet on the condition that Andrew resign.

Professor Andrew was devastated. His life was derailed, and his life goals were vanquished. He contacted two of his graduate school friends working in academic institutions, but no comparable positions were available.

Becoming desperate, Andrew called the student who had filed the complaint to demand she retract it. The graduate student instead went to the student newspaper, which published an article about Andrew's harassment. Later that day, the chairman called Andrew into his office and told him that his teaching and research careers were over and that he had himself to blame.

In the evening, Andrew tried to kill himself with sleeping pills. Usually prompt in answering his calls, one of his friends, worried by Andrew's unresponsiveness, went to his apartment. Andrew did not answer, and his friend called 911. When the police broke in, Andrew was lying on the floor unconscious. He was taken to a hospital and later transferred to an inpatient psychiatric unit.

Upon discharge from the hospital, Andrew resigned. While job searching, he saw an ad for a naturalist–lecturer on a cruise ship and decided to apply for the job. The cruise ship company hired Andrew. Andrew liked teaching, and the passengers very much enjoyed him.

At the end of his first contract with the shipping company, Andrew was surprised at how good he felt about his job. He renewed his contract for another year and then for many years afterwards. He still works as the cruise ship naturalist and is one of the major draws for customers.

Andrew's inability to change his career nearly cost him his life. Fortunately, he survived his suicide attempt, and his next job was a great fit for him, illustrating an ability to recover when a viable option presented itself.

PHASE 4: HUMILIATING PERSONAL OR SOCIAL DEFEAT

Human social structure is highly organized. Attaining a particular social position can be a major aspiration. Negotiation of social hierarchies and determining when to yield to others in social situations are universal human experiences. Whether one is born into nobility, fame, fortune, or poverty, there is always room for advancement.

According to the social rank theory (Price, Sloman, Gardner, Gilbert, & Rohde, 1994), the term *social defeat* applies to a failure or struggle to obtain a particular social status or to maintain it as a result of an external event or social circumstances. In both major and minor social conflicts, those who win the prize become victors and those who fail suffer a defeat. The ability to cope with social defeat is central to well-being, happiness, and, at times, survival.

From the evolutionary perspective, depression can be adaptive in circumstances of social defeat. When adjusting to the realities of social hierarchies, depression may help reduce the level of arousal, initiative, and activity generated by noradrenergic fight-or-flight responses. The latter are useful during a conflict over power because they help maximize intellectual, physical, and emotional resources, but they can be harmful afterwards, when a yielding approach is essential.

Depressed affect after a social defeat signals resignation and acceptance that can also be adaptive because it may reassure the social conflict victor that the depressed competitor is no longer a threat. Consistent with this theory, research indicates that acute suicidal states involve anxiety, panic, mental anguish, and desperation rather than depression (Fawcett et al., 1990).

A person's perception of his or her social defeat is a cognitive understanding of the outcome of the particular social conflict. As such, it is distinct from mood, hopelessness, and depression. A person who understands and appreciates a defeat experienced in a social conflict may not necessarily be depressed or hopeless and, in fact, could be hopeful for a victory or revenge. Research indicates that the acknowledgment of social defeat carries a near-term suicide risk, which is independent of depression and hopelessness (O'Connor, Gaynes, Burda, Soh, & Whitlock, 2013; Taylor, Gooding, Wood, & Tarrier, 2011).

The consequences of social defeat are as varied as the conflicts from which they arise. One aspect of social defeat is its objective magnitude. From an impartial perspective, the defeat of not getting on the debate team, not being invited to a birthday party, or being criticized at work would be considered relatively minor. On the more serious end of the spectrum are devastating losses such as being evicted from one's home, being fired from a job for fraud, or being exposed as a pedophile priest.

Importantly, the magnitude of a social defeat involves not only the size of the "prize" but also the extent of the emotional toll the defeat imparts on the person who has suffered it. The latter could take the form of public embarrassment, shame, indignity, and dishonor. The social defeats of eviction, a job loss, and a conviction of sexual molestation are devastating not only because of the income or social status loss but also due to disgrace and ostracism accompanied by the defeat.

Consequently, of many possible social defeats, those associated with public disgrace and humiliation dramatically increase near-term risk of suicide. The most common examples are suicides of tycoons who have lost their fortune and have been in the news (Herszenhorn, 2013), business owners who have lost or are about to lose their businesses and will have to face their friends or investors (Keneally, Nathan, & Collins, 2014), and men who have recently lost their homes (Serby, Brody, Amin, & Yanowitch, 2006).

Interestingly, suicides are often triggered by personal defeats that most people would consider trivial, such as getting a B+ on an organic chemistry exam as a college freshman. Strikingly, most people who have suffered life-altering defeats, such as being impeached from a public office for sexual misconduct, do not die by suicide (Feuer, 2008). Thus, in determining imminent suicide risk, the individual's perceived magnitude of the social defeat is more important than the objective magnitude.

Perception of failure and subsequent risk for imminent suicide can vary dramatically by one's culture, history, and personality. Cultural aspects of suicide risk include acceptability of suicide.

Receiving B's in college carries immeasurable meaning for students who equate good grades with success, whereas socially minded students consider B's to be good grades. For proverbial immigrant children who were raised to fulfill their authoritarian parents' expectations of success and higher social status, two B's in science courses may spell the end to their parents' dreams. The anticipated humiliation and fear of the parents' reaction to this failure may be so strong as to result in panic attacks and anguished turmoil, characteristics of the acute suicidal state.

The following case examples illustrate situations in which humiliating defeat was the core phase of the suicidal narrative.

Case 30

Dan was a 44-year-old, married, California wine distributor executive who was good at his job and rose quickly to the position of vice president of marketing. During the first Internet bubble in the late 1990s, he left the company to start his own online wine distributing company. He raised a large amount of money from his friends, added his own, and opened his business as sole owner, confident that he would succeed. However, soon his business was failing, and his friends' investments were lost. He tried to borrow more money but could not find new investors.

Dan's business failure was a terrible blow financially and psychologically. His savings were depleted, and he was in debt. His image of himself as an exceptional business visionary was shattered. More than anything, however, Dan was ashamed that he had let his friends down. Dan was a gregarious, athletic man, a team player, and a leader. His friends invested in his business because they trusted his business sense and knew that they could rely on him.

In a last-ditch attempt to raise funds, Dan flew to New York for a meeting with a new group of potential investors. On the eve of the meeting, an article about his failing business appeared in a local newspaper. Several of his friends read it and called him to ask about their investments. Feeling humiliated and unable to face his associates, Dan hung himself in his hotel room. He left a suicide note apologizing for letting everybody down and asking for forgiveness for being unable to live with his shame.

The most prominent feature of Dan's suicidal narrative is the feeling of humiliation after he squandered his friends' investments. Dan was a man known for his drive but also for his kindness, ethics, and morals. Losing his friends' investments shattered Dan. Telling them about it was a fate worse than death to him, making a very compelling humiliating social defeat phase of the suicidal narrative. If Dan had borrowed the money from venture capitalists, his life may have turned out differently.

Case 31

Adrianna was a 55-year-old woman who at the time of her death was unemployed and living in a psychiatric residence on disability income. She died of prescription opiate and benzodiazepine overdose after her son Luke called her residence administrators and demanded that they keep his mother away from him. Adrianna had previously reported that her son had died of heart failure years ago.

Adrianna had a history of severe borderline personality disorder. She had many psychiatric hospitalizations for depression and suicidal behavior. She had three suicide attempts resulting in medical intensive care unit (MICU) admission. On one occasion, she was intubated with a ventilatory support for days. Adrianna was obese, weighing more than 350 pounds. She was diagnosed with type I diabetes mellitus, and her blood glucose was poorly controlled. She had few friends and poor relationships with the residence staff and her neighbors.

A former sales representative, Adrianna was divorced three times and had two adult children. Luke, who was 28 years old at the time of her death, had a congenital heart malformation that carried a life expectancy of 25 years. He had an office job, was married, and had two children. Before his alleged death, he lived in rural Pennsylvania 100 miles away from his mother. Adrianna's other son lived on the West Coast.

The last known encounter between Adrianna and Luke took place during her last psychiatric hospitalization and was humiliating. Luke attended the family meeting and instead of being empathetic, he told Adrianna that he was tired of her manipulating him with her illnesses and said that he would never visit her in the hospital again. "I have been dealing with this since I can remember," he told the treatment team. "Imagine what it was like to call 911 because your mother threatened to kill herself starting in middle school all through high school," he said. "I have had enough."

Several days later, Adrianna was discharged. According to the residence staff, she and Luke sometimes talked on the phone, but he never visited. There was a lot of screaming. After their phone calls, Adrianna would say how she regretted her difficult relationship with him and that she wanted to see her grandchildren—another one was on the way. One day, Adrianna got off the phone crying and said that Luke had died of a heart attack. She took a day off, ostensibly to go to his funeral. The reality was that Luke's wife gave birth, and Luke told his mother that she was not invited to the christening and, if she came, she would never see her grandchildren again.

As in Dan's case, Adrianna's suicide was driven by humiliation. In her case, the humiliating event was personal. Facing the other residents, knowing that they were aware of her lies about her son's death and of her failure as a mother, was a fate worse than death to her. Adrianna's connections to others was based on a lie. Once that lie was exposed, there was nothing left.

PHASE 5: PERCEIVED BURDENSOMENESS

Joiner's interpersonal theory of suicidal behavior suggests that concurrent feelings of burdensomeness and thwarted belongingness increase an individual's desire for death. *Burdensomeness* is defined as the sense that one is a burden to his or her family or loved ones, whereas *thwarted belongingness* is akin to social alienation and isolation. This model has been implicated extensively in suicidal behavior, but the duration of these psychological states remains unclear. Further research is necessary to more precisely understand the role of burdensomeness and thwarted belongingness in the acute period.

In a 2009 study of patients referred to the hospital for "severe suicidal symptoms," "recent" suicide attempt (a specific time frame was not indicated), or serious suicidal ideation, burdensomeness and thwarted belongingness were significantly predictive of current suicide attempt, but only when combined with previous number of attempts. (Joiner et al., 2009). In a psychological autopsy study comparing the suicide notes of 20 people who attempted suicide and lived versus 20 people who died by suicide, those who died by suicide reflected greater levels of burdensomeness compared to those who survived. Their suicide methods were more lethal in nature than those who survived their suicide attempts (Joiner et al., 2002).

Failure to achieve unrealistic goals or failure to achieve financial gains anticipated either due to perfectionism or to expectations of others often involves financial hardship. The resulting financial difficulties may force a person to seek help from others. Asking friends or relatives for money or moving in with one's elderly parents can make many people feel like a burden. According to some suicide notes, suicidal individuals come to perceive themselves as a burden to the extent that they believe that their close others would be better off without them—that is, they are high on perceived burdensomeness (Joiner et al., 2002).

Perceived burdensomeness is a mental state characterized by apperceptions that others would "be better off if I were gone," which manifests when the need for social competence that is posited by frameworks including self-determination theory (Ryan & Deci, 2000) is unmet. Furthermore, greater perception of burdensomeness in suicide notes is associated with more lethal means of suicide. A person's perception that he or she is a burden to others is an independent predictor of suicidal ideation in a range of samples, including older adults (Jahn & Cukrowicz, 2011) and people with chronic pain (Kanzler, Bryan, McGeary, & Morrow, 2012). Perceived burdensomeness also has been shown to mediate the association between perfectionism and suicidal ideation (Rasmussen, Slish, Wingate, Davidson, & Grant, 2012) and to remain predictive of ideation even after controlling for factors such as depression and hopelessness. Perceived burdensomeness is the fifth phase of the suicidal narrative.

Case 32

Penny, a 28-year-old single woman, was diagnosed with bipolar disorder after an extensive prodromal state, which manifested as recurrent, mood lability, and impulsive behavior. Penny completed high school with good grades, was accepted into Emory University, but took a leave of absence after her freshman year to pursue activist work. She was active in feminist organizations, and she often worked through the night, constantly moving from place to place. At age 26 years, she fell in love with a woman. When her love was not reciprocated, she left the country and had her first manic episode in Europe. Severe, treatment-resistant depression followed. Penny moved in with her mother and left the house only for doctors' appointments. She stopped talking to friends. She was treated as an inpatient for depression with suicidal ideation and with post-discharge follow-up in dialectical behavior therapy (DBT) programs and by esteemed therapists. Despite the expensive treatments, her condition did not improve. She did not find group therapy helpful and did not connect with the other patients, who did not share her passion for social causes. After the DBT program let her go and after she got the "maximum" benefit from participation, her mother let her know that she would no longer pay for ineffective expensive treatment and that Penny should snap out of it and get a job. Feeling alienated from the world and knowing that she had become a burden to her mother, Penny attempted suicide by asphyxiation. She survived this attempt and was admitted to an inpatient psychiatric unit. She was later discharged to a long-term residential treatment facility.

Penny's suicidal narrative is complicated and has several components. Her goals of saving the world were unattainable, her return home from Europe and discharge from the day program were humiliating, and she withdrew from her friends in a typical response to shame of her current life situation. However, the most compelling phase prompting her suicide attempt was feeling like she was a financial and emotional burden to her mother and also an emotional burden to her friends. The latter feeling led to her self-imposed isolation, which worsened her feeling of alienation. She had no source of income. Her depression was so severe that she lacked the concentration and initiative to work or study. Her stress tolerance was too low to negotiate the conflict with her mother. As a result, Penny believed that her life had reached a dead end, and she attempted suicide.

Case 33

Craig was a married 47-year-old unemployed lawyer who ended his life by jumping in front of an oncoming train after his wife told him she was tired of borrowing money from her parents for living expenses while he chased crazy projects.

Craig was an Ivy League law school graduate who initially had a very promising career but later suffered several setbacks, resulting in increasingly severe depressions. Three years prior to his suicide, he was diagnosed with bipolar disorder (BD) II, and at the time of his death, he was being treated with lithium, aripiprazole, and bupropion. Craig's first job was a partner-track position at a large law firm. He was the hardest-working, brightest associate, who was nevertheless difficult to get along with because he had a big ego and responded poorly to feedback. Nevertheless, he did well until he antagonized the partner with whom he worked on an important case to the extent that Craig was let go just short of making partner himself.

Craig was depressed for months, but then he found a partner-track job in a smaller firm. He was initially happy with the firm, and the firm was happy with him until history repeated itself: Craig insulted a senior attorney and was fired. After a second depressive episode, Craig was able to find a short-lived job in the district attorney's office. He was soon let go.

After this third setback, Craig could not find another job. His wife Jackie was a homemaker caring for their daughter, who had a learning disability. Craig's third depressive episode was more serious than the first two. He changed psychiatrists twice and was finally diagnosed with BD II. Craig's bipolar depression was treatment resistant. The medications were not effective, and he refused electroconvulsive therapy. The longer he stayed unemployed, the more difficult it was for him to find another job. However, he was hopeful and resistant to taking just any job to survive.

Initially, Craig and his family lived off savings, but soon the money ran out and they had to borrow money from Jackie's parents. This was humiliating for Jackie, who was resentful of his failure to provide for the family, and for Craig, who felt like a burden. Jackie told Craig that he was a failure who could not even support his only daughter and that his BD was just an excuse for laziness. She told him to "snap out of it" and to do what all normal men do and get a job or they would have to take their daughter out of her school, which specialized in learning disabilities.

Although Craig was cocky when manic, during his depressions he was prone to guilty ruminations, blaming himself for his family's predicament. He felt especially guilty for not being able to pay his daughter's tuition. Pressed by Jackie, he searched for a lower-paying job but was unsuccessful because he was overqualified. The money they had borrowed from Jackie's parents was running out. They could either ask for another loan, take their daughter out of private school, or sell their apartment. The atmosphere at home was reaching a boiling point: Jackie told Craig she wanted out of the marriage. Craig killed himself the day he discovered Jackie had consulted a divorce lawyer. In his suicide note, he said that he was ending his life because he could not go on living feeling like a burden to his family.

Craig's suicidal narrative is driven by failure to disengage, humiliation, and perceived burdensomeness. His bipolar disorder likely had strongly contributed to his suicidal process. The goals he had set for himself during hypomanic phases were most likely unrealistic, and his grandiosity impaired his reality testing, making it rigid and inflexible. As a result, Craig had difficulty accepting feedback and could not redirect his efforts when necessary. Because he was fired during manic episodes, the humiliation of losing the job was buffered by his inflated self-image. However, when he developed his most serious depressive episode, his failure as a provider was amplified by feelings of worthlessness and intense guilty ruminations (see Chapter 7), resulting in feeling like a burden to his family.

PHASE 6: THWARTED BELONGINGNESS

The other main component of the interpersonal psychological theory of suicidal behavior (Joiner, 2005) is the fundamental human need to be socially integrated or to "belong." Individuals are at greater risk for suicidal behavior when this need is unmet, and those who attempt suicide often experience loneliness or thwarted belongingness leading up to their suicidal behavior (Van Orden et al., 2008).

Numerous studies have suggested that the sense of belonging associated with community involvement or participation in social events serves as a protective factor against suicidal ideation (Joiner, Hollar, & Van Orden, 2006; Joiner & Van Orden, 2008; Kessler, Galea, Jones, & Parker, 2006). Kleiman, Adams, Kashdan, and Riskind (2013) examined variations in suicidal ideation by college semester, isolating belongingness as a mediating factor. The sense that one is a burden to his or her family or loved ones has been shown to be a predictor of suicidal ideation in a number of samples, independently of reports of depression or hopelessness (Joiner et al., 2006).

People who have failed in their life goals and have been forced into a position of real or perceived financial and/or emotional dependency that makes them feel like a burden to others are rarely proud of their predicament. Often, they are embarrassed by their failures and ashamed to disclose them to others. As a result, such people, even though they desperately want support and companionship, often remain to themselves and avoid social contact. Staying isolated thwarts a human being's basic need to connect, to be accepted, and to belong.

In contrast to perceived burdensomeness, which originates in the self-determination theory, the construct of thwarted belongingness has multiple origins and is an amalgam of theories of the human need to connect. Thwarted belongingness is a psychologically painful mental state that results when the fundamental need for connectedness or the "need to belong" is unmet (Baumeister & Leary, 1995; see also Cacioppo & Patrick, 2008).

A number of theories suggest that the various indices of social isolation—living alone (Heikkinen, Aro, & Lönnqvist, 1994), loneliness (Koivumaa-Honkanen et al., 2001), and low social support (Qin & Nordentoft, 2005)—are associated with suicide across the life span because they are indicators that the need to belong has been thwarted. Retrospective studies showed that both men and women who were socially well integrated had substantially lower risk for suicide long term (Tsai, Lucas, & Kawachi, 2015), regardless of burdensomeness, which was not examined. Thus, the thwarted belongingness is a unique construct and in the narrative crisis model plays a prominent role in phase 6 of the suicidal narrative.

Thomas Joiner's (2005) interpersonal theory of suicide posits that when a person feels both hopelessly alienated from others and a burden to them, he or she starts to develop suicidal ideation. According to Joiner, suicidal ideation is a necessary but not a sufficient cause for suicide. Suicide takes place when a person with suicidal ideation loses fear of death, which prevents most people with suicidal ideation from taking their lives. Joiner's theory equates losing fear of death with acquiring the capability for suicide, attained through practicing increasingly lethal means of ending one's life and through habituation to death.

Joiner's two-step theory readily explains why the overwhelming majority of people with suicidal ideation do not attempt suicide and do not die by suicide. However, the interpersonal theory does not explain why the average time interval from the first thought of taking one's life to the suicide attempt is 15 minutes (Deisenhammer et al., 2009) and why some survivors of serious impulsive suicide attempts report having no prior suicidal ideation. Joiner's framework does not quite account for the state of desperation felt by many suicidal individuals, with suicide being an urge to escape the intolerable pain of the moment rather than a rational plan.

However, there is a substantial body of research indicating that the two central concepts of interpersonal theory of suicide—the thwarted belongingness and perceived burdensomeness predisposing individuals to the development of suicidal thoughts and attempts (Schneidman, 1998)—are associated with long-term suicide risk. Subjective perception of lack of social connections and of thwarted belongingness specifically is associated with suicide attempts (Fässberg et al., 2012; Hatcher & Stubberfield, 2013). Similarly, a person's perception that he or she is a burden to others is a predictor of suicidal ideation in the elderly and people with chronic pain (Kanzler et al., 2012). Consistent with the interpersonal theory of suicide, the interaction of perceived thwarted belongingness and burdensomeness is predictive of suicidal ideation independent of depression (Joiner et al., 2009).

The following two cases illustrate suicidal narratives defined by alienation and thwarted belongingness.

Case 34

Adam was a 22-year-old college senior who wanted to kill himself by jumping off a bridge near his campus but was talked out of it by a passer-by who then called the police.

Adam was a typical American college senior with an average GPA and $50,000 in student loans. He was on a debate team, a fraternity member, and joined several other clubs because he liked the feeling of belonging to his class, college, and generation. Adam's parents were helping to pay for his education as an investment in his future, but they expected him to support himself after graduation. Adam imagined a bright future and felt justified to receive his parents' support, never believing that he was a burden to his parents.

Unexpectedly after graduation, Adam, unlike his friends, was unable to find a job. His Facebook feed was full of entries of friends furnishing their new apartments and hanging out with coworkers and new friends. Adam, on the other hand, had to move back in with his parents. Time passed and still Adam could not find a suitable job. As Adam's friends seemed to move into the next phases of their lives, he seemed to move backwards. The only jobs available seemed menial and did not even require high school diplomas. Taking such a job symbolized defeat, social and otherwise. To add insult to injury, his parents, who worked hard to put him through college, wanted him to start doing "something."

This turn of events led to a drastic change in Adam's state of mind. His feeling of belonging to a cohort of people marching forward to happy futures had been shattered. Reading his friends' Facebook entries was making him depressed, so he stopped using Facebook altogether, telling everybody that he was taking a break from it because it was taking too much time. Time, however, was all he had, and he spent it smoking weed and playing video games.

Some of Adam's high school classmates never went to college and were living at home. Adam tried to hang out with them several times, but he never really fit in. That is when he made his attempt.

In Adam's case, getting a good job after college signified continued belonging in a group with the same socioeconomic status as him. His failure at this thwarted his attempt at continued belongingness. Adam's sense of thwarted belongingness became even more acute after his ill-designed attempt to belong to the "bad crowd" from his high school. His parents never explicitly told him he had become a burden, but Adam imagined that they must be thinking it, adding perceived burdensomeness to thwarted belongingness.

Over time, Adam fell into both thwarted belongingness and, to a lesser degree, perceived burdensomeness. For somebody without other risk factors, this change in mental state alone would not increase imminent suicide risk. However, Adam was led to believe that he was destined for success in life, and his entitlement to happiness further increased the intensity of his suicidal narrative. Moreover, Adam was competitive, perfectionistic, and conscious of his family's social status. This made him perceive his failure as a personal social defeat, increasing his suicide risk dramatically.

Case 35

Shirley was a 59-year-old divorced woman who jumped to her death from the window of her apartment building several weeks following the death of her only friend and a mother figure, Susan.

Shirley was diagnosed with borderline personality disorder and had a long history of depression, anxiety, and panic attacks. She graduated from a good college and obtained a law degree from a prestigious law school, but because she was never able to get along with her peers or supervisors, a career never manifested. After college, she had several failed jobs at law firms; these jobs never lasted long because she was soon fired or asked to leave.

Shirley's parents divorced when she was in elementary school, and she was estranged from her father, who remarried and had three more children. Her mother died single when Shirley was in her 40s. Shirley entered a legal battle for an inheritance that was left mostly to her sister, her mother's favorite. Shirley died before the endless lawsuit was settled.

Shirley's longest employment lasted 7 years, when she worked for a nonprofit organization. After she was asked to resign, she filed a discrimination lawsuit, which dragged on for several years before it was settled.

Shirley was married for a year when she was in her 30s. Her husband left her because she was "impossible to be around." This was the consensus of most of the people who knew Shirley. Shirley had no friends except for Susan, who made a life habit of helping people like Shirley survive. Shirley was chronically depressed and suicidal, and her wrists were covered with scars from self-inflicted razor wounds.

Shirley often talked to Susan about how she liked people and wanted to get along with them. When Shirley would meet a man on the Internet, or a potential girlfriend in a class she was taking, Susan coached her through relationship basics—be nice, ask questions, and give them space—but it never worked. Everyone Shirley met quickly became disturbed by her blend of aggression, possessiveness, and lack of boundaries. "If not for me," Susan would say, "she would be dead. She has nobody else."

That was not quite true. Throughout her life, Shirley saw many psychiatrists and therapists. After Susan died, Shirley's therapist wanted to hospitalize her, but Shirley refused, saying that she was not suicidal. Shirley's suicide followed a canceled dinner with Susan's daughter. Shirley left a note saying that she did not belong in this world.

It would be difficult to find a clearer illustration of suicidal narrative dominated by thwarted belongingness than Shirley's case. Borderline personality disorder is characterized by difficulty regulating emotions, which leads to unstable moods, impulsivity, and poor self-image with constant fear of abandonment. Repeated and frantic attempts to avoid abandonment come across as hostile and needy, resulting in stormy relationships. Borderline personality disorder often manifests in self-harm or suicide attempts. While Susan was alive, she was the only person who Shirley could trust to be there for her. Given her borderline personality structure, Shirley experienced Susan's death as her final abandonment, which she did not survive.

PHASE 7: PERCEPTION OF NO FUTURE

Entrapment may be most directly associated with imminent risk for suicide. People may have many negative experiences and emotions, but until they feel trapped in their misery with the door shut, there is always a chance that their circumstances may improve. It is the notion of suffering with no escape that creates the anguish that triggers suicide. The feeling of finality of being trapped in unbearable suffering results in an emergence of the suicide crisis syndrome (Yaseen et al., 2010), which may result in imminent suicide.

Defeat and entrapment have historically been implicated in social-rank theories of depression and were relatively recently implicated in the integrated motivational–volitional model of suicide and the feedback loop hypothesis of the role of panic in the suicide trigger state (Katz, Yaseen, Mojtabai, Cohen, & Galynker, 2011; Williams, 1997). The inability to escape from defeating circumstances provides a setting for the emergence of suicidal ideation (O'Connor, 2011; Williams, 1997). Together with defeat, entrapment distinguishes suicidal individuals from controls independently of depression and hopelessness. Both predict suicidal ideation and attempts over time (O'Connor, 2003; R. C. O'Connor et al., 2013).

The concepts of defeat and entrapment have similarities in that both foster negative affect and describe a loss that could be irreversible. Possibly because of this overlap, defeat and entrapment are often considered together in suicide research. There is even controversy regarding whether defeat and entrapment describe one or two different phenomena (O'Connor et al., 2013; Taylor et al., 2009). However, in clinical work, defeat and entrapment relate to different aspects of acute suicide risk and need to be assessed separately.

It is the social aspect of a defeat, rather the magnitude of the loss, that increases risk of suicide in the near future. A person can lose all of his or her possessions during a hurricane and may not become suicidal because the person's loss is understood, respected, and sympathized with by loved ones and the society at large. On the other hand, a fewer than expected number of "likes" on Facebook after a profile picture change designed to improve social acceptance can bring on a suicide attempt.

With regard to imminent suicide risk, the social aspect of entrapment plays a minor role. It is people's perception that the trap they find themselves in has no exit that may be one of the most critical factors in predicting whether they will attempt suicide in the immediate future. The word *entrapment* readily brings visceral images of caged animals and captured people. Accordingly, it is the acute and almost physical sense of being locked up in a bad situation that predicts imminent suicide.

The following cases illustrate the suicidal narrative's essential last phase, perception of no future.

Case 36

Peter was a 58-year-old married engineer with three adult children who shot himself in the head in front of his wife Carrie during an argument.

Peter married Carrie when they were both 19 years old because she was pregnant with their first child, a boy. They had two more boys. At the time of Peter's death, his oldest son was married and lived in another state with his family; his middle son was single, lived at home, and worked at a local bank; and his youngest son, Dan, who had a severe congenital disorder, also lived at home, requiring 24-hour care. Peter's insurance was paying for most of Dan's care, but his income was instrumental to keeping his ill son out of an institution.

Peter knew his marriage was unhappy and so did everybody else. His wife was viewed as selfish, prickly, and manipulative. The two met as freshmen in college and dated for several months. The relationship was rocky even then. When Peter decided to break up because he did not love Carrie and wanted to meet somebody else, Carrie told him she was pregnant. He stayed.

They got married 1 month later because Peter decided to "do the right thing." After they had their third son and learned that he was ill, the marriage became truly difficult. The couple decided to care for Dan at home, regardless of cost, and his care had drained their savings. Peter's income was barely sufficient, and Carrie did not contribute financially because she was Dan's full-time caretaker.

Peter had to take a second job. That solved the financial problem, but he was never at home, so Carrie essentially raised their sons on her own. With time, she became increasingly bitter. She believed that life has passed her by and blamed Peter for it. As time went on, Carrie became hostile and her treatment of Peter became harsh. She angrily berated him for being a poor provider, a miserable lover, and a failure in all aspects of life. There were shouting matches every evening. Their older son left the house for college and never came back. Their middle son moved to a friend's basement. Dan was nonverbal and did not react.

Peter finally decided to file for divorce. However, the divorce lawyer told him that if he did divorce, Peter would lose the house and would have to continue to support his son while paying his wife a hefty maintenance. Peter felt trapped. Vicious arguments at home continued. The atmosphere became so toxic that the two older sons would not come home for the holidays.

Being at home was so painful that Peter often stayed with friends, who urged him to leave Carrie. "Nobody would want me with a disabled son. I cannot leave Carrie to take care of him all alone. She is a good woman. I have not been there for her enough," Peter would respond. Carrie had gotten into his head.

When he finally went to a psychiatrist, he was diagnosed with major depression and prescribed an antidepressant. Peter had suicidal thoughts but no plans. However, he had visions of himself crashing the car into a wall when driving. With Peter in his office, the psychiatrist called Carrie and alerted her to Peter's state of mind and high suicide risk. He asked her to remove all firearms from the house and to come in for a family session. Carrie became defensive and said that she would not take the blame for Peter's failures.

The psychiatrist advised Peter to stay with his friends. Peter did so for 1 week, but when he returned home to do his laundry, an argument quickly ensued, and Peter shot himself in the head. His life insurance was valid and had enough coverage to pay for Dan's care for 20 years.

Peter's case is an example of somebody reaching the phase of "perception of no future" while having few other phases of the suicidal narrative. His life goals were realistic, he was not entitled, he did not perceive himself as a burden (just the opposite), and he was connected to many people. The only other significant phase in his suicidal narrative was the failure to disengage, in his case from his commitment to keeping Dan at home and to his toxic marriage. And yet, his enmeshed relationship with his wife had evolved into his perception that his life had reached a point with no options. His only perceived choice was to stay with the woman he did not love out of guilt and duty. His final argument with Carrie escalated the already present suicidal crisis to the unbearable state of entrapment and pain.

Case 37

Marissa, a 40-year-old separated woman diagnosed with bipolar disorder, was admitted to an inpatient psychiatric unit after she was found unconscious in a bathtub with cuts on her wrists. Marissa was recently removed from her position as CEO of a small start-up company after her main investor (with whose son she was having an affair) discovered that the bylaws of the company were in disarray and that she did not actually own the company product.

Although Marissa was diagnosed with bipolar disorder only recently, she always had mood swings. When she was down, she had difficulty getting out of bed and was unmotivated but was still very functional. During hypomania, she was incredibly charismatic, creative, and very fast. Since the beginning of her last hypomanic episode 3 years prior, she was able to start a company, raise millions in venture capital, hire a staff of 20 people, and create a prototype of her product. "This is what I always knew I was capable of," she told her friends, "and it is finally happening."

However, as she was building her company, Marissa made many mistakes, which led to the removal from her position. She failed to hire a legal team, used company funds for personal expenses, and had an affair with the principal investor's son, who was employed by the company as her assistant. When a competitor sued for the rights to the product, the investors discovered the improprieties, and she was removed from the company she had founded.

Her affair quickly ended. After learning about the affair, the young man's father swore that he would never work with Marissa again and would make sure that nobody else would either. He sought legal action to block Marissa's access to the company accounts. Removed from the company that was to become her life's success, heavily in debt, and depressed, Marissa attempted suicide.

Marissa's case is typical of a suicidal narrative of somebody with bipolar disorder. Her life goal of making it "really big" could be seen as unachievable, her company collapse could be considered a public humiliating defeat, and the end of her affair may fall under the heading of "thwarted belongingness." Nevertheless, it was the lack of good options out of her business crisis that brought on her first-ever suicidal behavior. Whether real or not, the lack of good solutions or exits out of painful life situations is perceived as real and brings on very real emotional pain and the desperate state of entrapment, which is at the heart of the suicide crisis and forms the defining component of the suicide syndrome.

CONSTRUCTING THE SUICIDAL NARRATIVE

The suicidal narrative interview portion of the imminent risk assessment consists of two parts. The first part is a systematic assessment of each of its phases in which the patient is asked whether and to what extent the constructs previously described are applicable to the story of his or her life. After the clinician obtains enough information to construct a formulation of the patient's suicidal narrative, the clinician discusses the formulation with the patient until both agree that it adequately reflects the patient's perception of his or her life. Once the agreement is reached, the clinician can use the table provided at the end of the chapter to examine the intensity of the narrative and to perform the risk assessment.

The seven phases of the suicidal narrative discussed in this chapter—unrealistic life goals, entitlement to happiness, failure to redirect to more realistic goals, humiliating personal or social defeat, thwarted belongingness, perceived burdensomeness, and perception of no future options—read like a general outline of a life story gone wrong. Published research supports the relationships of each of the concepts outlined in these phases with suicidal behavior, and research efforts to test the narrative as a whole are ongoing.

Life events of suicidal patients are different, and so are the details of their suicidal narratives. However, some generalizations apply to all or almost all individuals. For example, setting up unrealistic life goals will frequently result in failures. Entitlement to happiness makes it difficult to admit failure in chasing a life's dream, which in turn makes it difficult to disengage from the now hopeless undertaking and to re-engage in a pursuit of a more realistic goal. The more one persists in a failed endeavor, the more likely the failure will be experienced as humiliating defeat. Such defeats often result in financial losses and the unwanted dependence on others (often loved ones) for economic support, which could be perceived as burdensome and shameful. In addition, the reluctance and embarrassment of admitting the failure may result in feelings of thwarted belongingness and a perceived sense of having no future.

The previous summary is a general outline of a typical suicidal narrative. The goal of the narrative portion of the imminent suicide risk assessment is to establish to what extent the suicidal patient's perception of his or her life (or of the patient's life narrative) fits this outline. In a comprehensive clinical assessment, all seven domains must be assessed. However, the "end" of the suicidal narrative—the sense of having no future— carries the most weight and should be assessed most explicitly.

The assessment sequence does not need to follow the phases in order but should depend on the course of the conversational interview. For example, if a patient's presenting complaint is suicidal ideation because he or she has no good options, then one may start by exploring the patient's perception of entrapment, which is the end of the suicidal narrative. Alternatively, if a patient has not spontaneously expressed suicidal ideation or intent, one may start the narrative section of the interview by exploring the life goals and expectations of happiness—that is, the beginning of the narrative.

When conducting the suicidal narrative part of the imminent risk assessment, it is important to "translate" the terminology used in this chapter, including most of the phase titles, into accessible language. The terms "attainable or unattainable goals" and "failure to disengage or redirect" are neither intuitive nor familiar to the general public or, as a matter of fact, to many clinicians. Clinicians' use of psychiatric terminology (or "psychobabble") is often perceived as condescending, cold, and insensitive, and an effort should be made to use simple vocabulary accessible to all.

A good entry into a discussion of the realism of the patient's life goals and his or her ability or failure to achieve them is a simple question about the patient's life, such as "How are things working out in your life?" or "How has life treated your lately?" Any response is likely to mention either a work situation or a relationship and provide an opening for follow-up questions. For example, the answer "I have had trouble with my boss" could lead to follow-up questions about the patient's occupation and career goals and the realism thereof.

Occasionally, the patient may feel too tense or too distressed to answer the opening question or will give an evasive answer such as "Everything is fine," making a life goals discussion slightly more difficult. One interviewing strategy in these cases is to use some factual knowledge of the person's life and offer the interviewer's best guess on what the problem might be, such as "I know you had some issues with . . . (your boss, your boy-friend) lately." After the patient acknowledges the issue, the interviewer can start the discussion in earnest by saying, "Please tell me more about this." Usually, the following questions are sufficient to formulate a clinical opinion about the patient's life goals: "What are your life goals?" "What would you like to achieve in life?" "How close are you to achieving them?" "Are they realistic?" "What would your life be like if you fail?"

After the life goals are identified, a good second question is "How important are these to you?" An answer to this question could be pivotal for understanding both their impor-tance and the degree of the patient's investment in them. For example, the answer "I have been working there for 30 years, and this job has been my life" is quite revealing of potential difficulty in disengaging from a lifelong ambition. Alternatively, the answer "I thought he was the one" is revealing of how difficult it may be for the patient to give up and start searching for a new relationship. Once the aim is identified, the interview can explore how central and meaningful the issue is to the person's life and possible alternatives.

Because most patients know what they feel, discussing patients' entitlement to happi-ness is often easier than talking about their life goals, which some people may have never defined consciously. Usually, the following questions are sufficient to formulate a clinical opinion about patients' expectations of happiness: "Are you happy now?" "How happy did you expect feel at this point in your life?" "Did you expect to feel this bad?" "Do you deserve to feel the way you are feeling?"

Like unattainable goals, the notion of humiliating social defeat is an abstract concept foreign to most patients. Even those patients who are aware that they have just lost a social battle may not consciously appreciate to what degree their defeat has been humil-iating. Other patients may not even be aware that the stress and emotional turmoil they have been experiencing were brought on by a social defeat. Fortunately, whether patients did or did not suffer defeat can be deciphered from their recent histories.

Often, patients will spontaneously bring up their losses and embarrassments. Statements such as "I lost this lawsuit," "I got laid off," "I am getting C's, it is so com-petitive," and "this is so embarrassing" are explicit acknowledgments of a defeat or humiliating situation, and they should be interpreted as such during an interview. In these instances, to formulate the opinion about the intensity of the defeat phase, the clinician needs to assess the extent of defeat or humiliation by asking, "How bad is it?" When the patient does not respond, one option is to wait for the patient to identify the conflict—for example, "I have been going through a bad divorce"—and then ask about its implications. For example, the question "Do you feel like you are losing this battle?" frames the divorce as a social struggle and sets up a discussion of possible losses and humiliations.

States of thwarted belongingness and perceived hopelessness are often very labile and can change rapidly depending on life circumstances. A rejection letter from one's dream college or failure to land a good job can be perceived as a thwarted attempt to belong to a group of successful people and generate an acute sense of thwarted belongingness. If a person in one of the previously mentioned situations is financially dependent on others, perceived burdensomeness may follow.

Although the terms thwarted belongingness and perceived burdensomeness are very cumbersome, the corresponding themes may be easier to talk about and empathize with during a psychiatric interview than the other concepts discussed in previous chapters. Most people can relate to feeling alienated or like a burden. Hence, simply asking if the patient feels alone and if he or she feels like a burden will often provide enough information to assess the severity of these two phases of the narrative. Several follow-up questions from the interview algorithm presented later or from the sample cases are most often sufficient to complete the assessment.

Finally, the assessment of either thwarted belongingness or perceived burdensomeness can be transitioned to the discussion of perceived entrapment by asking if the patient thinks that anything can be done about the current situation, followed by a question about whether he or she feels trapped in the current situation. In situations in which patients are not aware of being trapped, it is often possible to assess a perceived sense of entrapment by asking simple questions about choices, options, and solutions to everyday problems.

For example, when a depressed and suicidal porter with limited English who must work for an abusive manager for 2 more years so he can retire with a full pension is asked if he feels trapped, he may respond with bewilderment. However, when asked about his choices at work, he will readily acknowledge that he does not have any, revealing the extent of his entrapment. In another case example, a suicidal woman with a history of drug abuse entangled in a mutually exploitative relationship with her alcoholic boyfriend may not be aware that she feels trapped. However, when asked if she sees any solutions to her life situation, she will reveal the state of entrapment by answering "no." In both cases, a clinician needs to ask several explicit follow-up questions assessing the severity of perceived sense of entrapment.

On the other hand, many patients at a higher risk of suicide will spontaneously report feelings of entrapment. In these cases, it is important not to miss an opportunity to follow-up and assess whether the patient thinks the trap has an exit by simply asking "Are there any exits to your situation?" "Is there anything that can be done to open some doors for you?" and "What if . . . X . . . happens?" The more negative the answers to the "What if?" questions, the likelier the patient is to attempt suicide in the near future.

PROBING THE SUICIDAL NARRATIVE: AN INTERVIEW ALGORITHM

Patients' openness about their suicidal ideation or intent depends on the clinical setting and the individual. Many patients coming to the emergency department for help and protection from their suicidal thoughts and impulses are open about their suicidal intent. Patients who are either invested in hiding their intent or unaware of it may be less forthcoming. The algorithm outlined here should be used for guarded patients who do not disclose their suicidality in the first minutes of the interview. For patients who answer the first question by acknowledging their entrapment, such as "I am suicidal and I am trapped in a horrible situation," the algorithm should be reversed. The interviewer should first explore the entrapment and suicidality and conclude by assessing perfectionism and entitlement to happiness.

All patients and clinical situations are unique. The guideline should be personalized for each patient according to his or her history and circumstances. The case examples that follow show how the algorithm can be adjusted depending on the course of the interview.

- Forming rapport
  - How are you feeling today?
  - What happened (or what has been happening)?
- Perfectionism and entitlement to happiness
  - You said you feel miserable. Is this fair that you feel this way?
  - Do you work hard to achieve what you want in life?
  - Are you a perfectionist?
  - Do you deserve to be happy?
- Attachment to unachievable goals
  - Can you tell me more about your (work situation or relationship)?
  - How important is this to you?
  - Can you find an alternative?
  - How hard would it be to live without it?
- Humiliating (social) defeat
  - How bad was it?
  - Was it humiliating?
  - Did (do) you feel defeated?
  - Is it possible that it just seemed that way to you?
  - Do many people know about this?
  - How hard would it be for you to face them?
- Belongingness
  - Do you feel alone (in this)?
  - Even when you are with people?
  - Do you feel disconnected even from people who are closest to you?
- Burdensomeness
  - Do you feel like you are a burden to them?
  - How bad a burden?
  - Would they be relieved if you were not there?
  - Will others miss you if you are gone?
- Perception of entrapment
  - Are there any good options in your situation?
  - Do you feel trapped in it?

- Do you see possible good solutions, ways out?
- Is there anything that can be done to improve the situation?
- Constructing suicidal narrative
  - It seems that (suicidal narrative created from answers to the previous questions).
  - Does this apply to you?
  - What does and what does not?

CASE EXAMPLES

Case 38: High Risk for Imminent Suicide

Gary is a 30-year-old single Jewish man with a history of bipolar mood disorder I and two previous psychiatric hospitalizations who is currently living in an apartment with his parents. He returned to the United States 6 months ago after teaching English in Croatia, and his parents referred him for a psychiatric assessment to a bipolar specialist "so he can get the best possible treatment because his is a difficult case." Gary has no previous suicide attempts, but his parents are concerned that he may kill himself because "there is just something scary about him that makes us very uncomfortable."

DR: How are you feeling today? (*Forming rapport*)

GARY: Not so great. Trying to adjust to living with my parents.

DR: What happened?

GARY: I had been living in Croatia for 2 years, tutoring college students in English, and it was going great but then they did not renew my contract, and I figured I needed to get back home to regroup. So I moved back in with my parents, temporarily, until I find a job.

DR: Is this making you upset?

GARY: Very. I am 35 years old. I did not expect to be living with my parents at 35.

DR: Did you think you would be happier at 35? (*Entitlement to happiness*)

GARY: Of course. Who expects to be miserable? Ten years ago I thought I would be on top of the world by now.

DR: Are you saying that from where you were 10 years ago, you should be feeling a lot happier than you are now?

GARY: Exactly. I graduated from Cornell, did all the right things, even after I was diagnosed with bipolar.

DR: Are you a perfectionist? (*Perfectionism*)

GARY: You could say so. I always try to do my best. Straight A's and all that.

DR: I am sorry, it must have been rough for you. Do you think from everything that you've done, you deserve to be happy?

GARY: I have put in more than enough effort, a lot more than other people I know. This is just so unfair.

DR: Are you saying that life has not been fair to you?

GARY: Isn't this what I just said? Do you think I planned on having a manic break in the first year of college?

DR: Can you tell me a little more about your life plans and your life goals?

GARY: I always wanted to be a writer and a professor. My father is a writer, my mother teaches at NYU. I was writing and publishing when I was in high school. I could not get an academic job after college, but I worked for a publishing house, and wrote two novels. I also tutored, until I got a university job in Croatia. It worked great for 2 years and then I got into a fight with the stupid administrator and they did not renew my contract. I thought I had good CV but I applied to several teaching jobs and nothing (*unrealistic life goals*).

DR: How important is this career to you? (*Failure to redirect from unachievable goals*)

GARY: I cannot see myself doing anything else. I am a great teacher—all my students say so. I am also a good writer, and I have been published. I should be in academics.

DR: Can you see yourself doing other things?

GARY: Like what? Driving a cab?

DR: Well, some people would do that, but maybe for you something more intellectual. Would you consider becoming a schoolteacher, or, say, changing careers and going to social work school?

GARY: After all that I have been through? All my college classmates have academic jobs or are doctors and lawyers. There is a job opening at Stony Brook I am a perfect fit for. I should hear from them this week.

DR: What if you are not able to get the right job? How hard would it be to live without it?

GARY: I must get it. There is nothing else out there and I cannot continue living off my parents, it is just too embarrassing.

DR: What part was embarrassing? Everybody goes through difficult times. (*Humiliating defeat*)

GARY: It would be a disaster. I have no money, my parents are sick of supporting me. They keep saying that I must get a job. My sister is a lawyer, and she is not as smart as I am. And here I am. I was not able to get an academic job in the states, I lost one in Croatia, and here I am again, living off my parents.

DR: You sound defeated. Is this how you feel?

GARY: Exactly.

DR: Is it humiliating?

GARY: It is beyond humiliating. I cannot take a girl out on a date—I have to ask my parents for money. And what will I tell her? That I am an unemployed writer at 35 living with my parents?

DR: Do many people know about this?

GARY: When my contract didn't get renewed in Croatia, it was pretty public. All my friends knew. My girlfriend dumped me—good riddance: She did not love me and she just wanted a green card. This is one of the reasons I came back to the US. And here—I am sure my parents are talking to their friends, unless they are ashamed to. I tried to call a couple of my old friends. Can't talk to any of them; I feel so small by comparison.

DR: Do you think you may be exaggerating?

GARY: I am not exaggerating. I went to a club last Friday. I had to go alone and no girl would even dance with me.

DR: Do you feel alone? (*Thwarted belongingness*)

GARY: Terribly.

DR: Even when you are with people?

GARY: What people? I told you I have lost all my friends, I have nothing in common with them. And girls wouldn't even look at me.

DR: This sounds worse than alone; this sounds like you feel alienated. Is there anybody or anything that you feel connected to? Maybe professionally?

GARY: Well, I should feel connected to other writers, or academics—but everybody is so self-centered. And successful. And I am not.

DR: How about people closest to you, your parents and your sister? (*Perceived burdensomeness*)

GARY: I cannot talk to my parents. My sister is too busy with her children and her Wall Street shark husband.

DR: Do you feel like you are a burden to them?

GARY: I know. My parents said they cannot support me forever, and that if I cannot find a job, I should go on disability. I can't ask my sister for money, it is too humiliating, and she needs it for her own family.

DR: How bad a burden do you think you are?

GARY: They are certainly acting like I am a burden. I am not asking them to support me "forever," just until I get a good teaching job. I will pay them back . . . I think they can afford it—look at their lifestyle!

DR: Would they be relieved if you were not there?

GARY: Probably . . . I don't think that they look forward to facing me every day.

DR: Do you think they would miss you if you weren't around?

GARY: Not sure.

DR: Are the any good options in your situation? (*Perception of no future*)

GARY: I need a teaching job, which looks more and more like a miracle. There are no jobs out there.

DR: Do you see other alternatives?

GARY: Like what? I can try to look for an editor job, but I have not done any editing for years. And they do not pay well. I can try to finish my novel, but that is not a job.

DR: Other choices? Maybe tutoring, even an administrative assistant job pays . . .

GARY: I can't stand tutoring! And I am not good at it—I get too impatient with stupid students. . . . Administrative assistant? At 35? After being a professor? I would rather kill myself!

DR: Have you been thinking about killing yourself? (*Suicide intent and plan*)

GARY: Yes, but I would never do it . . . I don't have the guts.

DR: I may come back to this a little later, if you do not mind, but now I have just a few questions about your life situation. Do you feel trapped in it?

GARY: Yes.

DR: Do you see any exits?

GARY: Not really.

DR: Is there anything that can be done to improve the situation?

GARY: Do you have a job for me?

DR: (*Constructing suicidal narrative*) Let me make sure I understand. From what you are telling me it seems that you are kind of trapped in your life situation because the only professional life goal you see—the academic career—is unreachable. You are a hard-working perfectionist, and you can't give up on your dreams because this would signify defeat. So you keep pondering, while living with your parents, who make you feel like a burden. This is humiliating and so you are ashamed to call your friends, which makes you feel alone. I condensed it a little, but does this ring a bell?

GARY: Yeah, I can identify with this, and the humiliation is just unbearable.

DR: What do you mean by unbearable?

GARY: I am not sure if I can take it much longer.

Suicide Narrative Risk Assessment Table

Component	Risk Level				
	Minimal	Low	Moderate	High	Severe
Unrealistic life goals				X	
Entitlement to happiness					X
Failure to redirect to more realistic goals					X
Humiliating personal or social defeat					X
Perceived burdensomeness					X
Thwarted belongingness					X
Perception of no future				X	
Total					X

Gary identifies with all seven aspects of the suicidal narrative: The goal of the academic career he is chasing is unattainable, he feels defeated and alienated, he believes that he is a burden to his parents, and, finally, he understands that he does not have good options. His false hope for a miracle job opening and even more miraculous interview is likely to be dashed soon. Gary's suicidal narrative suggests very high risk.

Case 39: Moderate Risk for Imminent Suicide

Bernie is a 53-year-old single gay man with a history of generalized anxiety disorder who came for treatment of his depression with suicidal ideation after he discovered that his just deceased partner of 20 years had a family and children. Bernie had a plan to kill himself with a barbiturate and alcohol overdose. He had just retired from his teaching job. He has one brother and a large circle of friends. He saw a therapist twice in the past following relationship breakups, but he was never on medications and had no past suicide attempts.

DR: How are you feeling today? (*Forming rapport*)

BERNIE: I am still in shock from everything that happened.

DR: What exactly has been happening?

BERNIE: Well, he was the love of my life, he died in my arms, it was a fairy tale. . . . Twenty years together, he would come home, I would make dinner. Twenty years . . .

DR: And?

BERNIE: He got diagnosed with liver cancer last month, it was really quick, and I took him home, he wanted to die in our bed. And I took care of the funeral, and then this Korean woman shows up I have never met, with two teenagers, and tells me she is his wife! He had a wife!

DR: Are you angry?

BERNIE: I am not angry, I love him.

DR: You said your relationship was perfect. . . . Let me ask you maybe a strange question, but trust me, it is not strange: Are you a perfectionist? (*Perfectionism and entitlement to happiness*)

BERNIE: Strange question, you're right. No I am not, am actually pretty easy-going. I do my job, but I don't go crazy about it, I am not too hard on my students.

DR: What about your relationship? You said it was perfect. . . . Were you a perfectionist about that?

BERNIE: I am not sure, it just happened. He was on a tour with this dance company, and we met in a bar. It was love at first sight, and then he defected, and we stayed together and it was perfect.

DR: Did you ever expect to be this happy?

BERNIE: Never. But after John and I got together among all my friends, I was the happiest.

DR: Do you deserve to be happy?

BERNIE: Everybody deserves to be happy and I am not sure if I will ever be happy again.

DR: It sounds like the life was hard on you lately. . . . Now, after all that happened, what are you plans in life? (*Attachment to unachievable goals*)

BERNIE: I don't have any. I just retired and we planned to spend the rest of our lives together, and now it is impossible. That's why I think that my life is pointless. I would rather kill myself.

DR: I will have to ask you more about that later, but now I need to talk about something else. It may sound like an insensitive question to ask, but when one comes in suicidal we must do everything, fair? Do you think you can ever get over his death, and maybe have another relationship?

BERNIE: You can't find another fairy tale. You are rationed just one in your lifetime, if any. I cannot have another fairy tale.

DR: Still, do you think that somewhere out there maybe somebody like John . . . but truthful?

BERNIE: What do you mean?

DR: Well it sounds he was not truthful with you for many years. . . . Some people would say that he betrayed your trust.

BERNIE: I am not sure what you mean. . . . We loved each other. I had coffee with his wife. I talked to her how I could help her with the kids.

DR: But what if it does not work?

BERNIE: I should make it work, it is his family, and I do not need anybody else.

DR: When you discovered that John was married . . . was or is this embarrassing for you? (*Social defeat*)

BERNIE: I understand why you would think so, but it was not. I have many friends, and they are all very supportive and sympathetic. Everybody is concerned; that's why I am here.

DR: What is everybody concerned about? Did you tell them about John's wife?

BERNIE: No, I didn't . . . I could not . . . I did not want them to think badly about him . . .

DR: What did you tell them?

BERNIE: That he died in my arms . . .

DR: Are you saying that telling them the truth would have been too humiliating for him? For his memory I mean.

BERNIE: Yes. . . . He was a saint.

DR: Do you feel alone in (this)? (*Thwarted belongingness*)

BERNIE: Not at all, as I said I have a lot of support.

DR: I heard what you said. I meant do you know anybody else who ended up in your situation—having lived with somebody for 20 years, who was leading a . . . double life?

BERNIE: How dare you call it a "double life?!" John was incapable of lying.

DR: But he got married and had two children while you were together, and he did not tell you about it . . .

BERNIE: He must have had his reasons. . . . . I can't think about it, I cannot talk about it.

DR: And you don't feel like you are a burden to them? (Perceived burdensomeness)

BERNIE: I try not to be a burden. I have enough friends and I am very considerate. Nobody complained. So far that is.

DR: Are there any good options in your situation? (*Perception of no future*)

BERNIE: Options in what?

DR: Well, you are here because you "lost a reason to live."

BERNIE: How can you go on living when your fairy tale has ended? There was no happy ending. . . . There cannot be—he is no longer with me. There is nothing I can do to bring him back. What is the point?

DR: Is there anything that can be done to improve the situation?

BERNIE: I am trying to get to know his wife and his children. . . . I don't even know what he told them about me. Probably that I was a roommate and that he was saving money that way. I don't remember much from the funeral, all this feels like nightmare . . . a horror movie, and everything is in a fog.

DR: How about the fact that John was not truthful to you for 20 years? How can you solve that?

BERNIE: I don't know, I feel no anger. . . . I only feel love and sadness. Nothing will ever match it. And I don't need anything. Or anybody (crying).

DR: (*Constructing suicidal narrative*) Let me make sure I understand the situation correctly. It seems that you wanted a perfect relationship and were incredibly lucky to have one for 20 years. It ended tragically and you learned some shocking things about John that put you in a bind: If your relationship was what you thought it was, a fairy tale, then nothing can ever match it, there is no point in living, and you want to kill yourself. Admitting that John was lying to you would ruin the fairy tale—and then what?

BERNIE: Nothing can ruin my fairy tale . . . I loved him so much.

DR: Fortunately, you have friends to support you and as a considerate person you try not to burden them too much. Does this sound right?

BERNIE: Most of it. Except he wasn't lying.

DR: How is this possible?

BERNIE: I don't know; he just wasn't. . . . I will never meet anybody like him, even if I try.

DR: Will you try?

BERNIE: I don't know.

Suicide Narrative Risk Assessment Table

Component	Risk Level				
	Minimal	Low	Moderate	High	Severe
Unrealistic life goals			X		
Entitlement to happiness			X		
Failure to redirect to more realistic goals					X
Humiliating personal or social defeat					X
Perceived burdensomeness			X		
Thwarted belongingness		X			
Perception of no future					X
Total			X		

In contrast to Gary, who does not volunteer suicidal thoughts or plans, Bernie's presenting complaint is active suicidal ideation and intent. Yet, at this moment, Bernie's narrative is less alarming than that of Gary. Bernie's drive for a perfect relationship is as strong as Gary's aspiration for an academic career, and he has seemingly achieved it in his 20-year fairy tale relationship with John, except, of course, it was based on a lie. Bernie's image of his life is as elusive as Gary's hope for an academic job, if not more. Acknowledging the truth to himself and to others for Bernie appears to signify a destruction of the only thing that made his life meaningful—his love for John. Bernie is also very conscious that he is trapped between a rock and a hard place with very few options: He will try to date, but he is not emotionally available and his dating is likely to lead nowhere. However, his social support is fairly strong, and he feels neither defeated, alienated, or like a burden. Hence, at this moment, he should be considered a moderate risk for imminent suicide. This risk will increase drastically if he is unable to come to terms with his past and move onto the next relationship.

Case 40: Low Risk for Imminent Suicide

Kate is a 28-year-old woman who was admitted to a psychiatric unit for a suicide attempt. Kate repeatedly cut her left arm and left thigh with a razor blade after she was let go from a nonprofit after a falling out with her supervisor. The cuts were deep enough for her thigh wounds to require sutures. Kate had a long psychiatric history and was diagnosed with attention deficit disorder as a child and with major depressive disorder, generalized anxiety disorder, panic disorder, and borderline personality disorder in high school. She was accepted to but never completed college, despite several attempts to do so. She worked only sporadically, mainly for environmental causes, and was supported by her father. During the interview, Kate was confrontational and provocative.

DR: How are you feeling today? (*Forming rapport*)

KATE: I am feeling awful.

DR: What is making you feel awful?

KATE: I was in Europe traveling, working for a cause, and then I met somebody who was nice at first, but then horrible to me, and I was in so much pain that I cut myself. I was bleeding and went to the ER, and they sutured me but then put me onto the psych unit. I don't know why.

DR: I will ask you about your suicide attempt a little later if you do not mind; Please tell me what cause were you working on?

KATE: The environment. We are sucking the life out of the environment. If we continue like this, soon there will be no resources left. We used up most of the oil already and so many species are endangered. We need to organize and stop this. I have been canvassing and organizing people.

DR: And what was so special about this person to you that you attempted suicide when things did not work out?

KATE: He also cared about environment and was working for this nonprofit . . . or pretended to care. . . . In either case, I volunteered for him and then he turned out to be a jerk—I always meet jerks. That hurts.

DR: I'm not sure I understand: Was this guy a perfect partner or supervisor in your fight for the cause. . . . Or . . . were you in love? (*Entitlement to happiness*)

KATE: It was the cause. . . . I just kind of started feeling for him, but then he fired me out of the blue. . . . And I thought we hit it off so well.

DR: I see, not yet romantic but with potential to grow. You said you were hurt; do you often get hurt and feel bad, or was this was an exception and you are mostly happy?

KATE: Hah, I wish I were happy. I am either unhappy or depressed.

DR: Do you think this will change?

KATE: It better—one can't live like this . . . I hope it does, but I have been on this depression rollercoaster for so long that it's hard to keep the hope.

DR: This question may feel strange to you, but bear with me: Do think that you deserve to be happy?

KATE: Everybody does . . .

DR: But at the moment I am not concerned with everybody, asking about you: Are you entitled to happiness?

KATE: In a fair world I would be: I am a fair person, I care for others, I fight for causes . . . I always do my best.

DR: Are you a perfectionist? (*Perfectionism*)

KATE: I always give it my best but it does not always work—my room is a mess.

DR: Can you tell me more about your causes? (*Unrealistic life goals*)

KATE: I only have one: the environment. Nobody understands how serious the damage is we are causing our planet. Do you want me to elaborate?

DR: Please do; that's why I asked.

KATE: Global warming is the biggest immediate problem. The climate has already changed, yearly temperature just keeps setting records. Hurricane Sandy was the worst ever, and then . . . there are the natural resources: We are running out of oil, and there's deforestation in the Amazon. People just don't understand how bad it is going to get. . . . Nobody listens . . . they just don't get it.

DR: How important is this cause to you? (*Attachment to unachievable goals*)

KATE: It is my whole life!

DR: If for some reason you can't champion this cause—will you champion another?

KATE: What can be more important than the environment? And I don't see why I would need to.

DR: You attempted suicide after a conflict with your supervisor.

KATE: There are other supervisors . . . I live for the environment.

DR: You said that people don't listen. Does this make you feel defeated? (*Social defeat*)

KATE: It can be frustrating, but I don't give up.

DR: You cut yourself after you were let go. Why? Was it humiliating?

KATE: It wasn't humiliating; it was infuriating. I felt so betrayed, and so angry, and did not know how to live—at that moment, and so I cut myself.

DR: Did the meeting with your supervisor make you feel defeated?

KATE: I am not defeated. I am a fighter. I will find another organization.

DR: Do many people know about this?

KATE: My family and friends; everybody knows!

DR: How hard was it for you to face them?

KATE: Well, it was not fun but I did, didn't I? That's why I am here . . .

DR: What do your friends think? I mean your close friends? (*Thwarted belongingness*)

KATE: I only have two close friends, and they think I should not be cutting myself and that I should get some help.

DR: So, do you feel disconnected even from people who are closest to you?

KATE: Sometimes. They get tired of me . . .

DR: Do you feel like you are a burden to them? (*Perceived burdensomeness*)

KATE: Not really . . . maybe emotionally . . .

DR: Not financially? I thought your job was a volunteer job.

KATE: They only pay my rent. I have inherited some money from my grandmother. It should last another year.

DR: And after that?

KATE: After that I will have to get a job.

DR: Have you ever had a paying job?

KATE: No, but my volunteer job was very important and I am very responsible.

DR: Did your supervisor feel that way?

KATE: He turned out to be a jerk.

DR: So, what are your plans now? (*Perception of no future*)

KATE: I will take some time off and maybe go on a yoga retreat.

DR: And then?

KATE: And then I will look for a job.

DR: What kind?

KATE: For the cause, of course . . . something to do with environment.

DR: What are your options?

KATE: I will find something.

DR: Do you have people you can ask for a reference letter? I suspect your supervisor is not one of them.

KATE: No, and I would not ask him if you would pay me. I will find somebody.

DR: (*Constructing suicidal narrative*) It seems that you met somebody who you thought had the same goals that you did and really understood you, but then he turned on you—unexpectedly—and that was so painful that you wanted to die. But then you didn't, and it sounds like you have a pretty good support system and that you still have options for how to volunteer for the cause . . . as long as you still have your inheritance. Does this sound right?

KATE: Sounds about right . . . you are very smart.

DR: Thank you. Does all this apply to you?

KATE: Even worse: I really started caring for the guy . . . I thought we were going to be a couple.

DR: Twice disappointed!

KATE: I have got to go back out there and start looking . . .

Suicide Narrative Risk Assessment Table:

Component	Risk Level				
	Minimal	Low	Moderate	High	Severe
Unrealistic life goals		X			
Entitlement to happiness			X		
Failure to redirect to more realistic goals					X
Humiliating personal or social defeat			X		
Perceived burdensomeness	X				
Thwarted belongingness		X			
Perception of no future	X				
Total		X			

Although Kate attempted suicide and may do so again in the future, her current suicide risk is relatively low, primarily because she does not feel trapped and thinks she has options for the future. However, Kate only has options because her inheritance shelters her from the need to support herself. She has few friends, her goals of converting everybody into an environmentalist are unattainable, and her approach to life lacks maturity. There is a good chance that once she runs out of funds, she will become a burden on her parents, with very few options. At that point, her life may take the shape of the suicidal narrative, and her risk for imminent suicide will increase.

Test Case

Test Case 2

Zhang is a 20-year-old Chinese student at Queens College who was admitted to a local hospital after being admitted to the emergency room for a suicide attempt by methanol poisoning. He was dialyzed in the MICU and was transferred to an inpatient psychiatric unit. Zhang was treated with medications, and the following interview was conducted on the eve of discharge:

DR: How are you feeling today?
ZHANG: Much better, I feel much better, I am ready to go home.
DR: You were admitted after a suicide attempt; what has changed? What is different now, after 2 weeks in the hospital?

ZHANG: My thoughts are better, and I don't think the same thing all the time. I am not depressed anymore.

DR: What was making you depressed when you came in?

ZHANG: I had these bad thoughts I could not stop.

DR: What were you thinking?

ZHANG: I cannot talk about them, it is private.

DR: Were these thoughts getting in the way of what you were trying to achieve in life?

ZHANG: I could not study, the thoughts were just too upsetting . . . and they just keep coming over and over . . . like in a loop. My grades dropped.

DR: Did your parents get upset?

ZHANG: Yes, I am pre-med, and they sacrificed everything for me when they came from China. They want me to be a doctor and they always ask about grades. I had good grades in high school.

DR: Are you a perfectionist?

ZHANG: I have to be, I don't have a choice.

DR: If you are a perfectionist, you must be working very hard. Are you a hard worker?

ZHANG: I am a hard worker, but I should work harder.

DR: In a fair world, for the effort you put in, do you deserve to be happy?

ZHANG: Not now, but if get into medical school, I do.

DR: How important is a medical career for you?

ZHANG: Very important. It is everything for me. I always wanted to be a doctor for as long as I can remember.

DR: Why?

ZHANG: I don't know. It is something I always wanted to do.

DR: Do your parents want you to be a doctor?

ZHANG: Yes, they are very supportive.

DR: Can you find an alternative?

ZHANG: I never thought of that. Like what?

DR: Like other medical professions. Like a PA, a nurse, or even a social worker. Social workers help people.

ZHANG: I don't know. Maybe. Not sure (silence, staring into space).

DR: You seem hesitant, why?

ZHANG: I don't think my parents would like it. They will be disappointed . . .

DR: After you saw your grades and thought that you may not get into med school you almost killed yourself. Can you go on living without med school?

ZHANG: Now I can, I feel much better than before.

DR: What is the worst thing about possibly dropping out of the pre-med program?

ZHANG: I just would not know how to tell my parents, I would let them down. I would let the whole family down. I would die of embarrassment.

DR: You almost did, would it be humiliating?

ZHANG: Very humiliating.

DR: Is it possible that these are just your fears, but they would actually understand?

ZHANG: No, they would be very upset. They are very proud of me. They always talk about me being a doctor to the rest of the family. They say, they immigrated for me, so I could be happy. If I don't get in they would tell me they immigrated for nothing . . .

DR: Your parents come to visit you in the hospital every day. Do they know about your grades?

ZHANG: No, I didn't tell them. They always compare me to Xu—he always gets straight A's and he is at Cornell, and I am in Queens College, I didn't get in.

DR: You sound like this is a race, and you have been losing even before you got any grades.

ZHANG: I did, but I thought if I get straight A's I could make up for not getting into an Ivy League.

DR: Are your parents supporting you?

ZHANG: Yes, they pay my tuition and they give me money for books and lunch. I also live at home and they pay for my food.

DR: Do you feel like you are a burden to them?

ZHANG: I know I am—they always talk about money, and they are in their grocery store 16 hours a day.

DR: Are you close to your parents?

ZHANG: I guess so.

DR: I mean, do you do things together, do you tell them about what is happening in your life; do they tell you what is happening in theirs?

ZHANG: Aah. This is, like, American. We do things together—like sharing work around the house, but we don't talk very much.

DR: What about your friends? Are you the type of person who always has many friends or one or two best friends?

ZHANG: One or two best friends.

DR: When is the last time you talked to one of them?

ZHANG: I don't know. Maybe a month. I am too busy at school and helping my parents around the house.

DR: Did you tell them you are here?

ZHANG: No, I can't. I am too ashamed.

DR: You must feel very alone; how about here, in the hospital?

ZHANG: Not here—there are always nurses and staff.

DR: You said earlier: I just would not know how to tell my parents, I would let them down.

ZHANG: I would let the whole family down. I would die of embarrassment.

DR: Does this mean you have not told them?

ZHANG: Yes.

DR: Are you planning to tell them?

ZHANG: I don't have a choice.

DR: Are there any good choices in your situation?

ZHANG: No.

DR: Have you thought about your possible options, when you are discharged? I mean if you were no longer a pre-med?

ZHANG: No. I don't want to think about it.

DR: But you will have to, right?

ZHANG: (*Silence, looks down*)

DR: (*Constructing suicidal narrative*) From what you are saying, it seems that your family planned for you to be a doctor and that you have been working toward this goal almost since you remember yourself. But not all goals are attainable, and it seems that you have not thought of any alternatives, Plan B, so-to-speak. So if pre-med does not work out, there does not seem to be any good choices for you. Dropping out of the pre-med program may feel like a defeat in the battle for med school you have been fighting; and also very hard on your parents, who will feel like they have failed in the eyes of your community. You also said that you feel ashamed to be a burden to them, and it also seems that you are kind of by yourself. Does this sound right?

ZHANG: Yeah . . . (*silence*)

Suicide Narrative Risk Assessment Table

Component	Risk Level				
	Minimal	Low	Moderate	High	Severe
Unrealistic life goals					
Entitlement to happiness					
Failure to redirect to more realistic goals					
Humiliating personal or social defeat					
Perceived burdensomeness					
Thwarted belongingness					
Perception of no future					
Total					

Zhang's whole life may be seen as one evolving suicidal narrative. Perfectionist since childhood, devoted to the goal of becoming a doctor to uphold the honor of his family, he does not have the mental aptitude to achieve his goal, nor does he have the flexibility to disengage from it. Abandoning a medical career will signify disgrace for his family and ostracism in his community. He is not even in a position to seek support from his family or friends, which leaves him isolated, internally humiliated and defeated, without any chance for support from others. His failure is about to become public, and he is at a very high risk of ending his life, either to avoid the pain of admitting his failure to his parents or after facing their inevitable extreme disappointment.

6

Suicide Crisis Syndrome

CHRONIC LONG-TERM SUICIDE RISK VERSUS ACUTE SHORT-TERM SUICIDE RISK

Ninety percent of those who complete suicide carry a psychiatric diagnosis (Chang, Gitlin, & Patel, 2011), and 50–70% of them have seen a clinician during the month preceding their attempt (Chang et al., 2011). As discussed in previous chapters, most serious mood and psychotic disorders carry a 4–20% risk for completed suicide (Appleby et al., 2012; Van Os & Kapur, 2009). Because these are measures of actual deaths, this range may seem wide; however, the 4% completion rate signifies substantial risk. In their daily work, clinicians face the difficult task of identifying high-risk patients among those who already are at elevated long-term risk for suicide.

In Fawcett's et al.'s (1990) investigation of time-related predictors of suicide in affective disorders, the researchers discovered that suicides within 1 year versus 2–10 years after the study intake had different clinical features of affective disorders. Three well-known suicide risk factors—severe hopelessness, suicidal ideation, and past suicide attempt—were predictive of suicide in years 2–10 of the follow-up but not predictive suicide within 1 year. Surprisingly, of the six clinical factors predictive of a suicide within 1 year, only one—severe loss of interest or pleasure (anhedonia)—was directly related to the symptoms of major depression (Fawcett et al., 1990). Panic attacks, psychic anxiety, diminished concentration, global insomnia, and moderate alcohol abuse were found as anxiety related.

From Fawcett et al.'s (1990) study, it was evident that an acute suicidal state and the role of anxiety in short-term suicide risk needed to be researched further. However, due to logistical and ethical difficulties in conducting prospective research on suicidal patients, a well-validated and universally accepted tool for the assessment of risk for imminent suicide has yet to be created.

SUICIDE WARNING SIGNS

Until relatively recently, the concept of "warning signs," although popular in other medical fields, had not been applied to suicide or other psychiatric crises. In 2006, Rudd et al. proposed that warning signs of imminent suicide might exist that would enable individuals to intervene to prevent suicidal behavior.

Recently, researchers have identified many suicide-specific risk factors. These include emotional, cognitive, behavioral, social, and demographic characteristics, although suicide research often isolates these domains, studying them separately. For example, a Medline search using the key words suicide + [negative affect] revealed that those most studied were depression and anxiety, which are both very common in suicide attempters. Most depressed and anxious people are not acutely suicidal; thus, these emotions are of little use in assessing suicidal states and imminent suicide.

On the other hand, negative affects predictive of imminent suicide risk and panic were studied the least, including insomnia, hopelessness, despair, entrapment, and desperation. To date, this body of research has provided very limited data on which of these emotions are the warning signs, their comorbidity, and which clusters confer incremental and additive suicide risk.

For instance, although some of these emotions have been linked with suicidal ideation (Kessler, Borges, & Walters, 1999), they do not differentiate people with suicidal ideation who have or have not attempted suicide (Klonsky & May, 2014). Moreover, no direct correlation has been found between the number of possible risk factors or warning signs endorsed by a patient and his or her degree of short-term risk (Moscicki, 1997).

The expert consensus of the American Association of Suicidology has condensed the available information into a list of 10 suicide warning signs, including purposelessness, hopelessness, withdrawal, and anger/aggression (Rudd et al., 2006). However, despite the intellectual appeal of such a framework, there is no clear evidence of its clinical usefulness.

Given these limitations, Fowler (2012) proposed that clinicians should not simply rely on risk factors or warning signs independently when assessing safety but, rather, use them together in a collaborative, patient-specific manner to facilitate the understanding of the unique suicidal mental processes. More prospective studies are needed to establish suicide warning signs as predictors for future suicidal behavior.

Suicide Warning Signs

These signs may mean someone is at risk for suicide. Risk is greater if a behavior is new or has increased and if it seems related to a painful event, loss, or change.

- Talking about wanting to die or to kill oneself.
- Looking for a way to kill oneself, such as searching online or buying a gun.
- Increasing the use of alcohol or drugs.
- Acting anxious or agitated; behaving recklessly.
- Sleeping too little or too much.
- Withdrawing or feeling isolated.
- Talking about feeling hopeless or having no reason to live.
- Talking about feeling trapped or in unbearable pain.
- Talking about being a burden to others.
- Showing rage or talking about seeking revenge.
- Displaying extreme mood swings.

Source: Substance Abuse and Mental Health Services Administration: http://store.samhsa. gov/shin/content/SVP11-0126/SVP11-0126.pdf.

SUICIDE CRISIS SYNDROME

As described in Chapter 2, the concept of the suicide crisis originated in Baumeister's (1990) notion of suicide as an acute mental process and also in Shneidman's (1998) construct of "psychache" as a specific state of mind leading to suicide. The term *suicide crisis* was first used by Hendin, Maltsberger, and Szanto (2007), who described the construct of a "suicide crisis" as an acute, high-intensity, negative affect state that may serve as a trigger for a suicide attempt.

Building on the work of Hendin and others, we have proposed that the mental state of the suicide crisis constitutes a distinct syndrome, the suicide crisis syndrome (SCS), which we initially termed the "suicide trigger state." Our initial research showed that SCS had three components: frantic hopelessness, an affective state of entrapment, dread, and hopelessness; ruminative flooding, a cognitive state of incessant and overwhelming rumination and a sense of one's head bursting with uncontrollable thoughts; and panic-dissociation, a state of strange somatic experiences in the context of severe anxiety and panic (Yaseen et al., 2012; Yaseen et al., 2010, 2014).

Our latest research indicates that SCS may include several other affective symptoms. One of them is emotional pain, which is a mental state of persistent inner anguish similar to psychache (Orbach, 2003b). Another is fear of dying or, rather, the fear of sudden death (Galynker et al., 2016)—a panic-like feeling that may be related to the sense of losing control over one's planned death by suicide. Both factors are predictive of suicidal behavior with 4–8 weeks after hospital discharge. The third symptom is acute anhedonia, or the inability to experience pleasure or to imagine past or future activities as pleasurable (Yaseen et al., 2012).

Based on these findings and other published work related to the acute suicidal state, we have formulated the proposed *Diagnostic and Statistical Manual of Mental Disorders* (DSM; American Psychiatric Association, 2013) criteria for the suicide crisis syndrome, which are listed here. Included in the criteria are two items reflective of unstable undifferentiated negative affect, which includes anxiety, depression, hopelessness, and depression, and that are often observed proximally to suicidal behavior: Frantic anxiety and depressive turmoil.

Proposed DSM Criteria for the Suicide Crisis Syndrome

Part A: The core feature of the SCS is persistent and desperate feelings of entrapment, which is an urgency to escape or avoid an unbearable life situation when escape is perceived as impossible. Thus death appears as the only achievable solution to unbearable pain.

Often present are persistent thoughts of wanting to die or kill oneself as a way to escape an unacceptable life situation, which is perceived as simultaneously painfully intolerable and inescapable. (Typical situations include terminal illness, humiliating failure at work, or rejection by a romantic partner.)

Part B: In addition, SCS involves the following:
1. Affective disturbance, which amplifies the desperate need to escape
2. Loss of cognitive control, which amplifies the perception of the impossibility of escape
3. Hyperarousal, which fuels action to achieve the escape through suicide

At least one symptom from the following three categories must be present simultaneously:

1. Affective disturbance as manifested by the following:
   a. Emotional pain distinct from anxiety and depression
   b. Rapid changes in emotions or extreme mood swings
   c. Extreme anxiety or panic with possible dissociative symptoms and sensory disturbances
   d. Acute anhedonia (inability to experience, remember, or imagine experiencing things as enjoyable)
2. Loss of cognitive control as manifested by the following:
   a. Intense and persistent ruminations about one's own distress and the life events that brought it on
   b. Inability to deviate from a repetitive negative pattern of thought (cognitive rigidity)
   c. Repeated unsuccessful attempts to suppress negative or disturbing thoughts
   d. An experience of pain or pressure in the head from loss of control of one's negative thoughts impairing the ability to process information or make a decision (ruminative flooding)
3. Disturbance in arousal as manifested by the following:
   a. Agitation—a state of extreme arousal, physical restlessness, hypervigilance, or of heightened irritability
   b. Global insomnia

The remainder of this chapter describes the SCS symptoms in detail, in the order they are listed in the proposed DSM criteria. The next section is devoted to suicidal ideation and intent, followed by entrapment, affective disturbance, loss of cognitive control, and abnormal arousal.

SUICIDAL IDEATION AND INTENT

Suicide cannot occur without a wish to die and a suicidal act, which could be either conscious or unconscious. A self-inflicted shooting death with a suicide note is an example of a conscious and planned suicide, whereas deaths by unintentional overdose or due to reckless driving while intoxicated could result from an unconscious wish to die without a plan. Thus, questions about suicidal ideation and intent have always been central to any suicide risk assessment.

Accordingly, Part A of the suicide crisis syndrome identifies persistent suicidal thoughts as the central feature of the suicide crisis syndrome as follows:

> Persistent thoughts of wanting to die or kill oneself as a way to escape an unacceptable life situation, which is perceived as simultaneously painfully intolerable and inescapable. (Typical situations include a loss or impending loss of self, status, or attachment, such as terminal illness, humiliating failure at work, or rejection by a romantic partner, respectively.)

Although questioning a patient about his or her suicidal ideation and intent is an essential part of the assessment, the answers may not be as indicative of the short-term risk as clinicians would like them to be.

Suicidal Ideation

Suicidal ideation refers to thoughts about suicide and encompasses a wide range of cognitions, from fleeting and infrequent to persistent and unrelenting. *Suicide intent*, which refers to suicidal ideation that includes the purposeful plan to act, implies a more serious suicide risk and is considered separately. Suicidal ideation can vary in severity from vague ideas with no plan to a detailed plan. Suicidal ideation also ranges greatly in intensity from infrequent thoughts that are noted with faint curiosity and leave no lasting impact to thoughts that can be easily suppressed and thoughts that are constant and uncontrollable.

Although seemingly essential for any suicidal act, self-reported suicidal ideation (as elicited in the assessment) contributes to near-term suicide risk modestly at best. In teenagers and young adults (aged 15–24 years), suicidal ideation severity and intensity (i.e., frequency and controllability) are significant independent predictors of future suicide attempts over a period of 9 months, above and beyond the predictive power of past suicide attempts. However, this increase in suicide risk is minor in comparison to the sixfold increase in suicide risk due to history of suicide attempt(s). Moreover, the duration of suicidal thoughts is associated with higher risk only in males (Horwitz, Czyz, & King, 2015).

Self-reported suicidal ideation was even less useful in predicting imminent suicidal behavior in suicidal callers to crisis hotlines. In this setting, self-reported suicidal ideation and plans are likely very reliable, but disclosure of suicidal ideation did not predict either suicidal ideation or suicide attempt(s) in the following 2–8 weeks (Witte, Gordon, Smith, & Van Orden, 2012).

When suicidal ideation is measured using structured psychometric scales rather than clinical interviews, its value as a predictive tool for future ideation or behavior is only marginally better. The Scale for Suicidal Ideation (SSI), Hamilton Depression Scale (HAM-D) item 3, Beck Depression Inventory item 9, and simple questioning on whether patients had seriously considered suicide all have different (poor) predictive value for suicidal ideation and attempts during a 6-month follow-up period. In structured interviews, an SSI score >8 seems to be best at predicting future suicide attempt over a period of 6 months, with a predictive value of 32% (Valtonen et al., 2009).

Despite these findings, suicidal ideation is one of the most frequent warning signs of suicide and must be assessed. However, it must be concluded that this cornerstone of suicide risk assessment is not as useful in predicting imminent suicidal behavior as clinicians we like to believe, and it should not be relied on when making clinical decisions.

Suicide Intent and Plan

The term *suicide intent* refers to a conscious desire to end one's life and, importantly, a resolve to act. The most prominent instrument for the assessment of the intensity and seriousness of suicide intent is the Suicide Intent Scale (SIS) (Beck, Schuyler, & Herman, 1974). The SIS consists of an objective component based on history (isolation, precautions against discovery, suicide note, and final preparations before death) and a subjective component based on self-report. Because patients with the most severe suicide intent usually go on to complete suicide, the SIS was designed for retrospective use immediately following a suicide attempt.

Generally, patients who make medically serious suicide attempts have higher total SIS scores. The objective component of the SIS is highly correlated with the lethality of the most recent suicide attempt, as well as with communication difficulties in recent suicide attempters. The subjective component is associated with various mental pain variables, and this component is related to the intensity of SCS. Suicide attempters with intense mental pain and communication difficulties have higher scores on the objective component of the scale (Horesh, Levi, & Apter, 2012).

The same strong relationship between the lethality of the attempt and the degree of suicide intent holds true in clinical assessments of intent and for many cultures with diverse suicide statistics. On the other hand, the association between the degree of suicide intent and the degree of lethality of the attempt is dependent on the accuracy of expectations about the likelihood of dying as a result of the attempt: Higher levels of suicide intent were associated with more lethal attempts, but only for individuals who had more accurate expectations about the likelihood of dying from their attempts (Brown, Henriques, Sosdjian, & Beck, 2004).

However, although the association between the suicidal intent and potential lethality of past suicide attempts appears strong, repetition of suicide attempts in the future is not related to the seriousness of the intent of the original episodes. Thus, the relationship of lethality and suicidal intent to further suicidal behavior does not appear to be straightforward (Haw, Hawton, Houston, & Townsend, 2003), and suicide intent, just like suicidal ideation, is not a reliable predictor of suicidal behavior in the near future.

The following are case examples of patient interviews assessing suicidal ideation and intent.

Case 41

Alina is a 17-year-old female with schizoaffective disorder, incorrectly diagnosed with bipolar disorder during her first manic episode. Alina had substantial negative symptoms, interpersonal deficits, was socially isolated, lacked initiative, and also admitted to having hallucinations since age 11 years. In high school, she had several psychotic episodes requiring hospitalization, which prevented her from graduating from high school with her classmates and disrupted her social life.

As a result, as a high school senior, Alina was a year behind and was trying to get her GED through an individualized tutoring program. She always appeared unhappy but denied being depressed. When asked about her state of mind, she would say that she was always thinking painful thoughts about how she was lazy and not trying hard enough to be successful.

One day, after returning from an Easter visit with her cousins, she came to her therapist's office looking particularly unhappy. Alina's mother texted the therapist that Alina had told her that she did not want to live anymore.

Alina's office interview with her therapist

Suicidal ideation

DR: Alina, your mother texted me that you told her you did not want to live anymore. Was she telling the truth?

ALINA: Yes

DR: What's going on?

ALINA: I am just in so much pain, it's not worth it.

DR: Are you thinking about suicide?

ALINA: I just want to be gone. I don't want to suffer.

DR: And how long have you been having these thoughts? Days, weeks?

ALINA: All week.

DR: Are you having these thoughts now?

ALINA: Not now.

DR: These thoughts about not wanting to live, are they with you all the time?

ALINA: Almost.

Suicide intent and plan

DR: Have you thought about how you would kill yourself?

ALINA: Yes. I would take my mother's pills. She has like 10 bottles in her medicine cabinet.

DR: And what would happen if you take them?

ALINA: I would die and won't feel anything anymore. Life just is too painful.

DR: What prevents you from taking these pills tonight?

ALINA: She is with me all the time. And it would upset her. A lot.

DR: Can you picture yourself actually taking the pills?

ALINA: I can, but I don't think I would do it. I am too scared.

DR: What would it take for you to actually take the pills?

ALINA: To know that nobody cares.

DR: Did you pick the pill bottle you will use?

ALINA: I will use her sleeping pills.

DR: Did you hold the bottle in your hands?

ALINA: Yes.

DR: Did you open it?

ALINA: No.

The therapist is able to elicit Alina's persistent suicidal ideation. Moreover, she acknowledges having conditional suicide intent with a specific plan, preparatory actions for suicide, and even practicing. Alina's description of her intent and plan is indicative of a high short-term risk. She has specific intent to end her life and has decided on a method. The self-report of suicidal ideation by itself is not predictive of short-term risk, but in Alina's case, it is very congruent with her intent and plan, and it makes her admission of suicidality more credible.

Case 42

Richard is a 73-year-old retired dentist with a history of bipolar disorder and agoraphobia. He was depressed for several months as a freshman in college and had difficulty leaving his room and attending classes. He had prolonged undiagnosed hypomania through dental school and residency, followed by a second episode of depression after several years in practice. He was hospitalized, treated with electroconvulsive therapy (ECT), and after discharge worked in a city hospital. He married a nurse, and they had two children. The couple divorced when he was 60 years old, and he married his 35-year-old dental hygienist.

When Richard was 65 years old, he was caught drinking alcohol at work, and the ensuing investigation uncovered that he was abusing sedatives. He was hospitalized with psychotic depression and was treated with ECT. At the time of the suicide risk assessment, he was in individual treatment for residual depression and severe agoraphobia. He and his wife were also in couples therapy because his symptoms were interfering with their social life. At the time of the interview, he was taking two antidepressants, a stimulant, and a low-dose antipsychotic. Richard's daughter called his psychiatrist after Richard stated to her about his wife that he was tired of "all her crap." Richard's daughter also alerted the psychiatrist that Richard was very angry at his wife for flirting with younger men.

Richard's office interview with his psychiatrist
    Suicidal ideation
        DR: Hello Richard, how are you feeling?
        RICHARD: Annoyed.
        DR: Annoyed at what?
        RICHARD: My wife is driving me crazy. She just keeps coming on to men right in front of me.
        DR: What are you going to do?
        RICHARD: I don't know, kill myself!
        DR: Have you been thinking about suicide?
        RICHARD: Sometimes.
        DR: How frequently?
        RICHARD: Not once a day but not once in a blue moon either. Maybe once a week.
        DR: And what exactly do you think?
        RICHARD: That I want to kill this flirt, my wife that is. And since I don't want to spend the rest of my life in jail, I would rather shoot myself.
        DR: How persistent are these thoughts? Do they last seconds, minutes, days?
        RICHARD: Not long. Minutes.
        DR: Is it hard to suppress these thoughts? Does it require effort, or do they just go away?
        RICHARD: They go away. Unless she is flirting right in front of me. Then it's pretty hard.
        DR: Do you have a gun at home?
        RICHARD: Somewhere. Not sure.

DR: Do you have bullets at home?

RICHARD: Somewhere, not sure. But, doc, don't worry, these are just thoughts.

DR: When was the last time that you held your gun?

RICHARD: I don't remember. Two years ago, maybe.

DR: And what did you do with it?

RICHARD: I took it out of the box and put it back in.

DR: Where was it?

RICHARD: In the attic.

DR: Were you looking for it?

RICHARD: No I was just organizing stuff.

DR: Was the gun loaded?

RICHARD: No.

DR: Did you load it?

RICHARD: No.

DR: Did you look for the bullets?

RICHARD: No.

DR: Did you aim the gun at yourself?

RICHARD: No.

DR: Did you aim it at anything?

RICHARD: No, I just looked at it and put it back.

DR: Were you thinking of shooting yourself at the time?

RICHARD: No.

DR: Where you thinking of shooting your wife?

RICHARD: No.

Richard's suicidal ideation is less severe and persistent than that of Alina, and by his description, holding the gun in his hand may not be considered preparatory suicidal behavior. However, although flippant and impulsive, his description of losing control and shooting himself if his wife flirts too much is a conditional suicide plan, which carries with it a homicide or double homicide potential. This interview warrants an immediate intervention and removal of the firearm from the house.

ENTRAPMENT

Part A of the proposed DSM criteria for SCS identifies entrapment as the central feature of the acute suicidal state:

> The core feature of SCS is thus persistent and desperate feelings of entrapment, which is an urgency to escape or avoid an unbearable life situation when escape is perceived as impossible. Thus, death appears as the only achievable solution to unbearable pain.

As discussed in Chapter 1, entrapment has been proposed as a central psycho-logical element of several models of suicidal behavior, notably the arrested flight/ cry of pain model by Williams and Pollock, as well as O'Connor's integrated motivational–volitional theory (O'Connor, 2011; Williams, 1997). The narrative crisis model separates the cognitive perception of no exit/future from the emotional state of entrapment. The cognitive perception of no future constitutes the last phase of the suicidal narrative, whereas the affective state of entrapment is the key element of the suicide crisis and of SCS.

Frantic hopelessness is the SCS factor similar to or identical to entrapment, as identified in our early studies of short-term suicide risk using the Suicide Trigger Scale (STS-3) (Yaseen et al., 2012; Yaseen et al., 2010, 2014, 2016). Because in our subsequent studies it became clear that entrapment and frantic hopelessness are essentially the same symptom (Tucker, O'Connor, & Wingate, 2016), in 2015 we started using the more accepted term, "entrapment," for both constructs.

Desperation is another symptom that suicidal individuals often feel prior to attempting suicide. Desperation is a state of mental anguish so intense that it requires immediate relief, and any relief in the future appears irrelevant. In most cases, an unbearable life situation (entrapment) is likely to cause mental anguish (desperation), and whether the two belong to the same syndrome remains an open question for future research.

Entrapment

The suicide crisis syndrome is an acute, panic-like state that can culminate in a suicide attempt (Fawcett et al., 1990; Hendin et al., 2007), sometimes over a time period as short as 10 minutes (Deisenhammer et al., 2009). In the narrative crisis model, entrapment serves as the main affective component of SCS, more dominant than emotional pain, panic–dissociation, and fear of dying (Katz, Yaseen, Mojtabai, Cohen, & Galynker, 2011; Yaseen et al., 2012; Yaseen et al., 2010, 2014).

Entrapment as a psychological symptom is defined as urgency to escape or avoid an unbearable life situation when escape is perceived as impossible. The SCS entrapment factor is a complex mixture of feelings of entrapment, desperation, hopelessness, the need for escape, and loss of control to change the situation, which is associated with depression and anxiety but differs from both by its sense of urgency.

Although a sense of entrapment may be associated with either objective or subjective stressful life events or circumstances (Brown, Harris, & Hepworth, 1995), Gilbert and Allan (1998) suggested that entrapment could be divided into two subclasses: (1) external entrapment relating to external events or circumstances and (2) internal entrapment relating to internal thoughts, feelings, and perception. Thus, individual experiences of entrapment can emerge from a wide range of external hardships (Gilbert & Gilbert, 2003; Gilbert, Gilbert, & Irons, 2004; Williams, 1997), and clinical assessment of entrapment should highlight how stressful life events are viewed (Lazarus & Folkman, 1984).

For example, perceptions of defeat have been found to predict suicidality even when controlling for depressive symptoms (Taylor, Gooding, Wood, & Tarrier, 2011), whereas perceptions of entrapment have been found to predict anxiety when controlling for depressive and psychotic symptoms (Birchwood et al., 2007). Moreover, there was a stronger relationship between entrapment and suicidality, relative to the relationship between defeat and suicidality, and a stronger relationship between defeat and depression compared to the relationship between entrapment and depression (Siddaway, Taylor, Wood, & Schulz, 2015).

In agreement with these and other findings in cross-sectional and retrospective studies, our work has shown that, prospectively, among the SCS factors, entrapment has the strongest association with short-term suicidal behavior, and the predictive validity of the entrapment subscale of the SCI for post-discharge suicidal behavior in high-risk psychiatric inpatients (odds ratio [OR] = 10) is just short of that of the full scale (OR = 13). Moreover, in acutely suicidal inpatients, entrapment fully mediates the relationship between the ruminative flooding, panic–dissociation, and fear of dying and suicidal ideation, suggesting that it is related to suicide more intimately than the other SCS factors. In contrast, entrapment is only a partial mediator of the relationship between emotional pain and suicidal ideation, suggesting that entrapment and emotional pain may be closely related.

Desperation

In a suicidal crisis, the mental processes leading from the states of emotional pain and entrapment to suicide may be mediated in part by desperation. Hendin et al. (2007) define desperation as a state of anguish accompanied by the need for relief so urgent that any wait becomes unacceptable. The need for relief is so acute that the urge to relieve the pain becomes "the urge to end it all"—that is, the urge to end one's life by suicide. For a person in a state of desperation, the future possibility of relief from the current pain is so remote that it becomes irrelevant.

In the suicidal crisis, desperation, like entrapment, is intertwined with the last phase of the suicidal narrative: the perception of no future. The cognitive realization of being in a life situation with no good options does not automatically lead to desperation. However, such perception is likely to worsen the emotional pain with concomitant frantic anxiety and depressive turmoil—that is, to bring on the suicidal crisis and, with it, the dreadful urge to use suicide as the only perceived means to escape the dead end.

Evidence that desperation is a critical component of the mental state preceding imminent suicide derives primarily from interviews of clinicians with patients who died by suicide while in psychiatric treatment. For example, the following is an illustrative case of a 53-year-old clergyman with bipolar disorder (Hendin et al., 2007):

> This patient's erratic behavior had caused him to be removed from his parish which humiliated and enraged him. Despite receiving treatment, which included hospitalization, his bipolar illness was not well controlled. His temper tantrums aimed at his wife and child and his irresponsible handling of money threatened his marriage. Feeling that his life was falling apart, his anguish became intense and intolerable. Emotionally out of control, the patient appeared to have killed himself impulsively when he encountered frustration in getting started in a day treatment program.

As can be seen from the description, the case described a man, demographically in a cohort with the highest suicide risk, suffering public humiliation, which led to a trap-like life situation with no good options. As a result, he fell into a state of emotional instability, experienced as emotional disintegration, characteristic of depressive turmoil (discussed later). His emotional instability was worsened by his bipolar disorder. The patient killed himself impulsively after reaching a state of desperation when his anguished turmoil became intolerable. The final blow was when, in his mind, his last option for improvement, the day treatment program, failed him.

Note that desperation is often present in the context of hopelessness. However, desperation is sometimes seen where hopelessness is not, and when they do coexist, hopelessness is long-standing, whereas desperation is more acute. The same is true about the relationship between desperation and almost any other symptom, except acute physical pain. For patients who feel intensely desperate, the issue is not whether and when they would feel better but, rather, that they can no longer tolerate their present state.

The intense and brief states of desperation and urge to escape leading to suicide may leave no opportunity to evaluate the suicidal person and intervene. However, levels of desperation fluctuate, and of course not every bout of desperation leads to suicide. On the other hand, the mere fact that a person is desperate dramatically increases his or her risk of imminent suicide. Thus, every imminent suicide risk assessment must probe the degree of the patient's desperation.

Case 41—Continued

Entrapment

> DR: When you are having these thoughts that nobody cares or that you don't want to be here, do you feel trapped?
>
> ALINA: Last weekend I did.
>
> DR: Or putting it differently, do you feel trapped by the pain?
>
> ALINA: Yes! Often . . .
>
> DR: Was this when you were with your cousins? And now?
>
> ALINA: With them, yes. Now, not as much.
>
> DR: How bad is the feeling of being trapped? Do you see any good options in your situation?
>
> ALINA: Not really . . .
>
> DR: If you think really hard . . . maybe medications?
>
> ALINA: I have been sick for so long. Nothing seems to be working.
>
> DR: I see. . . . I want to know more about how you felt last weekend when you were visiting your cousins. Did you feel so overwhelmed that you were losing control of your feelings?
>
> ALINA: Yes, I felt so bad. . . . I don't want to remember how bad I felt, because I do not want to feel like that again.
>
> DR: Does this feeling make you restless?
>
> ALINA: Yeah . . . moving around helps. Last weekend I put my headphones on and went for a walk.

DR: Does listening to music make you feel better?

ALINA: Yes. And TV.

Desperation

DR: How long can you tolerate being this upset?

ALINA: I do not know. Last weekend I was having suicidal thoughts.

DR: And now?

ALINA: Now not as much as last weekend but still pretty bad.

DR: Tell me about the last weekend. How painful was it?

ALINA: As painful as it gets. Somehow I managed to go to sleep and woke up feeling better. We need to do something, because if I feel like that again, I am not sure I will make it.

DR: What would you do?

ALINA: I don't know. I told you, I thought of taking pills. There are a lot of pills in the house. I need to feel better. I can't have another weekend like that.

DR: Medications should help, if not now, in the future.

ALINA: I can't wait for the future.

Alina's answers show that she feels both trapped in her current life situation and desperate to escape it. She sees no good options or treatments for her illness, which makes her feel anguished, isolated, and hopeless for the future. She has already rehearsed her suicidal actions, and her short-term risk is high.

Case 42–Continued

Entrapment

DR: When you think about your situation—your wife's flirting, her out-of-control spending, your limited funds, your fixed income—do you feel trapped?

RICHARD: I told you I do—I can't talk to her about the money and she just keeps buying designer outfits. I can't talk to her about her flirting either.

DR: What if you just don't give her the money?

RICHARD: Then she will leave, and spend and flirt to her heart's desire. . . . And how am I going to be alone at 72 with agoraphobia? I can't leave the house by myself.

DR: Can you think of any good solutions to the problem?

RICHARD: I wish I could work, but I have been retired for a while. I can't start over.

DR: What about working for somebody else? Less headache managing the office . . .

RICHARD: I was never good with the bosses.

DR: What about talking to her about the finances, and how she makes you feel when she flirts?

RICHARD: Do you think I have not tried? I only feel worse afterwards.

Desperation

DR: How long can you tolerate this mental state that you are in?

RICHARD: It has been 3 years, and I will soon be at the end of my rope.

DR: How soon?

RICHARD: I don't know . . . 6 months maybe.

DR: Six months is good. I will take 6 months. Good couples' therapists can accomplish a lot in that time.

RICHARD: I hope so.

DR: Do you have hope that the pain will soon get better?

RICHARD: It has to, because if it does not somebody will get hurt.

DR: Like who?

RICHARD: I do not know . . .

DR: The two of you are in therapy now, it may still help. You may just need to wait a little bit.

RICHARD: I am trying . . . I like Dr. K. She is good.

Although the causes of Richard's sense of entrapment are different from those of Alina (romantic relationship conflict vs. mental illness), their feelings of entrapment are similar in intensity. Neither Alina nor Richard sees any good options in their respective life situations. In contrast to Alina, however, Richard is not desperate, and he can tolerate his pain a little longer before, in his estimate, he may lose control and act out dangerously using the gun he has at home. This lack of desperation may give the interviewing doctor a feeling of confidence that Richard's life and that of his wife are not in imminent danger and that he has several weeks to remove the weapon and initiate couples' therapy.

AFFECTIVE DISTURBANCE

Individuals in a suicidal crisis frequently experience extreme affective disturbance, which is a complex state of fluctuating negative affect. Four of the five SCS factors describe distinct aspects of aversive affect. They are entrapment, emotional pain, panic–dissociation, and fear of dying (the fifth, ruminative flooding, represents loss of cognitive control) (Yaseen et al., 2012; Yaseen et al., 2010, 2014, 2016). These symptoms can be present alone, in combination with each other, or simultaneously with other related symptoms, primarily anhedonia, extreme anxiety, or depressive turmoil (Fawcett, 1988).

Of these, entrapment represents the most dominant feature of the suicidal affective state. The other aspects of the aversive negative affect constitute the first item of Part B of the proposed DSM criteria for SCS, affective disturbance. When suicidal individuals develop this highly aversive negative affect, it amplifies their desperate need to escape what has become an unbearable life situation.

Part B divides affective disturbance into four categories, which include all of the previously discussed negative affects, and combines all anxiety symptoms into one category:

- Emotional pain distinct from anxiety and depression (i.e., emotional pain)
- Rapid changes in emotions or extreme mood swings (i.e., depressive turmoil)

- Extreme anxiety or panic with possible dissociative symptoms and sensory disturbances (i.e., all anxiety-related symptoms, such as frantic anxiety, panic–dissociation, and fear of dying)
- Acute anhedonia—inability to experience, remember, or imagine experiencing things as enjoyable (i.e., acute anhedonia)

In the following discussion, however, for the sake of conceptual clarity and completeness, frantic anxiety, panic–dissociation, and depressive turmoil are discussed separately. The same structure is retained in the case interviews.

Emotional Pain

Emotional pain (also called "mental pain" and "psychological pain") is a mixture of poorly differentiated but intense negative emotions such as guilt, shame, hopelessness, disgrace, and rage. It arises when the essential needs to love, have control, protect one's self-image, void shame, guilt, and humiliation, and feel secure are frustrated (Williams, Barnhofer, Crane, & Beck, 2005). Emotional pain is similar to entrapment and is strongly correlated with, but distinct from, anxiety and depression. It can be so intense that the individual seeks to escape by committing suicide (Orbach, 2003b; Shneidman, 1993). Compared to entrapment, emotional pain may lack desperation due to the realization that all escape routes are blocked. Accordingly, although emotional pain and entrapment have equally immediate relationships to suicidal ideation, in a multivariate analysis, entrapment was a stronger predictor of short-term suicidal behavior compared to emotional pain (Galynker et al., 2016).

An evaluation of emotional pain is a good starting point for the SCS part of the suicide risk assessment.

Depressive Turmoil

The term *depressive turmoil* describes a state of affective instability with rapid changes in negative moods, primarily depression and anxiety. Fawcett (1988, p. 7) defined depressive turmoil as "rapid switching of mood from anxiety to depression to anger, and accompanied by agitation and perturbation." It is a state of affective instability with rapid changes in negative moods distinguishable from anxiety and depression by psychomotor agitation and anger, which are reflective of entrapment. Depressive turmoil is common in recently discharged depressed psychiatric inpatients and has been shown to be associated with increased risk of suicide (Angst, Angst, & Stassen, 1999).

Depressive turmoil resembles several other clinical entities, particularly those with the suicide warning sign of "extreme mood swings." In fact, the intense turmoil of mixed and undifferentiated emotions that a suicidal person experiences may be better described as "anguished turmoil."

Because of its strong anxiety and agitation component, depressive turmoil also resembles depressive mixed states (Benazzi & Akiskal, 2001; Dilsaver, Benazzi, Akiskal, & Akiskal, 2007). A depressed mixed state is observed predominantly in patients with bipolar depression, particularly those with bipolar II disorder (Akiskal & Benazzi, 2005; Takeshima & Oka, 2013), and it may be one of the strongest risk factors for suicidality (Valtonen, Suominen, & Haukka, 2008).

Finally, depressive turmoil has many common features with activation syndrome (AS), which at times emerges during antidepressant therapy. As described in Chapter 4, AS consists of anxiety, agitation, panic attack, insomnia, irritability, hostility, aggressiveness, impulsivity, akathisia (psychomotor restlessness), and hypomania/mania. AS is similar to bipolar mixed states, but the fluctuating AS symptoms of agitation, insomnia, and hostility overlap with the affective disturbance and the depressive turmoil in SCS.

Extreme (Frantic) Anxiety

Frantic anxiety is a particularly severe form of anxiety frequently elicited in interviews with acutely suicidal individuals. It is characterized by psychic and somatic symptoms and restlessness. The psychic anxiety is characterized by worries, anticipation and expectation of the worst, irritability, and fears of what "the worst" may bring. Patients also complain of a state of inner restlessness, trembling, inability to relax, and being easily startled and overreactive. Anxious fears are diffuse and free-floating, and they are directed at whatever a person is encountering at any time in his or her daily life: being alone or being in crowds, strangers, animals, traffic, heights, trains, and so on. At the time of the suicidal crisis, the anxiety can be so severe that most or all of the previously mentioned symptoms are experienced simultaneously and coalesce into a coherent, intense, and frantic dysphoric state.

Depending on their culture, history, and suicidal narrative, suicidal patients may label frantic anxiety differently. However, all or nearly all will identify with the sense of feeling so vulnerable that it is as if they "have no skin." Together with "franticness," as discussed later, the raw sensitivity of "having no skin" differentiates the suicidal anxiety from situational anxiety and that of generalized anxiety disorder (GAD). In the words of eminent suicide expert Jan Fawcett, "There is anxiety and then there is suicidal anxiety; if you measure anxiety level on a 1 to 5 scale, the intensity of the suicidal anxiety is at 11."

A person in a suicidal crisis who has "no skin" feels defenseless before the outside world, where anything or anybody around them can hurt them unpredictably. Even the most insignificant events, such as a mother changing the TV channel or a coworker canceling a business lunch, are perceived as hurtful. Being alone is perceived as abandonment, and being in crowds is experienced as surveillance and judgment for an irreparable flaw. A person with "no skin" knows on some level that his or her fears and concerns are blown out of proportion, and yet the person's normal defenses against such perceived insults are down.

Many formerly suicidal patients with GAD or major depressive disorder (MDD) describe the experience of responding to antidepressant treatment as "growing a thicker skin." They often state that their life has not changed very much—the work is still difficult, the boss still shows no appreciation, the wife/husband is still not supportive, and yet, all the events that did not let them sleep at night do not bother them as much or not at all. Although treatment of suicidality is beyond the scope of this guide, the "skin thickness" could be a useful gauge to use to measure for the ongoing acuity of the suicidal crisis.

The "franticness" associated with SCS is the mental equivalent of severe physical agitation and gives the mind its feverish hectic quality. Suicidal anxiety can be so intense and frenzied that it may reach the disorganized and undifferentiated state, in which it fuses with other negative affects described in this section—anhedonia, emotional pain, and depressive turmoil—and reaches the level of desperation, when the promise of relief even in the near future becomes irrelevant because the pain is too great to bear even for another second.

Some well-known anxiety rating scales used in research, such as the Hamilton Rating Scale for Anxiety (HAM-A), include these less specific items, which are present dimensionally in a broad range of psychiatric disorders. For the clinical purpose of imminent suicide risk assessment, it is more practical to keep a categorical approach and, when assessing anxiety, to focus on the core symptoms specific to anxiety, assessing the rest with the diagnoses or constructs to which they are most directly related.

Most tellingly, in a retrospective study of 100 inpatient suicide attempts, 90% of imminent attempters reported high anxiety compared to 85% who reported symptoms of depression (O'Connor et al., 2013). Several other observational studies have reached similar conclusions, which were also supported by many epidemiological studies. Finally, recent prospective studies of acute suicidal states show that increased anxiety predicts suicidal behavior in the 2 months following the assessment (Kanwar et al., 2013; Lim, Ko, Shin, Shin, & Oh, 2015; Nam, Kim, & Roh, 2016; Nock et al., 2014; Rappaport, Moskowitz, Galynker, & Yaseen, 2014).

Fear of Dying

Fear of dying describes one of the morbid cognitions during panic. It has been shown to mediate the transition from latent to active suicidal ideation and to suicide attempt in some depressed subjects (Katz et al., 2011; Siddaway et al., 2015; Yaseen et al., 2012). Among subjects with panic attacks, specifically experiencing fear of dying during a panic attack increases the odds of subsequent suicide attempt sevenfold, even after controlling for comorbid disorders, demographic factors, and other panic symptoms (Yaseen et al., 2013).

Although fear of dying has been repeatedly linked to suicide risk (Lester, 1967; Yaseen et al., 2013), it remains to be explained why fear of dying and not fear of losing one's mind, or "going crazy," predicts future attempt. One possible explanation for this seemingly paradoxical association is that in our minds, both fear of death and suicidal ideation/suicide attempt exist in the conscious realm of "death by distress." As described in Chapter 1, in depressed patients, conditions of psychosocial stress elicit a separation distress response in the form of panic, which is amplified through a positive feedback model (see Figure 1.2). In patients with suicidal ideation, in which panic symptoms do not trigger any death-related thoughts, the "death by distress" notion remains compartmentalized in the subconscious and panic cannot trigger a transition from suicidal ideation or suicide attempt. In contrast, in patients for whom panic attacks occur with fears of death, "death by distress" enters the conscious realm and may trigger suicidal behaviors.

This interpretation is consistent with Rudd's psychodynamic model of depression in that panic attacks with fear of dying and depression are connected by a negative view of the self. During a panic attack with fear of dying, negative cognitions about the self result in the desire to self-impose punishment, which feeds the positive feedback cycle of the panic attack. Thus, thoughts of death in depression-associated panic attacks would emerge from the negative self-view associated with depression, resulting in a simultaneous fear of fatal punishment ("I am doomed") and belief in its deservedness ("I don't deserve to live").

Panic–Dissociation

The panic–dissociation factor describes an intense anxiety state of altered sensorium and de-realization associated with panic. Unlike the head pressure experienced during ruminative flooding, panic–dissociation involves the somatic experience of unfamiliar sensations felt all over the body, especially involving the skin. Having panic–dissociation as part of SCS is consistent with a number of reports that have linked increased risk for suicide with affectively intense panic attacks (Katz et al., 2011; Yaseen et al., 2013).

Thus, panic–dissociation is characterized by the experience of somatic symptoms commonly associated with a panic-like dissociative state. The inclusion of panic–dissociation in SCS is supported by previous reports linking a specific subset of panic attacks with increased suicide risk (Ozturk & Sar, 2008; Yaseen et al., 2012).

Panic attacks are a heterogeneous syndrome comprising affective symptoms—primarily fear, cognitive symptoms congruent to fear, and symptoms of autonomic nervous system activation such as sweating and changes in heart rate (Fowles, 2007). Comorbid panic attacks aggravate the course of any psychiatric disorder, from severe and debilitating schizophrenia to relatively mild conditions such as social phobia. Panic attacks are significantly more frequent in those who go on to die by suicide than in those who do not (Fawcett et al., 1990). This is particularly true for patients with panic attacks and MDD, who are 50% more likely to have suicidal ideation and two times more likely to have attempted suicide than patients with MDD without panic attacks (Katz et al., 2011). Moreover, depressed patients with suicidal ideation and panic attacks are two times more likely to attempt suicide.

Of note, in a prospective study, some panic symptoms, most notably catastrophic cognitions (fear of dying and fear of "losing control" or "going insane"), were more strongly and specifically associated with suicide attempt, whereas others were more related to suicidal ideation (Yaseen, Chartrand et al., 2013). Another study, however, indicated that the somatic symptoms of tingling, hot flushes or chills, and nausea were associated with past suicidal behavior, whereas dissociation was linked to suicidal ideation (Rappaport et al., 2014).

The SCI data reliably indicate that somatic, panic-like symptoms predict future suicidal behavior. The most prominent panic and dissociative symptom predictors are fears of being physically ill or damaged, sweating, nausea, problems breathing, and rapid heartbeat. Other strong predictors are strange sensations in the body or on the skin and a perception that the body may be changing. Finally, in depressed individuals, a dissociative symptom that the world feels different or unreal also increases short-term risk for suicide (Yaseen et al., 2012; Yaseen et al., 2014).

Acute Anhedonia

Anhedonia is defined as the inability to experience joy from activities that are normally found pleasurable, and it has long been considered primarily as one of the symptoms of major depression. Only relatively recently was anhedonia recognized as a transdiagnostic syndrome, which is present in many disorders and is subserved by dopaminergic reward circuitry involving the nucleus accumbens (Wise, 1980). The severity of anhedonia appears to be associated with a deficit of activity of the ventral striatum (which includes the nucleus accumbens) and an excess of activity of the ventral region of the prefrontal cortex (including the ventromedial prefrontal cortex and the orbitofrontal cortex), with dopamine playing a pivotal, but not exclusive, role. The imbalance in neuronal activity is present in all major psychiatric disorders: schizophrenia, bipolar disorder, MDD, and borderline personality disorder (BPD). All carry a high risk for suicide, estimated to be 4–15% (Van Os & Kapur, 2009).

In schizophrenia, until recently anhedonia had been subsumed by the broader term "negative symptoms," which pertain primarily to the lack of motivation to embark on potentially rewarding activity—that is, the anhedonia motivational component. The consummatory component of anhedonia in schizophrenia manifests as the inability to both experience joy and remember joy experienced previously (Treadway & Zald, 2011). Anhedonia as emptiness is most often seen in BPD, in which "chronic feelings of emptiness" are one of the criteria for the BPD diagnosis and are listed as criterion 7 in DSM-IV.

Whereas anhedonia in MDD and schizophrenia has a strong motivational component that reduces activity level, anhedonia in BPD is mostly consummatory, with motivation remaining relatively intact. As a result of this consummatory–motivational imbalance, patients with BPD engage in frantic activity to escape their inner emptiness, searching for intense experiences that may include self-injurious behavior. Patients with BPD often state that they cut themselves to feel "something" because they feel empty. Paradoxically, the emptiness of BPD can be a quite intense and painful undifferentiated negative emotion, very similar to the concept of emotional pain. This mental pain can be so intense that patients with BPD seek the physical pain of self-injury to escape and find relief from the intolerable pain of inner emptiness.

Both emotional pain and anhedonia are frequently experienced by drug- and alcohol-addicted individuals in the course of acute and, more important, protracted withdrawal. Drug addiction directly engages the reward circuitry and nucleus accumbens, and it results in what is called an allosteric shift in the neurobiology of the brain, which adjusts to the drug of abuse so the addicted state is perceived as neutral or normal. The absence of the drug is experienced as intense dysphoria and decreased ability to experience any positive emotions, including pleasure. The drug-seeking behavior shifts from craving euphoria in a euthymic state to craving normalcy in a dysphoric, anhedonic state.

Regardless of the categorical diagnosis, anhedonia, as a dimensional transdiagnostic entity, has been extensively correlated to suicidal ideation in adolescents and adults

(Gabbay, Ely, Babb, & Liebs, 2012). As a state, intensifying anhedonia is a component of the suicidal crisis and needs to be examined when assessing risk for imminent suicide.

As the intensity of suicidal crisis increases, the specific negative feelings attached to individual endeavors and activities converge into a state of psychic pain. Some people experience psychic pain physically as "head pain." This generalized intense sense of dysphoria must be assessed in depth during the assessment for imminent suicide risk.

The following case examples describe comprehensive assessment of the affective disturbance aspect of SCS.

Case 41—Continued

Emotional pain

DR: Alina, how are you feeling right now? You look like you are in pain.

ALINA: Yeah, I feel really awful. .... Everybody keeps asking me about school, and which schools I have applied to and I have nothing to say.

DR: Is that depression that you are feeling?

ALINA: It's not that; I am always depressed. It's like everything hurts, like I have the flu. My legs hurt, my back hurts, and my brain hurts. When they ask me questions, I can't think. It's too much pain and my mind goes blank.

DR: Are you anxious?

ALINA: I am always anxious. It's not that. It's like I have a headache, but it's different. It's excruciating. Like all my feelings need Tylenol or something.

DR: Do you feel that this pain is too much to live with?

ALINA: Sometimes.

DR: Do you feel that for you to go on this pain must be stopped right now?

ALINA: Sometimes.

Depressive turmoil

DR: You said that you feel better now. .... Do these feeling of being trapped in your pain, and being raw, and having no skin, can they appear suddenly? Do they come in waves?

ALINA: I could be fine one moment and then it just hits me. Out of the blue. And I start drowning.

DR: Like when Dorothy smirked?

ALINA: Yes. I was pretty OK until then, and then it was like somebody hit me. I could not catch my breath. And I got so angry I could not even talk anymore. I had to walk away.

DR: So is it like a wave or like a punch?

ALINA: It can be ether. It's more like a punch when there is a trigger. Like Dorothy with her smirk, or my mother telling me to be like somebody I could never be. When there are no triggers, it comes and goes in waves.

DR: How do you feel when the wave passes?

ALINA: Better usually.

DR: Do you feel happy?

ALINA: Not happy; hyper.

Frantic anxiety

> DR: When you felt trapped, did you feel emotionally raw?
>
> ALINA: Yes! (Emphatically, as if recognizing something)
>
> DR: Did you feel like even the smallest things were bothering you, that normally would not?
>
> ALINA: Yeah, after I told Dorothy that I will take a gap year before college, she kind of smirked, like I was so inferior to her, and I kept thinking about it all evening. And then I dreamt about it. . . . Can you believe it, I had a dream about Dorothy's smirk!
>
> DR: Do these feelings make you feel restless and make you want to escape?
>
> ALINA: Yes! Escape and never come back . . .

Panic-dissociation

> DR: Last weekend after Dorothy smirked at you and you felt like a wave of a bad feeling hit you, did you feel that something was wrong with you physically?
>
> ALINA: My skin was crawling. I wanted to leave but my mother didn't let me.
>
> DR: How about later that evening, when you felt trapped in your pain?
>
> ALINA: I felt nauseous, and also my whole body was aching. I could barely move.
>
> DR: It may sound like a strange question, but did your body or your body parts feel different?
>
> ALINA: Yeah. . . . Now that you asked, my stomach was squashed.
>
> DR: Did the world around you feel any different?
>
> ALINA: Yes, the sounds were muffled, like from behind a wall, and everything was tilted.
>
> DR: What do you mean?
>
> ALINA: Like I would walk and the ground felt tilted and rubbery.

Fear of dying

> DR: Were you scared?
>
> ALINA: I thought I was going to die. I did not know how much of this I could take.
>
> DR: (Gently) But you did not answer my question.
>
> ALINA: I was scared I was going to have a heart attack. That's not how I want to die.
>
> DR: How?
>
> ALINA: I told you, I would take the pills.
>
> DR: Are you scared now?
>
> ALINA: I am OK now, just a little nauseous and my hands are tingling.

Acute anhedonia

> DR: What makes you feel good, usually?
>
> ALINA: Watching TV or reading.
>
> DR: Have you been doing that?
>
> ALINA: There is nothing on. I watched *Game of Thrones* twice and read it twice.
>
> DR: What about doing something with Sara? She called you a couple weeks ago if I remember.
>
> ALINA: It hurts me even to think about this. And I am boring. I have very little to say. She is still on vacation anyway.

DR: What about going for a run with your mom? You used to like that.

ALINA: I used to like running in middle school, with my friend. I don't like it anymore. And my mother runs faster than me, she is all about winning. Just thinking about this is giving me a headache.

DR: Are you able to feel anything positive?

ALINA: Like what? Ice-cream tastes good. There is only so much ice cream I can eat.

Alina's mental state at the time of the interview shows all aspects of affective disturbance. She clearly feels mental/emotional pain and distinguishes her "awful" state of mind both from depression and from anxiety. Her emotional pain is not constant but, rather, fluctuates in intensity, which represents depressive turmoil. The pain intensity depends on Alina's contact with the real world, which makes her feel damaged and inadequate. The pain comes in characteristic waves, and at their peak Alina feels the emotional rawness of frantic anxiety. The fantasy worlds of TV and fiction, which do not talk back, are her nonsuicidal escapes that make her feel good.

Alina describes both frantic anxiety and several essential panic–dissociation elements of SCS, such as nausea, skin crawling, and tingling. Her experiences of sounds being muffled and the world being tilted, as well as the ground feeling rubbery, are typical dissociative experiences. She spontaneously says that she thought she was going to die, which means that the "death by distress" notion was very much in her consciousness and was also very intense.

Alina's lack of interest in searching for new shows on TV or for new books, as well as her lack of desire to shop for clothes and makeup and to dress up (activities she used to enjoy), is an example of motivational anhedonia. Her lack of pleasure when going to the gym and to the movies with her mother is an example of consummatory anhedonia.

Case 42–Continued

Emotional pain

DR: Richard, how have you been feeling lately?

RICHARD: Not so good.

DR: Are you depressed?

RICHARD: No, not depressed. It's like I am anxious, which is more painful than the depression.

DR: Would you say regardless of how you label it, you feel emotional pain?

RICHARD: Yes, you could say that.

DR: Is it too much to bear?

RICHARD: Sometimes.

DR: How about right now?

RICHARD: Right now also.

DR: Do you feel that for you to go on it must be stopped?

RICHARD: It better be.

Depressive turmoil

DR: This fear you just mentioned, that she would leave and you will be all alone in the end, is it there all the time or does it come in waves?

RICHARD: In waves.

DR: Waves of what? What feeling?

RICHARD: I just get very angry. I gave her everything I had, she spent all my money, and then she is going to leave. She makes me so mad.

DR: Mad or scared also?

RICHARD: Mad and scared. Nobody wants to be alone at the end.

DR: Do these feelings come out of the blue?

RICHARD: Sometimes. But mostly, it is when she is around. It gets so bad, I am afraid that if I speak, I will just scream.

Frantic anxiety

DR: Do you feel like you've lost control over the situation?

RICHARD: I never had any control, I just had the money.

DR: It sounds like you feel helpless to change the situation.

RICHARD: You could say so.

DR: Do you feel emotionally raw?

RICHARD: What do you mean?

DR: I mean, like having a very thin skin or no skin, like whatever she says will drive you crazy.

RICHARD: It does but I cannot show it. She will pick a fight and it will cost me.

DR: Does she get under your skin so much that you're afraid you will lose it?

RICHARD: She does, and I do lose it. I don't know what to do anymore. She just won't listen.

DR: Are you scared that she will leave?

RICHARD: Terribly. I can't stop thinking about this, particularly at night.

Panic–dissociation

DR: When you are in the middle of a wave of bad feeling, anger, or anxiety, do you feel like something is wrong with you physically?

RICHARD: My eyes are hurting, and my stomach.

DR: Any strange sensations in your skin?

RICHARD: My eyelids are burning.

DR: Do you feel like something strange is happening in your body?

RICHARD: I feel my stomach shake in the morning and that I am disconnected from the world.

Fear of dying

DR: Does all this feel scary to you?

RICHARD: Very.

DR: Are you scared that you might die?

RICHARD: Yes.

DR: What do you mean?

RICHARD: I mean my body will just give in and something will happen.

Anhedonia

DR: Does this pain make it difficult for you do things that you like?

RICHARD: Yes, it's hard.

DR: What is your most favorite thing to do?

RICHARD: I like watching movies.

DR: Have you been able to lately?

RICHARD: Not for a while. I can't make myself do it and when I try it feels like a chore.

Like Alina, Richard has most of the symptoms of SCS affective disturbance, but he is not very skilled at examining his feelings or talking about them. Richard acknowledges having emotional pain, which is distinct from anxiety and depression. Thinking about his wife's spending gives Richard frantic anxiety, mixed with waves of anger (depressive turmoil), and his state of mind is so painful that he cannot stand it much longer (frantic anxiety). His hurting eyes and burning eyelids are somatic symptoms of panic, and his feeling of being disconnected from the world is a dissociative symptom. He admits to fear of dying—so scary that he does not want to think or talk about it. Finally, his anhedonic symptoms are demonstrated by his lack of pleasure from his favorite activities.

LOSS OF COGNITIVE CONTROL

Cognitive dysfunction is arguably the most studied and the most understood aspect of suicidal behavior. We and others have shown that the suicidal crisis is characterized by a ruminative and rigid thought process (Halari et al., 2009), difficulties in decision making and judgment (Leykin, Roberts, & DeRubeis, 2011), problems with recall bias (Patten, 2003), and unsuccessful attempts on unwanted thought suppression (Van der Does, 2005).

In the proposed DSM definition of SCS, loss of cognitive control is the second of the three Part B criteria. In suicidal individuals who experience the loss of cognitive control, the thought patterns identified in Part B may amplify the perception of impossibility of escape from the unbearable life situation. These thought patterns are ruminations, rigidity, thought suppression, and ruminative flooding. In the proposed criteria, they are defined in the colloquial clinical terms as follows: Loss of cognitive control as manifested by

- intense and persistent ruminations about one's own distress and the life events that brought it on (i.e., ruminations);
- inability to deviate from a repetitive negative pattern of thought (cognitive rigidity);
- repeated unsuccessful attempts to suppress negative or disturbing thoughts; and
- an experience of pain or pressure in the head from loss of control of one's negative thoughts impairing the ability to process information or make a decision (ruminative flooding)

Of the four loss of cognitive control symptoms, ruminative flooding (RF) stands out as the most severe. RF is characterized not only by uncontrollable perseverative thinking involving continual thoughts about the causes, meanings, and consequences of one's negative mood (Katz et al., 2011; Yaseen et al., 2013; Yaseen et al., 2012;

Yaseen et al., 2010, 2014, 2016) but also by somatic symptoms, including headaches and head pressure.

Ruminations

Ruminations can be defined as repetitive thoughts focused on one's own distress. The distress can be symptomatic, such as anguish, suffering, or guilt, or it can be factual, relating to difficult life situations and stressors. The more recently developed term "repetitive negative thinking" (RNT) also describes the ruminations and worry present in anxiety and depression, and it was hypothesized to be a transdiagnostic symptom present in many other disorders, including post-traumatic stress disorder, social phobia, obsessive–compulsive disorder, insomnia, eating disorders, panic disorder, hypochondriasis, alcohol use disorder, psychosis, and bipolar disorder (for a review, see Ehring & Watkins, 2008).

Ruminations have repeatedly been associated with suicidal thoughts and attempts (Morrison & O'Connor, 2008). Ruminations about one's own symptoms, or brooding ruminations, are more strongly associated with suicide attempts compared to ruminations about the events of one's life, or reflective pondering (Morrison & O'Connor, 2008). Brooding ruminations are very similar to and may be identical to RNT, although this remains to be proven through rigorous research.

Patients at risk for imminent suicide believe that they are trapped in an endless loop of repetitive thinking from which there is no escape. Not surprisingly, in acutely suicidal people, ruminations are often focused on the perceived dead-end life situation from which there is no exit. The more they ruminate about their own failures, the more convinced they become that there are no viable solutions to improve their lives. Hence, suicide becomes the only remaining option.

In a sense, acutely suicidal patients find themselves trapped in their own circular thinking about their own entrapment. When they try to break out of the loop with a willful effort, they either fail or succeed for only a very short period of time. Some patients with particularly intense ruminations experience them as a vortex rather than a loop, and they liken their attempts to stop their ruminations to trying to climb out of the vortex. This imagery indicates that the ruminations have escalated to the level of ruminative flooding, which is a sign of a suicidal crisis and a symptom of SCS.

Cognitive Rigidity

Anecdotal accounts and the clinical experience of numerous clinicians over many years, as well as recent research data, indicate that the thought process in acutely suicidal individuals is often inflexible and rigid.

Clinical experience repeatedly shows that acutely suicidal patients have difficulty changing their thinking patterns, becoming locked into inflexible repetitive thought patterns affixed to various aspects of their suicidal narrative: failure to meet their own expectations, real or imagined social defeat or defeats, alienation, perceived burdensomeness, and, finally, increasingly desperate perception of no future. These thoughts are ruminative; circular ruminative thinking about the same matter is inflexible almost by definition. Note that rigidity in thinking may be present even in impulsive suicide attempters, who may not develop ruminations. Thus, clinicians may attempt preventive interventions aimed at improving flexibility in thinking before these patients decide that suicide is their only option.

In research studies, cognitive rigidity in patients with suicidal ideation or history of suicide attempts has been shown many times through testing rigidity in set-shifting— that is, the ability to change thinking and behavior in response to a changing environment (Marzuk, Hartwell, Leon, & Portera, 2005). In the assessment of imminent suicide risk, cognitive rigidity can be evaluated following the assessment of ruminations by testing whether the patient can change his or her mind when presented with a hypothetical alternative interpretation of the patient's current life situation. If the patient is unable to do so, the clinician can offer an alternative interpretation. The patient's ability or inability to accept the proposed and less pernicious interpretation of his or her life will then reveal the degree of cognitive rigidity.

Thought Suppression

Thought suppression is the deliberate attempt to not think of something. It is often used as a strategy of conscious cognitive control when unpleasant thoughts need to be diminished or eliminated (Wegner, 1989). Research shows that this natural and intuitive strategy is counterproductive and achieves the opposite result. Thought suppression works for only a very short period of time, and when the strategy fails, unwanted thoughts return with both higher frequency and increased intensity (see reviews by Abramowitz, Tolin, & Street, 2001; Wegner, 1989). Remarkably, individuals with a greater tendency to suppress unwanted thoughts react to emotional thoughts more strongly and have a more difficult time regulating their emotions (Wegner & Zanakos, 1994). Conversely, those with less thought suppression are much more adept at regulating their emotions.

Thought suppression is a common strategy utilized by suicidal patients to reduce the thought pressure from unwanted ruminations. However, as with all thought suppression, these willful attempts paradoxically increase the frequency of intrusive thoughts and amplify the intensity of suicidal thinking (Wegner, Schneider, Carter, & White, 1987). Findings from several studies showed that a tendency to suppress unwanted thoughts was associated with past suicidal ideation and attempts (Pettit et al., 2009) and that thought suppression was a mediator of the relationship between emotion reactivity and the occurrence of self-injurious thoughts and behavior (Najmi, Wegner, & Nock, 2007).

Ruminative Flooding

As articulated in Chapter 2, the RF component of SCS encompasses the uncontrollable onslaught of repetitive automatic and affectively charged, negative thoughts characterizes by ruminations and rigidity. However, unlike simple ruminations, RF includes negativistic cognitive distortions with paranoid flavor, which amplify with failed attempts on thought suppression, resulting in somatic symptoms in the brain. RF is distinguishable from simple ruminations by the presence of headaches or head pressure—migraine-like somatic symptoms in the head, which confer increased risk of suicidal ideation and past suicide attempts (Yaseen et al., 2013; Yaseen et al., 2012; Yaseen et al., 2014, 2016).

Thus, in RF, the thought process disturbances reach such power and intensity that only suicidal thoughts remain possible. The rigidity and the obsessive single focus of the suicidal thought process amplify the intensity of ruminations. As ruminative intensity increases, the subject matter narrows further, stultifying the thought process even more. In RF, the endless feedback loop of ruminations and rigidity reaches a point at which the thought process in itself becomes unbearably painful. The pain of uncontrollable ruminative negative thinking experienced by suicidal patients is distinct from that of a normal headache and is often described as "head pain" or "pressure in the head" that can be directly linked to the vortex of unwelcome thoughts.

In their loss of control over their own thought process, ruminating patients are similar to patients with tangential thinking, looseness of associations, and flight of ideas, which are essential components of thought disorder. Hence, arguably, suicidal ruminations can be considered a variant of thought disorder or psychosis. Although not all ruminations reach delusional intensity, almost all could be categorized as "overvalued ideas." Of possible relevance, overvalued ideas are very common in patients with BPD (Zanarini, Frankenburg, Wedig, & Fitzmaurice, 2013), and meta-analyses show that low-dose neuroleptic is the only treatment that appears to be beneficial for patients with BPD (Vita, De Peri, & Sacchetti, 2011). Low-dose antipsychotics could be considered in suicidal individuals with loss of cognitive control as well.

The following continuing case examples illustrate the comprehensive assessment of the loss of cognitive control aspect of SCS.

Case 41—Continued

Ruminations

DR: I want to talk a little bit more about last weekend, when you felt your worst. Was it after you thought that Dorothy smirked at you?

ALINA: Yes, but then I fell asleep.

DR: Well, do you remember, while you were alone in your room, before you fell asleep, did you keep thinking the same thoughts again and again?

ALINA: Yes.

DR: Were thoughts running, or was your head quiet?

ALINA: Running.

DR: What were you thinking exactly?

ALINA: I was trying to think of what to say to her so I would sound smart.

DR: Were you able to come up with anything?

ALINA: No, and then I started thinking about how miserable I was.

Rigidity

> DR: Why are you so sure that Dorothy is happy in college?
>
> ALINA: She looks happy. And she must be, she got into a very good school, what is there to be unhappy about?
>
> DR: There are all kinds of reasons: difficult courses, too much work, stiff competition, no friends. I can go on.
>
> ALINA: Why does she look happy then?
>
> DR: Just good social skills. Never compare your insides with other people's outsides.
>
> ALINA: You are just making things up. She said that college was great and she loved it.

Thought suppression

> DR: These are pretty upsetting thoughts. What happens when you try not to think them?
>
> ALINA: It does not work very well.
>
> DR: What happens?
>
> ALINA: They just keep coming back.
>
> DR: Does it work even a little? I mean, when Dorothy with her smirk comes back, is her smirk the same, better or worse?
>
> ALINA: Worse.

Ruminative flooding

> DR: Was your thinking clear or foggy? Did it feel noisy in your head?
>
> ALINA: Noisy. Sometimes.
>
> DR: Is it hard to figure out sometimes what exactly you are thinking?
>
> ALINA: Sometimes.
>
> DR: At those times when you were thinking so hard that your head was noisy and confusing, did you feel pressure in your head?
>
> ALINA: Yes.
>
> DR: Were these thoughts and images of Dorothy smirking giving you a headache?
>
> ALINA: My brain hurt.
>
> DR: Did you feel that your head could explode from having too many bad thoughts you could not suppress?
>
> ALINA: Yes.
>
> DR: Did you feel that these thoughts and images were like a vortex pulling you in, and you try to climb out but you can't?
>
> ALINA: I wasn't even trying to climb out. I gave in.

Although at the time of the office interview Alina is not acutely suicidal, the therapist's assessment of her state of mind during the last weekend reveals most of the loss of cognitive control symptoms of SCS. Alina describes negativistic ruminations about her being inferior to Dorothy; she cannot even consider alternative, less toxic interpretations of Dorothy's behavior (rigidity); she describes unsuccessful attempts at thought suppression (Dorothy's smirk coming back with a vengeance); and she acknowledges the ruminative flooding (vortex). Thus, over the weekend, although Alina did not attempt suicide, she was in the midst of a suicide crisis.

Case 42—Continued

Ruminations

>   DR: Richard, you seem distracted to me; is your thinking right now clear or foggy?
>
>   RICHARD: I have a lot on my mind. It is hard to focus.
>
>   DR: Are you thinking about your wife and her spending?
>
>   RICHARD: That is all I can think about.
>
>   DR: Do you keep thinking the same thoughts again and again, like in a loop?
>
>   RICHARD: Yes.
>
>   DR: Is it worse at night before you fall asleep?
>
>   RICHARD: I have a hard time falling asleep.

Cognitive rigidity

>   DR: You know, there may be other approaches you could use to deal with you financial situations.
>
>   RICHARD: I can't think of any, I have tried. I am on a fixed income.
>
>   DR: Maybe she does not fully understand the situation. Did you try talking to her? Will you ask her to come in for a session?
>
>   RICHARD: No, she will leave. She thought she had married a rich man. I can't tell her we have no money.

Thought suppression

>   DR: You look distracted, like you are back in your endless thinking loop. What happens if you try to suppress these thoughts and think about something else?
>
>   RICHARD: I can't stop thinking about this; there is no point in thinking about anything else until I find a solution.
>
>   DR: What happens if you do try?
>
>   RICHARD: Nothing, the thoughts just come back.
>
>   DR: Worse, the same, or better than before you tried?
>
>   RICHARD: Worse.

Ruminative flooding

>   DR: Does all this thinking, these endless thoughts you cannot suppress, make you feel pressure in your head?
>
>   RICHARD: Yes. And pain in my skull, actually.
>
>   DR: Some liken their ruminative thoughts to a vortex, which just keeps getting deeper and deeper, and is sucking them in. Is that how you feel?
>
>   RICHARD: Kind of.
>
>   DR: Does it feel that you are trying to climb out but you can't, and it is just pulling you back in?
>
>   RICHARD: Yes, this is exactly how it feels.
>
>   DR: For how long can you bear this head pressure or pain?
>
>   RICHARD: I can't. I have just about had it.

In contrast to Alina, who has somewhat recovered from the previous weekend's suicide crisis, Richard's crisis is very much present and could be worsening. An outside observer may notice that he is internally preoccupied. His thinking is dominated by ruminations he is powerless to control or suppress, and he admits to ruminative flooding. This loss of cognitive control in combination with Richard's affective disturbance, revealed by the first part of the previous interview, indicate that Richard is at high short-term risk for suicide.

AGITATION AND INSOMNIA

Hyperarousal is the third and final category of Part B symptoms required for the proposed DSM diagnosis of SCS. This disturbance in arousal could be manifested either by agitation—a state of extreme arousal, physical restlessness, hypervigilance, or heightened irritability (Ballard et al., 2016; Bryan et al., 2014)—or by global insomnia. Hyperarousal is the energy that may fuel suicidal behavior.

On the surface, agitation may appear to be an uncomplicated symptom. It can be conceptualized in at least two different abnormal states: a state of extreme arousal or a state of heightened irritability and anxiety. The first definition of agitation, as an unpleasant arousal, places it in the same domain as other disturbances of arousal, such as lethargy, insomnia, and hypersomnia. On the other hand, the second definition of agitation, as a state of anxious excitement or disinhibition, consigns agitation to the spectrum of moods, together with anxiety, anhedonia, and anguish.

In the course of short-term suicide risk evaluation, agitation is usually assessed as an objectively observed psychomotor behavior—that is, an abnormal state of arousal rather than a self-reported mood state (we rarely, if ever, ask patients if they feel agitated). Regardless of which definition is used, agitation has been repeatedly linked with suicidal behavior (Fawcett, Busch, Jacobs, Kravitz, & Fogg, 1997). Agitation has been hypothesized to be one potential mechanism through which bipolar disorder, medical illness, and the prescription of certain psychiatric medications might increase the risk of suicidal behavior (Henry & Demotes-Mainard, 2006). This hypothesis remains to be tested, but it appears to be consistent with clinical experience: By definition, bipolar manic and mixed states involve increased arousal. Agitated delirium, which is common in medical illness, also involves increased arousal as well as akathisia, which is a side effect of many antipsychotics and some antidepressants.

Insomnia is another aspect of disturbed arousal reported in the literature to precede suicidal behavior (Hochard, Heym, & Townsend, 2016). Preceding completed suicides and serious suicide attempts, acutely suicidal individuals may experience difficulty falling asleep, waking up at night after initial sleep, or sometimes waking up every hour. Dreams, nightmares, night terrors (which could be nocturnal panic attacks), and being exhausted in the morning even after sleeping several hours were all reported to doctors or noted by relatives (Hochard et al., 2016). These clinical reports are consistent with the research findings of disturbed arousal in suicidal patients (Hochard et al., 2016; Ribeiro, Silva, & Joiner, 2014).

Insomnia is a very prevalent condition and is not specific to the acute suicidal state, which is also true of anxiety, ruminations, and panic—all of which are very common symptoms experienced by those with or without mental illness. However, prior to the suicide attempt, insomnia may escalate sharply, particularly in adolescents, for whom it is the second leading acute symptom, after emotional pain, that precedes high-lethality suicide attempts (Wong, Brower, & Craun, 2016).

Although agitation and insomnia are risk factors for suicide in their own right, other components of SCS may have agitation or insomnia as a part of their clinical presentation. Agitation defined as extreme anxious arousal overlaps with frantic anxiety. The symptoms of emotional pain and the ups and downs of depressive turmoil, desperation, and entrapment all include some elements of agitation and are frequently concomitant with insomnia.

Reports of withdrawal and hypersomnia in relation to suicide are less consistent. Some parents of adolescents who went on to die by suicide described their children as staying in their rooms and in bed prior to their death. Veterans Administration clinicians who treat suicidal veterans have reported the gradual withdrawal from life by suicidal veterans who would not answer phone calls or would skip their appointments prior to their fatal suicide attempts.

The following continuing case examples describe the assessment of the agitation and arousal aspects of SCS.

Case 41–Continued

DR: You said that you did not know if you would make it last weekend but then you fell asleep. Was it hard to fall asleep?

ALINA: Yeah, I just kept thinking the same thoughts, just as you said.

DR: What where you doing as you were thinking? Were you lying in bed?

ALINA: I tried. I could not. I could not stay in bed.

DR: What did you do?

ALINA: I tried to watch TV, but I could not concentrate. I could not sit still. So I walked around the room.

DR: How did you fall asleep?

ALINA: I had two beers.

DR: Did you sleep through the night?

ALINA: No. I woke up 2 hours later when my mother came.

DR: Then?

ALINA: She tucked me in. Then I slept on and off. It was nice to have my mother next to me.

Last weekend, Alina had both agitation (pacing around) and early and late insomnia. This adds to the evidence that she was in the midst of a suicidal crisis.

Case 42–Continued

DR: You seem restless; did you notice your leg is jumping up and down?

RICHARD: Not until you said it. You notice everything don't you?

DR: Am I irritating you? Why are you getting up?

RICHARD: You make me feel like I am under a microscope. And I just can't sit still. There is too much on my mind.

DR: Do you feel restless inside, like you need to move?

RICHARD: No, I just feel like standing.

DR: You also look tired. Did you sleep well last night?

RICHARD. I always wake up a couple of times to go to the bathroom.

DR: Last night after you went to the bathroom, did you fall asleep right away?

RICHARD: No. I walked around a bit, and then I watched TV.

DR: Did pacing around help calm down your thoughts?

RICHARD: Not really. I just did not know what else to do.

In this interview in his doctor's office, Richard shows signs of psychomotor agitation (leg restlessness and jumping up). He is also irritable, telling the doctor he feels like he is under a microscope. His has also developed insomnia, not being able to fall asleep in the middle of the night and pacing. Richard's psychomotor activity further confirms that has developed a suicide crisis syndrome.

SUICIDAL CRISIS ASSESSMENT ALGORITHM

The assessment of SCS is more straightforward than the assessment and the construction of the suicidal narrative because it is an expansion of the familiar Mental Status examination to include the items describing mental processes of acutely suicidal individuals. Here, the suggested SCS interview algorithm is presented. It was used in case examples 15 and 16, in the case examples presented later in this chapter, and in the test cases. It does not include rapport building, which usually has been accomplished earlier, in the course of the suicidal narrative part of the assessment.

The algorithm used is structured according to the proposed DSM criteria. In real clinical situations, in order to minimize misleading self-reports by individuals who have made up their minds to die by suicide and would like to hide their intent from the interviewing clinician, the direct explicit questioning about the patient's suicidal ideation and intent should be reserved until the end of the interview. This change in the order of the assessment also applies to the overall interview strategies discussed in detail in Chapter 8.

Although during the course of a conversational interview the question order can be flexible and determined by the patient's answers, it is suggested that the interviewer evaluating the SCS severity follows roughly the same order as in the guide and starts with the assessment of affective disturbance, followed by loss of cognitive control and arousal (for a detailed discussion of complete interview strategies, see Chapter 8). The affective disturbance part of the SCS assessment contains questions about the emotional state that, when asked sensibly, reveal concern and care. They should be asked before the questions about loss of cognitive control and arousal because they are more clinical and, if asked first, may seem uncaring and create a misperception of the clinician "just doing a job."

In "real life," when asking about affective disturbance, it is suggested that the interviewer start with the most intuitive and easy to understand questions about emotional pain, followed by more intrusive and specific questions about different aspects of entrapment and concluding with the most intrusive questions about fear of dying. Similarly, when assessing loss of cognitive control, it makes sense to start with questions about less severe pathology, such as ruminations, and then elaborate on the more severe and distressing pathology, such as ruminative flooding.

Interview Algorithm

Part A
    Suicidal ideation
        Have you been thinking about suicide? (. . . death? . . . ending your life? . . . not being alive?)
        How often?
        When was the last time you thought about suicide?
        What was your exact thought?
        How did you respond to this thought?
        Have you thought of a way to end your life?
    Suicide intent and plan
        Have you made a plan to end your life? (. . . to die? . . . to kill yourself? . . . to commit suicide?)
        How long have you been planning it?
        What is it?
        Please tell me the specifics? (Which pills? Which gun? Which bridge? Which rope?)
        Have you obtained the means? (Bought the pills, the gun, the rope?)
        Have you practiced? (Opened the bottle? Put a gun to your head? Drove over the bridge? Made a noose?)
        What stopped you?
        What will it take for you to go through with it?
        Who knows about your plans?
    Entrapment
        When you think about your current (unbearable) life situation,
            . . . do you feel trapped?
            . . . do you see possible exits from your condition?
            . . . do you see possible good solutions or ways out of your problem?
            . . . do you see ways of improving the situation?
            . . . do you see ways of solving your problem?
    Desperation
        When you think about the (unbearable) life situation,
            . . . how long can you tolerate living like this?
            . . . is there hope that your life (your pain, your illness, your condition) will improve?
            . . . can you wait for it to improve?

. . . how long can you wait?

. . . for you to go on, do you need for the pain to stop now?

. . . do you feel the urge to escape your situation now?

. . . is suicide an escape?

Part B

1. Affective disturbance

Emotional pain

Do you feel like you are in pain?

Is this pain emotional?

Is it too much to bear?

Do you feel it needs to be stopped?

Do you feel this pain can get better?

Will it only get worse?

Depressive turmoil

Do you feel waves of bad feelings or that your mood is even?

Do you feel waves of anxiety, anger, fear?

During these waves, are you afraid you might die or lose your mind? Which one?

Do these feelings come in waves out of the blue?

Do they make you feel restless and agitated?

Frantic anxiety

Do you feel that you have no control?

Do you feel that you have lost control to change things?

Do you feel powerless?

Do you feel helpless?

Do you feel overwhelmed with negative emotions?

Do you feel emotionally raw?

Do you feel like you have no skin?

Do you feel like the smallest things are bothering you, as if your life lies in the balance?

Do you feel so nervous that you are on the verge of losing control?

Panic–dissociation and sensory disturbances

With the waves of bad feelings, do you feel something is wrong with you physically?

Do you also have physical symptoms such as sweating? (Nausea? Problems breathing? Rapid heartbeat?)

Do you feel strange sensations in your body or skin?

Do you feel something happening to (in, on) your body?

Do you feel that the world around you is different?

Fear of dying

Do you also worry about bad things that may happen to you?

Do you have nightmares about death? (Which ones?)

Do you wake up at night in a sweat, so scared you might die it is hard to breath?

Do you fear for your life?

Acute anhedonia
   What makes you feel good usually?
   Has this activity become a burden to you?
   Has this activity become painful?
   Does it feel like torture?
   Are you able to feel anything positive?
   Is it hard to try to feel positive? How hard?

2. Loss of cognitive control
   When you think about
      ... being trapped in your current life situation
      ... possible exits from your condition
      ... possible good solutions, ways out of your problem
      ... improving the situation
      ... solving your problem
   Ruminations
      Is your thinking clear or foggy?
      Are your thoughts racing, running fast, or is your head quiet?
      Is it hard to figure out exactly what you are thinking?
      Do you have unpleasant thoughts in your head that keep running again and again?
      Do these thoughts come mostly at night before you go to sleep?
      Do you think these thoughts also during the day?
      Are you having these thoughts right now?
      Do you feel pressure in your head from having too many thoughts?
      Are you having headaches from having too many thoughts?
      Do you feel like your head could explode from having too many thoughts?
   Cognitive rigidity
      You know, these negative thoughts you have been having about your life—this is not the only way to look at things. For example, here is an alternative interpretation ...
      But really—many people are happy doing this; can you see your life from this point of view?
      How hard is it to see your problem in a different light?
      Do you succeed? How often?
      How long can you think other thoughts before you come back to the ones that bother you?
   Thought suppression
      Do you try to forcefully suppress these thoughts?
      Can you?
      Is it working?
      Is trying to suppress your thoughts only making them worse?
   Ruminative flooding
      Do the out-of-control bad thoughts make you feel pressure in your head?
      Does this make you feel like your head could explode?

For some people, this endless thinking feels like a vortex, which just keeps getting deeper and deeper. Is that how you feel?

Does it feel like you are trying to climb out but you can't?

3. Agitation and insomnia

You seem agitated to me. Is this how you feel?

Do you feel agitated inside?

Is it hard to stay calm?

Does this agitation prevent you from sleeping?

Have you had problems falling asleep? Waking up in the middle of the night? Too early?

When you have problems sleeping, do these thoughts we talked about a minute ago bother you?

CASE EXAMPLES–CONTINUED FROM CHAPTER 5

Case 38: High Risk for Imminent Suicide, Continued

Gary is a 30-year-old single Jewish man with a history of bipolar mood disorder I and two previous psychiatric hospitalizations who is currently living in a two-bedroom apartment with his parents. He returned to the United States 6 months ago after teaching English for 2 years in Croatia, and his parents referred him for a psychiatric assessment to a bipolar specialist "so he can get the best possible treatment because his is a difficult case." Gary has no previous suicide attempts, but his parents are concerned that he may kill himself because "there is just something scary about him that makes us very uncomfortable."

During the suicidal narrative part of the assessment, Gary revealed all five aspects of the suicidal narrative: He could not give up on a unrealistic expectation of an academic career; his professional and personal failures made him feel defeated and alienated, as well as a burden to his parents; and with the next job application rejection, he would find himself at a dead end with no good options, which would make him a very high suicide risk.

The Suicidal Crisis Syndrome Assessment

Part A

Suicidal ideation

DR: Have you been thinking about suicide? (. . . death? . . . ending your life? . . . not being alive?)

GARY: Yes.

DR: How often?

GARY: Daily.

DR: When was the last time you thought about suicide?

GARY: When I was sitting in the waiting room.

DR: What was your exact thought?

GARY: That if I don't get this job I am going to kill myself.

DR: How did you respond to this thought?

GARY: I tried to think positive, like about what I would do after I get the job offer.

Suicide intent and plan

DR: Have you made a plan to kill yourself, if you do not get the job offer?

GARY: Not specifically. I have an idea.

DR: How long have you had an idea?

GARY: For a while . . . years.

DR: What is it?

GARY: I wouldn't want to fail—I have failed at many things in my life. And I want it to be quick.

DR: Please be more specific. What is quick? Guns? Jumping?

GARY: Falling down is too scary . . . I would use a gun.

DR: Which gun?

GARY: Something cheap I could get in a shop. Legally.

DR: Have you bought it?

GARY: No. It's not difficult, I researched it out online; I can do it any time.

DR: Where would you aim?

GARY: In my mouth.

DR: Why?

GARY: I don't want to blow my face off, and you can't really miss.

DR: Have you held a gun?

GARY: Yes.

DR: Have you put it in your mouth?

GARY: Yes.

DR: Was it loaded?

GARY: No.

DR: Have you told anybody about this plan?

GARY: No. I am not crazy. They will put me away.

Entrapment

DR: When you think about your life situation, living with your parents, being supported by them, looking for a job, everything you told me about choices, do you want to escape?

GARY: Yes, it's close to intolerable . . .

DR: Do you feel an escape is possible?

GARY: Not sure. I need a miracle. I need a teaching job.

DR: Other than that, do you see any other good options?

GARY: None. I feel trapped. I feel horrible and I feel trapped.

Desperation

DR: How long can you tolerate the mental pain you are in?

GARY: I don't know—sometimes I think I can't.

DR: Do you have hope that the pain will soon get better?

GARY: Yes—when I get a job.

DR: Can it get better if you do not?

GARY: I doubt it.

DR: I know you are expecting to hear from "College A." What if they say no?

GARY: That is going to be pretty bad. I am not sure I will be able to take it.

DR: What do you mean by that?

GARY: Don't worry doc, I am not going to kill myself now. There is still hope.

Part B

1. Affective disturbance

    Emotional pain

    DR: Gary, you came to see me because you were feeling bad. You told me earlier that you were in pain. Is it emotional pain that you are in?

    GARY: Yes, although at times everything hurts, even my legs.

    DR: How bad is it?

    GARY: Sometimes it feels unbearable. It can get so bad, I do not know how long I can take it.

    DR: How long can you take it?

    GARY: I don't know. That's why I am here. Maybe you will be able to stop it. I can't go on like this.

    DR: Do you feel it all the time or it comes and goes?

    GARY: It comes and goes. But when I have it, it is relentless. It's torture.

    DR: Does anything make it better?

    GARY: Nothing of late.

    Depressive turmoil

    DR: Do the bad feelings that you feel come and go or is your mood even?

    GARY: They come and go.

    DR: Could these be waves of anxiety? Or fear?

    GARY: Maybe.

    DR: When they do come, do they come in waves out of the blue, or there is usually a reason?

    GARY: Sometimes there is a reason ... well, there used to be a reason, now they just come.

    DR: During these waves, are you afraid you might die or lose your mind?

    GARY: I feel like I am going crazy.

    DR: Do you also have physical symptoms such as sweating? Nausea? Problems breathing? Rapid heartbeat?

    GARY: All of these.

    DR: Do you sometimes wake up at night—just like that, nauseous, heart beating, short of breath and in a sweat, so you get scared you might die?

    GARY: That too.

Frantic anxiety

> DR: Do you feel scared of what is happening in your mind?
>
> GARY: Yes I do, sometimes it is really scary.
>
> DR: Do you feel emotionally raw?
>
> GARY: I don't know what I feel. I just know it feels like hell. Like I am in hell, that is.
>
> DR: Are you able to make yourself feel differently? Or talk yourself into feeling differently?
>
> GARY: It does not work. Still feel like sh . . .
>
> DR: Do you feel like the smallest things that should not be bothersome, really get to you?
>
> GARY: Yes, and they make me jumpy.
>
> DR: Making you anxious, like you have no skin?
>
> GARY: Like I have no skin.
>
> DR: Do you feel anxious and scared of losing control?
>
> GARY: I do, and I do lose it with my parents. And when I do, they look really scared of me.
>
> DR: Do you become frantic when that happens?
>
> GARY: You can say that, and this is what scares them, I guess.

Panic–dissociation

> DR: When this happens, do you feel strange sensations in your body or on your skin?
>
> GARY: Yes, how did you know?
>
> DR: Experience. Tell me what they are, please.
>
> GARY: It is hard to describe. I have not felt anything like that until recently.
>
> DR: Please try.
>
> GARY: It's crazy. I can feel blood going through my veins, and I can feel my nerves.
>
> DR: How?
>
> GARY: The blood is kind of buzzing and the nerves are burning. I can also feel my stomach move inside.
>
> DR: Really? Anything else you could add?
>
> GARY: Yes. At those times everything feels different. The world looks different.

Fear of dying

> DR: When this happens to you, do you ever get scared that you might die?
>
> GARY: Yes.
>
> DR: Literally, like your life is going to end?
>
> GARY: Yes.
>
> DR: Please explain.
>
> GARY: I feel so bad mentally and physically that I am afraid that something must be at a breaking point somewhere inside me. One moment it will just snap and kill me.
>
> DR: How frightening.
>
> GARY: You are telling me.

Anhedonia

> DR: What is your favorite thing to do for fun that usually makes you feel good?
>
> GARY: Reading. I read a lot. And writing short stories. I used to be good at that.
>
> DR: Have you been reading lately?

GARY: Only newspapers. And they are full of crap.

DR: Does it help relieve the emotional pain you have been feeling?

GARY: Not reading newspapers.

DR: Is reading newspapers painful to you?

GARY: It's never been fun. I like reading good fiction. Classics. Newspaper writers are illiterate.

DR: Have you been reading classics?

GARY: No. I have read and re-read most of them . . . I thought I could learn how to be a good writer that way.

DR: And now?

GARY: Just opening the book makes my head hurt.

2. Loss of cognitive control

Ruminations

DR: Is your thinking clear or foggy?

GARY: Yeah, a little foggy. I never thought I would say something like this. I think well—usually that is.

DR: Are your thoughts racing, running fast, or your head is quiet?

GARY: It is not that they are racing, it's like they are fragmented. Frequently flying fragments (smiles).

DR: Are these fragments hard to read?

GARY: They can be confusing.

DR: These fragments, are they repetitive? Do they keep running again and again? In circles?

GARY: Again and again, but not in circles.

DR: Do these thoughts come mostly at night before you go to sleep?

GARY: That's why I cannot sleep, I just keep thinking.

DR: Do you think these thoughts also during the day?

GARY: During the day too, and in the morning. I wake up thinking about this stuff.

DR: What stuff?

GARY: What is going to happen if I lose this job. I can't not think about that.

DR: Do you feel pressure in your head from having too many thoughts?

GARY: No, they give me headaches.

DR: Do you feel like your head could explode from having too many thoughts?

GARY: That's too dramatic . . .

DR: Do you worry mainly about what's happening in your head, or trying to find a solution?

GARY: A solution—what's the point of worrying about worrying?

Cognitive rigidity

DR: Your thoughts about your life are pretty negative. You blame yourself a lot. Things may not be as black as they seem to be and not all the blame in the world lies with you.

GARY: How so?

DR: Well, you are a really smart guy, you are good at teaching. The academic jobs you are looking for are highly competitive and political. Your talents may be better used elsewhere.

GARY: You're kidding right? (Smirks)

DR: No I am not. You have been traveling a lot, which gives you a different perspective on life. You could teach high school, you could teach college ESL courses, you could tutor. You have a lot to offer.

GARY: Teaching ESL as a career? That's a great career goal. My parents would be really proud.

DR: Let's forget about your parents for a minute. There are quite a few happy ESL teachers. You could really make a difference.

GARY: Nice try, doc. You can't call teaching English at night a success.

Thought suppression

DR: What happens when you try to shut down these negative thoughts?

GARY: I can't.

DR: Do you try?

GARY: Of course I try, it just does not work. They keep coming back.

DR: Does trying to suppress your thoughts make them worse?

GARY: I never thought of this. Maybe it does. It certainly does not make them any better.

Ruminative flooding

DR: For some people this endless irrepressible thinking feels like a vortex, which just keeps sucking you in deeper and deeper. Is that how you feel?

GARY: Yes, actually now you got it. A vortex.

DR: Does it feel that you are trying to climb out but you can't?

GARY: Yes.

DR: Like you are drowning?

GARY: Yes

3. Agitation and insomnia

DR: You seem agitated to me, is this how you feel?

GARY: I don't know how you can feel agitated.

DR: I meant, not being able to sit still, needing to move, getting up and pacing, the way you have been doing as we were talking.

GARY: Yes, I have been feeling kind of restless, not sure about agitated.

DR: Do you feel agitated inside?

GARY: Do you mean like stirred up? Yeah . . .

DR: Is it hard to stay calm?

GARY: It is very hard to stay calm, particularly around my parents.

DR: Does this agitation prevent you from sleeping?

GARY: I have a hard time falling asleep.

DR: Are you waking up in the middle of the night? Too early?

GARY: In the middle of the night. I have a hard time waking up in the morning.

End of the SCS part of the interview.

Gary's Suicide Crisis Syndrome Intensity Assessment Table

Symptom	Symptom Severity				
	Minimal	*Low*	*Moderate*	*High*	*Severe*
Part A					
Suicidal ideation				X	
Suicide intent and plan					X
Entrapment					X
Desperation				X	
Part A summary					X
Part B					
Affective disturbance					
Emotional pain					X
Depressive turmoil					X
Frantic anxiety					X
Panic–dissociation					X
Fear of dying					X
Anhedonia					X
Affective disturbance summary					X
Loss of cognitive control					
Ruminations					X
Rigidity					X
Thought suppression			X		
Ruminative flooding					X
Loss of cognitive control summary				X	
Overarousal					
Agitation					X
Insomnia				X	
Part B summary					X
Overall summary					X

Gary has suicidal ideation that is persistent but not constant, and he also has a plan. Although his plan is conditional, it is lethal, and Gary has already engaged in preparatory actions and rehearsals. He has an intense sense of entrapment and is just short of being desperate due to his hope of getting an unlikely job offer. Gary's psychic pain is nearly intolerable. His fear of losing his mind and his anxiety are so expansive, they scare his parents. His anhedonia is painful and paralyzing, and his mood is unstable.

Despite his subjective feeling of being mostly in control of his thinking process, Gary has lost most of his capacity for rational thinking, which is reduced to reflective pondering. Gary appears to be dead set on his goal, incessantly thinking about becoming an academic; his looping thoughts cannot be derailed or suppressed, and he identifies with the experience of being flooded with these thoughts. The only component of ruminative flooding still missing is brooding ruminations about his loss of cognitive and emotional control of himself. Gary also exhibits signs of motor agitation while feeling agitated mentally inside. Overall, Gary's SCS symptoms are severe, and his short-term risk for suicide is high.

Case 39: Moderate Risk for Imminent Suicide–Continued

Bernie is a 53-year-old single gay man with a history of generalized anxiety disorder who came for treatment of his depression with suicidal ideation after discovering that his recently deceased partner of 20 years had a family and children whom Bernie knew nothing about. Bernie had a plan to kill himself with a barbiturate and alcohol overdose. He had also just retired from his teaching job. He has one brother and a large circle of friends. He saw a therapist twice in the past following relationship breakups, was never on medications, and had no past suicide attempts.

Part A

Suicidal ideation

DR: Bernie, you told me it has been hard for you to picture your future without Peter. Have you been thinking about ending your life?

BERNIE: It crossed my mind.

DR: How often?

BERNIE: Quite a bit actually. My life without him is meaningless.

DR: What was your exact thought?

BERNIE: That I want to join him. I would rather be dead with him than alive without him.

DR: How did you respond to this thought?

BERNIE: I got scared.

DR: When you were thinking about not being alive without him, have you thought of a way you may end your life?

BERNIE: Yes, in general terms.

DR: And?

BERNIE: Probably pills. I would read the *Final Exit* for specifics. I don't want to leave a mess, so no blood.

Suicide intent and plan

DR: Did you make a specific plan?

BERNIE: No. Just vague thoughts.

DR: And what were they?

BERNIE: Just pills. Maybe a bottle of good cognac and pills.

DR: Have you thought of what cognac and what pills?

BERNIE: I like Hennessey, so Hennessey. I always have a bottle or two at home. I don't know about the pills . . . sleeping pills. Something painless, just to go to sleep.

DR: Do you also have the sleeping pills?

BERNIE: Just what you prescribed.

DR: What will it take for you to go through with it?

BERNIE: Hopelessness I guess. And a realization that I will never meet anybody like him again.

DR: Who knows about your suicidal thoughts?

BERNIE: I told some friends that life seems pointless.

Entrapment

DR: When you think about your situation, about what Peter's death has revealed—his other family, his double life—do you feel trapped?

BERNIE: I do not feel trapped, but I am in pain. I do not understand what happened. I cannot reconcile this reality, when he is gone, and he has a wife and children, and our life together, when we only had each other.

Desperation

DR: How long can you tolerate the condition you are in?

BERNIE: Until you help me feel better. I don't have a choice, do I?

DR: Your pain should get better with time. Time heals, medication and psychotherapy help. Do you have the strength to wait?

BERNIE: I am a pretty strong person.

DR: You still did not answer my question: How long do you think you can wait?

BERNIE: I don't know. Several weeks . . . months . . .

DR: And then? If you don't feel better?

BERNIE: And then, I don't know. We'll cross that bridge when we get there. Hopefully never.

Part B

1. Affective disturbance

Emotional pain

DR: You must be in a lot of pain.

BERNIE: I am not sure the word "pain" describes it.

DR: Please describe what you feel inside, if you can.

BERNIE: It feels like a piece of me was ripped out . . . all that's left is a bleeding wound.

DR: It is emotional though, isn't it?

BERNIE. Yes, it is my soul that is bleeding.

DR: Do you feel that for you to go on, this pain must be stopped?

BERNIE: That's why I am here . . .

Depressive turmoil

DR: When you say you feel on edge sometimes, do your bad feelings come in waves?

BERNIE: Yes.

DR: What are the feelings, besides "having no skin?"

BERNIE: Fear. Fear of the future.

DR: Depression?

BERNIE: Yes, depression.

DR: What about anger?

BERNIE: No anger. I am not an angry person. I can't feel angry at him. He was my life.

DR: Do these waves come out of the blue, or do you have some control over them?

BERNIE: These are two different things. The waves come without warning, but when they do, I can bear down and ride them out until I start feeling better.

Frantic anxiety

DR: Does thinking about the two irreconcilable realities make you feel unhinged?

BERNIE: Yes, it makes me feel on edge.

DR: When you feel on edge, do you feel like the smallest things are bothering you? As if you have no skin?

BERNIE: Sometimes.

DR: When you feel at your worst, do feel like you may lose control?

BERNIE: Not really. I am pretty levelheaded; always have been.

Panic–dissociation

DR: I understand. Let's come back to the waves for a moment. When a wave of anxiety comes, do you feel any strange sensation in your body or skin?

BERNIE: I feel like my face is burning.

DR: The skin on you face?

BERNIE: Yes.

DR: How about inside your body?

BERNIE: Sometimes I feel like I am just one walking burning wound. It feels like all my insides are burning.

Fear of dying

DR: Does it ever feel so bad that you fear for your life?

BERNIE: No, not that bad.

DR: Do you have nightmares about dying?

BERNIE: No, I have nightmares, but they are not about dying.

DR: What are they about?

BERNIE: Trains. Going into tunnels which never end.

Anhedonia

DR: What are the things you enjoy that usually make you feel good?

BERNIE: I like listening to Jazz.

DR: Have you been doing that lately?

BERNIE: I tried, but I had to force myself.

DR: And how does it feel when you do?

BERNIE: It feels just OK. Even Miles is just OK.

DR: Are you able to feel anything positive at all?

BERNIE: Only the memories of our life together. We had a fairy tale life you know.

2. Loss of cognitive control

Ruminations

DR: When you think about your situation, are your thoughts racing or is your head quiet?

BERNIE: Neither. The thoughts are orderly but just very persistent.

DR: Are you thoughts repetitive? Do they run in circles?

BERNIE: It is hard to think about anything else, but him, and how perfect it was.

DR: Do these thoughts come mostly at night before you go to sleep?

BERNIE: All the time, but worse at night.

DR: Are you having these thoughts right now?

BERNIE: Yes, although talking to you is distracting me.

Cognitive rigidity

DR: You know, these ruminations about the perfect fairy tale life you had . . . do you literally believe your life was perfect? Is it possible to have a perfect life? Most of us would gladly settle for "very good."

BERNIE: Well—you don't believe me, but ours was perfect.

DR: Really? Flawless?

BERNIE: Flawless. I loved him. He loved me. I loved his flaws. He had perfect flaws.

DR: "Perfect" is hard to match. Is it possible that he was not perfect? That maybe there were things about him you did not know?

BERNIE: When I think about this, my head feels like it would explode. He was perfect. And then this: his wife, his children . . . let's talk about something else.

Thought suppression

DR: What happens when you try to forcefully suppress these thoughts, or try not to think them?

BERNIE: It only works for a short while. Peter is all I can think about.

DR: Is trying to suppress your thoughts only making them worse?

BERNIE: Not sure. Trying to suppress thoughts about Peter does not make them better. It's not a very good strategy.

Ruminative flooding

DR: Do you feel that you can't really control your thoughts about Peter, that they come and go as they please?

BERNIE: If you put it this way, then yes.

DR: Do these out-of-control thoughts about Peter and about how to make sense of what happened make you feel pressure in your head?

BERNIE: Sometimes, mostly at night when I can't fall asleep.

DR: Does this make you feel like your head could explode?

BERNIE: It's not that dramatic.

DR: At those times, do these thoughts feel like a vortex pulling you in?

BERNIE: Yes they do.

DR: And when they do, do you try to climb out? Can you?

BERNIE: Sometimes I can, and sometimes I can't.

3. Agitation and insomnia

DR: Have you had problems falling asleep?

BERNIE: Yes. Scotch helps.

DR: Are you waking up in the middle of the night?

BERNIE: Yes.

DR: And what happens?

BERNIE: I lie in bed thinking. Then I have another scotch.

DR: Do you wake up earlier than usual?

BERNIE: Yes, but that's OK. I try to exercise.

DR: When you tell me your story you seem remarkably calm. Do you actually feel calm, or are you a good actor and in reality you feel agitated inside?

BERNIE: I am far from calm, but I do not believe in burdening others with my feelings.

DR: Including doctors?

BERNIE: Including doctors.

End of the SCS part of the interview.

Bernie's Suicide Crisis Syndrome Intensity Assessment Table

Symptom	Symptom Severity				
	Minimal	Low	Moderate	High	Severe
Part A					
Suicidal ideation			X		
Suicide intent and plan			X		
Entrapment		X			
Desperation		X			
Part A summary			X		
Part B					
Affective disturbance					
Emotional pain					X
Depressive turmoil			X		

Frantic anxiety	X				
Panic–dissociation					X
Fear of dying		X			
Anhedonia			X		
Affective disturbance summary			X		
Loss of cognitive control					
Ruminations					X
Rigidity				X	
Thought suppression			X		
Ruminative flooding				X	
Loss of cognitive control summary				X	
Overarousal					
Agitation			X		
Insomnia			X		
Part B summary			X		
Overall summary			X		

Bernie's short-term suicide risk is lower than that of Gary, but it may increase if he is unable to reconcile his idyllic past with Peter with the reality of his partner's long deception. He has episodic suicidal ideation and a mental picture of a plan he would use if he does not feel better. His emotional pain is severe, but his frantic anxiety, depressive turmoil, and desperation are not very significant. He has substantial symptoms of panic and dissociation, and his fear of dying is revealed symbolically in his dreams but is not yet explicit. With regard to loss of cognitive control, his is very high on ruminations and rigidity, but he does not have ruminative flooding. He is also able to contain his state of inner agitation so that it is not visible to the outsider. Overall, at the time of the interview, Bernie manifested an SCS of moderate intensity.

Case 40: Low Risk for Imminent Suicide–Continued

Kate is a 28-year-old woman who was admitted to a psychiatric unit for a suicide attempt. Kate repeatedly cut her left arm and left thigh with a razor blade after she was let go from a nonprofit after a falling out with her supervisor. The cuts were deep enough for her thigh wounds to require sutures. Kate had a long psychiatric history and was diagnosed with attention deficit disorder as a child and with MDD, GAD, panic disorder, and borderline personality disorder in high school. She was accepted to but never completed college, despite several attempts to do so. She worked only sporadically, mainly for environmental causes, and was supported by her father. During the interview, Kate was confrontational and provocative.

Part A

Suicidal ideation

> DR: Please show me the cuts on your arms. No stitches, but still pretty deep. You told the doctors in the ED that you wanted to kill yourself. When was the first time you thought about suicide?
>
> KATE: In high school. I was not a happy teenager. I was picked on.
>
> DR: And how often do you think about ending your life?
>
> KATE: Every day.
>
> DR: Have you been thinking about suicide since you were admitted?
>
> KATE: Once in a while.
>
> DR: When was the last time?
>
> KATE: Yesterday.
>
> DR: What was your exact thought?
>
> KATE: That one day I am going through with it.
>
> DR: How did you respond to this thought?
>
> KATE: I tried to distract myself—I went to the dayroom and watched TV.

Suicide intent and plan

> DR: When you cut yourself, was your intention to hurt yourself or to die?
>
> KATE: I don't remember. Both, I guess. I was confused.
>
> DR: Were you following a thought-out plan or was your attempt sudden and not planned in advance?
>
> KATE: I did not plan it.
>
> DR: What about now?
>
> KATE: I am not planning anything now.
>
> DR: Why?
>
> KATE: Because it is not the time. I would have succeeded if it were. It was a wrong thing to do. My boss is a psychopath and an idiot.
>
> DR: What do you think it will take for you to go through with it?
>
> KATE: If I hit a dead end.

Entrapment

> DR: I thought this is how you felt when you got fired from the nonprofit.
>
> KATE: It felt like that at the time.
>
> DR: When you think about your fight for the cause and all the frustrations involved, do you feel trapped?

KATE: I did before I came in. It is very frustrating, but I think once I feel better I can still volunteer and be useful.

Desperation

DR: How impatient are you for your emotional pain to get better?

KATE: I would like to feel better, of course, but I could be patient.

DR: How long can you tolerate the condition you are in?

KATE: Until I feel better, I guess. I hope not too long.

DR: It seem that before you came in, the pain was so strong you wanted it to stop then. Do you feel the urge for it to stop now?

KATE: I feel an urgent need, but I am not going to cut myself.

DR: Do you have an urge to escape it now?

KATE: Not anymore. The pills have helped.

Part B

1. Affective disturbance

Emotional pain

DR: You just told me a lot about how you came to cut yourself so deeply that it required stitches and about what brought you to the hospital. Your cut seems to have healed. Do you still feel like you are in a state of emotional pain?

KATE: I do, because I still believe in my cause.

DR: Do you feel that this inner pain is too much to bear?

KATE: No, after this admission, I can handle it. It makes me angry. It makes me work harder.

DR: What if the pain becomes worse?

KATE: I hope it does not. But if it does I hope you will help me.

Depressive turmoil

DR: OK. The way you are right now, is your mood even or could you have waves of anxiety or other bad feelings?

KATE: It's mainly anxiety. It was pretty bad earlier today before I took the pills.

DR: What about anger? You came in pretty angry at the world.

KATE: I am still angry.

DR: Were you angrier in the morning before you took the pills?

KATE: I guess . . . definitely, now that you say so.

DR: It sounds like you are still in a bit of turmoil. Do these feelings make you feel restless and agitated inside?

KATE: Yes.

Frantic anxiety

DR: You still sound pretty frustrated and anxious. Is this how you feel inside?

KATE: Yeah, I am pretty anxious but it's OK.

DR: How anxious do you feel, exactly? Do you feel emotionally raw?

KATE: Not as much as I did when I was admitted—that was really bad. Now I am almost my usual self.

DR: With you being so sensitive, does it sometimes feel like the smallest things bother you, like you have no skin?

KATE: Most of the time.

DR: Even now?

KATE: Even now. I am always like that.

DR: Like the smallest things make you feel off balance?

KATE: Kind of . . . but not as bad as before.

DR: Did you feel like you were losing control?

KATE: Then, but not now. I am pretty good now.

Panic–dissociation

DR: Coming back to the waves . . . when the wave of bad feelings is at its peak, do you feel something is wrong with you physically?

KATE: I feel tightness in my chest; it's hard to breathe.

DR: Do you also feel strange sensations in your body or skin?

KATE: My fingers get numb.

DR: Do you feel something happening to your body?

KATE: I feel my nerves ring under my skin. . . . It sounds crazy, but I do. I just know where they are.

DR: And when you can sense your nerves, or at any other time, do you feel that the world around you is different?

KATE: No, it's always the same. Good old bad world that needs to change.

Fear of dying

DR: When you can't breathe, do you get scared that it may get so bad that you die?

KATE: No, I know this is anxiety.

DR: Regardless of shortness of breath, can your waves of anxiety and anger feel so bad that you fear for your life?

KATE: Not really. It's not life threatening.

Anhedonia

DR: What do you do for fun that usually makes you feel good?

KATE: I like food. I have a sweet tooth. I know it's not good for you, but that's the truth. The food here is awful.

DR: What about the food that your family brings?

KATE: They brought Dunkin' Donuts. It made my day.

2. Loss of cognitive control

Ruminations

DR: When you think about your fight for the cause and all the frustrations that led to your suicidal behavior, is your thinking clear or foggy?

KATE: Pretty clear.

DR: Though clear, are your thoughts racing, running fast, or is your head quiet?

KATE: My head is never quiet, and my thoughts are always fast. I'm not sure about racing.

DR: Are the thoughts still persistent, running in your head again and again?

KATE: Yes I still think about my causes all the time.

DR: Are these thoughts worse at night when you try to go to sleep?

KATE: Yes, sometimes it is hard to fall asleep.

DR: And you are having these thoughts right now, as we speak?

KATE: Yes, I confirm!

Cognitive rigidity

DR: You know, with all due respect, many people would disagree with your point of view on the environment. The mineral depletion may not be as catastrophic as you say.

KATE: What do you mean? You can't be serious.

DR: I am not saying that this is my point of view, but one can argue that mankind has an inventive mind, and will find other materials to create from and other sources of energy. Do you think this is possible, at least in theory?

KATE: I can't believe my ears, so you too are saying we can continue destroying our planet.

DR: I never said that. I just asked if you thought an alternative was possible.

KATE: I guess it is possible but very unlikely. It is very clear that mining and carbon emissions are the two main causes of global warming.

Thought suppression

DR: Do you ever try to forcefully suppress these thoughts?

KATE: Not particularly, why?

DR: They are not very comfortable thoughts to have.

KATE: It's OK, I have been living with these ideas for years.

Ruminative flooding

DR: Do you ever feel pressure in your head from having too many thoughts like these?

KATE: Not right now. When I was admitted I did.

DR: Were you also having headaches from having too many thoughts?

KATE: No headaches. Well, maybe slightly, but not for a while.

DR: For some people this kind of endless thinking may feel like a vortex, which just keeps getting deeper and deeper. Have you ever felt like that?

KATE: Not quite . . . maybe a little, when I was admitted.

3. Agitation and insomnia

DR: How are you sleeping?

KATE: Pretty well now, with the new pills. It takes me a while to fall asleep, but once I am asleep I sleep through the night.

DR: You seem a little restless. Is this how you feel?

KATE: I am always restless—this is just me.

DR: So, you are back to your usual self?

KATE: Pretty much. I want to be discharged.

End of the SCS part of the interview.

Kate's Suicide Crisis Syndrome Intensity Assessment Table

Symptom	Symptom Intensity				
	Minimal	Low	Moderate	High	Severe
Part A					
Suicidal ideation		X			
Suicide intent and plan		X			
Entrapment	X				
Desperation		X			
Part A summary		X			
Part B					
Affective disturbance					
Emotional pain			X		
Depressive turmoil			X		
Frantic anxiety			X		
Panic–dissociation		X			
Fear of dying	X				
Anhedonia	X				
Affective disturbance summary		X			
Loss of cognitive control					
Ruminations			X		
Rigidity		X			
Thought suppression	X				
Ruminative flooding		X			
Loss of cognitive control summary		X			
Overarousal					
Agitation		X			
Insomnia		X			
Part B summary		X			
Overall summary		X			

Although Kate was admitted with serious self-injurious behavior, currently she is not in a suicide crisis, and her short-term suicide risk is low. From the interview, it can be gleaned that Kate's SCS severity at admission was moderate. Currently, Kate has random suicidal thoughts and denies a plan. She has both anxiety and mood disorders, and at the time of the interview she reports emotional pain, waves of panic, depressive turmoil, and ruminations. However, she has virtually no entrapment or thought suppression, and her other SCS symptoms, including disturbance in arousal, are minimal. Thus, overall, her SCS symptoms are mild, and her short-term risk is low.

Test Case

Test Case 3

Jackie is a 19-year-old woman who was referred for an evaluation after she told her parents she would kill herself if they would not allow her to see her friends (who her parents believed were a bad influence on her). Jackie was recently discharged from an inpatient psychiatric unit where she had been admitted 2 months prior with confusion following an overdose with her stepmother's Klonopin. She was diagnosed with attention deficit hyperactivity disorder (ADHD) and a learning disability as a child, with depression and bulimia as an adolescent, and with borderline and narcissistic personality disorder during her recent psychiatric hospitalization. Of relevance, Jackie's mother died of suicide by hanging when Jackie was 12 years old.

Part A

Suicidal ideation
> DR: Jackie, you told your parents that you would kill yourself if they don't let you see your friends . . . what did you mean?
> JACKIE: I meant that my friends are the only thing I have, and I can't live without them.
> DR: How often do you think about suicide?
> JACKIE: Every day. You know what happened to my mother.
> DR: That must have been devastating for you. Every day—how often?
> JACKIE: It comes and goes, depending on what else is going on.
> DR: Did you think about suicide today?
> JACKIE: Yes.
> DR: And what was your exact thought?
> JACKIE: That if my parents don't let me see my friends, I am going to kill myself.
> DR: Have you thought of how?
> JACKIE: Pills. I am not going to do what my mother did. That was horrible, just horrible.

Suicide intent and plan
> DR: I know you tried to overdose before. Have you planned how you would do it this time?

JACKIE: (Angrily) I will take more pills this time than last time.

DR: How long have you been planning it?

JACKIE: (Sarcastically) All my life. What is there to plan?

DR: Do you know which pills you are going to use this time?

JACKIE: I can't use mine—they only give me what I need to take every day, like I am in the hospital. And I can't use my stepmother's, she now locks them up.

DR: And?

JACKIE: I will use my friends' pills. They are all on meds. They're all damaged, like me.

DR: Which friend's?

JACKIE: Olivia. She is bipolar. She is on Klonopin, Depakote, lithium, and Seroquel. A nice cocktail.

DR: Do you know where she keeps the pills?

JACKIE: In the bathroom and in the kitchen. I borrow them sometimes when I feel anxious.

DR: What will it take for you to go through with it?

JACKIE: If my parents take my phone away and try to lock me up like they did last time, I will kill myself, I swear.

Entrapment

DR: When you think about your life situation, do you feel trapped?

JACKIE: Not if I can see my friends.

DR: Your parents seem to think that your friends are a bad influence on you. They drink and they do drugs and . . .

JACKIE: You don't know my friends, and neither do my parents. They are the only ones who don't put me down. They are the only ones who make me feel good.

DR: It's a problem, though, that your parents feel otherwise. Do you see any possible solutions to this problem?

JACKIE: Not with my parents. They never listen to me, and they always only see bad in me. Nothing I do is good enough.

DR: Do you have other friends?

JACKIE: What? I am not going to betray my friends to please my parents!

Desperation

DR: How do you feel right now?

JACKIE: Miserable, angry, and frustrated.

DR: How long can you take feeling like this?

JACKIE: I don't know.

DR: To help your situation, we may need to do some family therapy with you, your father, and your stepmother. It may take some time. Can you live with your pain and frustration during this time?

JACKIE: As long as I can continue to be with my friends.

DR: And if not?

JACKIE: I will kill myself.

Part B

1. Affective disturbance
   Emotional pain

   DR: Can your state of mind be described as emotional pain? Does this ring a bell?

   JACKIE: Yes. I am in pain.

   DR: Do you feel that this emotional pain is too much to bear?

   JACKIE: Sometimes.

   DR: How about right now?

   JACKIE: I am bearing it right now.

   DR: Do you feel this pain can get better?

   JACKIE: Yes—I told you already. I am fine when I am with my friends.

   Depressive turmoil

   DR: Does your emotional pain come in waves or is your mood even?

   JACKIE: Neither. I am not sure what you mean.

   DR: Do you feel waves of anxiety?

   JACKIE: Yes.

   DR: Do these feelings come in waves out of the blue?

   JACKIE: Yes, they are not predictable.

   DR: Do you feel bouts of anger?

   JACKIE: Yes. I am trying to regulate that though.

   DR: Do you feel waves of fear?

   JACKIE: No.

   DR: Do the waves of anxiety and anger make you feel restless and agitated?

   JACKIE: Sometimes.

   Frantic anxiety

   DR: Do you feel that you have lost control?

   JACKIE: I am in control.

   DR: I mean: Do you feel that you have lost control to change things?

   JACKIE: I hope not.

   DR: Do you feel overwhelmed with negative emotions?

   JACKIE: Not now.

   DR: Do you sometimes feel emotionally raw, like you have no skin?

   JACKIE: What do you mean?

   DR: Like the smallest things are bothering you as if your life lies in the balance?

   JACKIE: No, that's too dramatic.

   Panic–dissociation and sensory disturbances

   DR: When you have waves of anxiety coming over you, do you feel something is wrong with you physically?

   JACKIE: No.

   DR: When you have waves of anxiety, do you also have physical symptoms such as sweating? Nausea? Problems breathing? Rapid heartbeat?

   JACKIE: Do you mean panic attacks? I have panic attacks.

   DR: When you have panic attacks, do you feel strange sensations in your body or skin?

   JACKIE: No.

DR: Do you feel something happening to (in) your body?

JACKIE: Other than nausea, no.

DR: When you panic, do you feel that the world around you is different?

JACKIE: I feel disconnected sometimes, like I am in a movie.

Fear of dying

DR: Do you worry a lot about bad things that may happen to you?

JACKIE: Not usually.

DR: Do you have nightmares about death?

JACKIE: I have nightmares about my mother.

DR: Tell me about them.

JACKIE: I would rather not. Thinking about it makes me feel bad.

DR: Do you wake up at night in a sweat, so scared you might die that it is hard to breath?

JACKIE: Once or twice.

DR: Were you scared you may suddenly die?

JACKIE: Yes.

Acute anhedonia

DR: What makes you feel good usually?

JACKIE: Being with my friends.

DR: What else?

JACKIE: I like Chipotle, it's the best.

DR: Does it taste good?

JACKIE: Great! And they serve only "happy meat."

2. Loss of cognitive control

Ruminations

DR: When you think about this impasse with your parents and your friends, is your thinking clear or foggy?

JACKIE: My thinking is always clear.

DR: Even when you took the overdose?

JACKIE: Yes.

DR: Right now, are your thoughts racing, running fast, or is your head quiet?

JACKIE: Quiet. My thoughts can be fast though. I have ADHD. Sometimes it is hard to concentrate.

DR: In the last couple of days, did you have unpleasant thoughts in your head that kept running again and again?

JACKIE: Yes—like what to do about my parents.

DR: Do these thoughts come mostly at night before you go to sleep?

JACKIE: No.

DR: Do you think these thoughts also during the day?

JACKIE: Yes.

DR: Are you having these thoughts right now?

JACKIE: Yes, you are asking me all these questions.

DR: Do you feel pressure in your head from having too many thoughts?

JACKIE: No.

DR: Are you having headaches from having too many thoughts?

JACKIE: No.

DR: Do you feel like your head could explode from having too many thoughts?

JACKIE: No. That's crazy.

Cognitive rigidity

DR: You know, you are saying that your friends are the only people in the world that have ever liked you and will ever like you. It can't be this black and white.

JACKIE: That's how it is though.

DR: Well, for example, did you make friends with other patients in the hospital?

JACKIE: There was one girl I liked.

DR: And? Did she like you?

JACKIE: Yeah we talked. She cut herself.

DR: Well, that's another thing altogether. She liked you. People care about you more than you think, Jackie.

JACKIE: Hmm . . .

Thought suppression

DR: When you have the thoughts about taking pills, do you try to suppress them?

JACKIE: Not sure what you mean.

DR: People often try to suppress the disturbing thoughts that make them feel bad. Do you?

JACKIE: Not consciously.

Ruminative flooding

DR: It sounds that you feel the worst when your parents don't let you see your friends, in fact you feel so bad you think about suicide. Do these bad thoughts make you feel pressure in your head?

JACKIE: No.

DR: Do these thoughts make you feel like your head could explode?

JACKIE: No.

DR: For some people thinking about suicide like a vortex, which just keeps getting deeper and deeper and can suck you in.

JACKIE: Not really.

3. Agitation and insomnia

DR: A while back you said you felt miserable and angry to me. Is this how you still feel?

JACKIE: Yes, pretty much.

DR: Do you feel agitated inside?

JACKIE: Kind of.

DR: Is it hard to stay calm?

JACKIE: It's OK. I can stay in control.

DR: Have you had problems falling asleep? Waking up in the middle of the night? Too early?

JACKIE: I am online a lot at night, talking to my friends.

DR: When you have problems sleeping, do these thoughts we talked about a minute ago bother you?

JACKIE: I sleep OK.

End of the SCS part of the suicide risk assessment.

Jackie's Suicide Crisis Syndrome Intensity Assessment Table

Symptom	Symptom Intensity				
	Minimal	Low	Moderate	High	Severe
Part A					
Suicidal ideation					
Suicide intent and plan					
Entrapment					
Desperation					
Part A summary					
Part B					
Affective disturbance					
Emotional pain					
Depressive turmoil					
Frantic anxiety					
Panic–dissociation					
Fear of dying					
Anhedonia					
Affective disturbance summary					

Loss of cognitive control

    Ruminations

    Rigidity

    Thought
    suppression

    Ruminative
    flooding

*Loss of cognitive
control summary*

Overarousal

    Agitation

    Insomnia

Part B summary

Overall summary

Jackie's mother's death by suicide increases her suicide risk long term, whereas her recent overdose increases her suicide risk both long term and short term. Her Part A SCS assessment shows clear and intense suicidal ideation and intent with a moderate lethality plan, as well as entrapment, which, however, is conditional on external circumstances. In contrast, her Part B assessment shows only minimal and low-intensity symptoms of affective disturbance, loss of cognitive control, and overarousal. Thus, Jackie's overall short-term risk is moderate. The divergent Part A and Part B symptom levels illustrate both the inconsistent relationship between the self-reported suicidal ideation and suicide risk and the usefulness of the full SCS assessment for short-term risk determination.

7

Emotional Response

EMOTIONAL RESPONSE AS A DIAGNOSTIC TOOL

Clinicians' emotional responses to patients (or countertransference) have increasingly been recognized as an important factor in treatment outcome (Bruck, Winston, Aderholt, & Muran, 2006). Until recently, however, they have received little attention with regard to suicide risk. Rather, acute suicide prediction has focused largely on patient risk factors, such as precipitating events (Bagge, Glenn, & Lee, 2013; Foster, 2011; Maltsberger, Hendin, Haas, & Lipschitz, 2003; Pompili, Innamorati, et al., 2011), behavior changes (Deisenhammer et al., 2009; Hendin et al., 2001), and intense affective states (Hendin, Haas, Maltsberger, Szanto, & Rabinowicz, 2004; Hendin, Maltsberger, & Szanto, 2007; Katz et al., 2011; Yaseen et al., 2010; Yaseen, Chartrand et al., 2013; Yaseen, Fisher, Morales, & Galynker, 2012; Yaseen et al., 2012; Hendin, Al Jurdi, Houck, Hughes, & Turner, 2010). Yet, even though they are easily identified retrospectively, such factors may be difficult to utilize clinically; these markers may be masked or minimized by the patient or misinterpreted by the therapist (Hendin, Haas, Maltsberger, Koestner, & Szanto, 2006; Marcinko, Skocic, Popovic-Knapic, & Tentor, 2008). In some cases, over-zealous efforts at intervention, which push an unready patient toward independence and may be misperceived as abandonment, even appear to precipitate patient suicide (Maltsberger et al., 2003).

A potential factor contributing to these difficulties, in addition to the difficulty of predicting behavior and constraints of the current health care system (Mojtabai & Olfson, 2008), may lie in clinicians' own emotional responses to the suicidal patient. Whereas clinical judgment is a conscious process, the suicidal patient may elicit powerful unconscious emotional responses (Kernberg, 1965; Maltsberger & Buie, 1974). These emotions, which are often negative, are difficult for clinicians to recognize and accept explicitly. Indeed, neuroimaging studies suggest activation of brain regions subserving unconscious processing during emotional compared to cognitive empathy tasks (Nummenmaa, Hirvonen, Parkkola, & Hietanen, 2008). Unaided conscious integration of unconscious emotional responses is likely to fail regardless of clinicians' experience (Van Wagoner, Gelso, Hayes, & Diemer, 1991). A systematic assessment of these responses, however, has the potential to ameliorate the inherent distortions of the clinician's judgment.

In qualitative studies of physician-assisted suicide, clinicians confronted with patients' desire for death experienced mostly anxious, helpless, and overwhelmed responses (Groenewoud et al., 1997). Maltsberger and Buie's (1974) seminal paper elaborated an array of emotions and behaviors rooted in different defenses to negative countertransference toward the suicidal patient, which they combined under a construct of "countertransference hate." Later research confirmed negative countertransference and feelings of anxiety and hostility as those prominently elicited by suicidal patients (Varghese & Kelly, 1999). Because the management of the clinicians' emotional response is correlated with therapeutic outcome (Bruck et al., 2006; Marcinko et al., 2008; Modestin, 1987), identifying emotional responses may reduce suicide risk.

Our own research showed that clinicians treating imminently suicidal patients recall somewhat positive feelings toward these patients, with hopes for treatment, while simultaneously finding themselves overwhelmed by, distressed by, and avoidant of them. Furthermore, we found that the paradoxical combination of optimism and distress/avoidance discriminated between suicidal patients and those who had unexpected non-suicide deaths. In addition, despite feeling slightly more positive in their responses preceding low-lethality suicide attempts, clinicians may also experience more sadness prior to either successful or highly lethal attempts. The latter emotional response may be characteristic enough that, if recognized and appreciated, it could aid in assessing suicide risk. Thus, self-assessment of emotional responses may have potential clinical utility in the treatment of suicidal patients.

Alternatively, poorly managed emotional responses to suicidal patients can result in harm. Research suggests that negative emotional responses correlate with negative patient outcomes (Marcinko et al., 2008), and the clinician's failure to control hostility, hate, and aggressiveness may even help push patients to suicide (Varghese & Kelly, 1999).

Of note, emotional responses to suicidal patients are different from both rational judgments and conscious "guesses" of suicide risk. Conscious clinical judgment is a poor predictor of both suicide (Ægisdóttir et al., 2006) and violence (Veilleux, 2011). It appears that, conscious or not, emotional responses are better predictors (Kernberg, 1965; Maltsberger & Buie, 1974). The following sections describe techniques for systematic qualitative assessment of these responses. Research efforts are underway to develop quantitative assessments that may potentially augment suicide risk assessment.

EMOTIONAL DIFFERENTIATION

To use our emotions as tools in the assessment of patients' risk for imminent suicide, we must be able to identify them. Emotions are essential to the human experience and have tremendous influence over our behavior. We seek positive emotions (e.g., happiness, fulfillment, and satisfaction) and avoid negative ones (e.g., shame, humiliation, and abandonment). The ability to recognize and identify one's emotions is not a skill that we are born with but, rather, a complex learned task that requires near-continuous conscious and unconscious judgments. This task is most complicated when one's professional occupation requires one to ignore emotions; in medicine, clinicians must care for patients regardless of their feelings about the patients.

Emotional experiences are life's essential sources of information (Farmer & Kashdan, 2013; Keltner & Kring, 1998), which may be both clear (e.g., falling in love) or confused (e.g., a general sense of unease). The ability to classify felt experiences into discrete categories is termed *emotion differentiation* (Barrett, Gross, Christensen, & Benvenuto,

2001; Tugade, Fredrickson, & Barrett, 2004). People's capacity to differentiate emotions varies widely (Kashdan, Ferssizidis, Collins, & Muraven, 2010; Tugade et al., 2004). Those skilled at emotion differentiation are able to feel and identify dozens of emotions and are capable of experiencing and naming several emotions simultaneously. At the opposite end of the spectrum are those whose descriptions of their emotional states are broad and nonspecific, often limited to feeling "good" or "bad."

The capacity to differentiate emotions from thoughts also differs from person to person. People often say "I feel" when they mean "I think." For example, when clinicians say, "I feel that this person is going to recover because the treatment is working," they are expressing a thought and an opinion rather than an emotion. One may think that the thoughts–feeling distinction is only semantic and carries no consequences. However, in medicine in general, and in assessment of imminent suicide risk in particular, distinguishing thoughts from emotions is the first essential step toward emotion differentiation.

Those who are better able to differentiate their emotions are more skilled in using them to guide their behavior (Barrett et al., 2001). The identification of negative emotions may be particularly important for clinicians who are trained to behave positively regardless of what they feel. Psychiatrists' emotions toward their patients may change dramatically both from encounter to encounter and within each session. Clinicians who are able to differentiate negative emotions may also be able to employ emotion regulation strategies to their advantage (Barrett et al., 2001) rather than suppressing them (Tugade et al., 2004). This ability is essential for using one's emotions as a tool to identify those at risk for imminent suicide.

MINDFULNESS

Gauging one's emotional response to a suicidal patient requires the ability to attend to one's inner experiences, such as thoughts and emotions, without judgment and with acceptance. This skill is called "mindfulness" (Baer, Hopkins, Krietemeyer, Smith, & Toney, 2006; Bishop et al., 2004; Brown & Ryan, 2003; Germer, Siegel, & Fulton, 2005; Hill & Updegraff, 2012), and it has gained popularity during the past two decades in therapies that reduce emotional distress, such as dialectical behavior therapy (DBT; Linehan, 1993a, 1993b), mindfulness-based stress reduction (Kabat-Zinn, 1990), and mindfulness-based cognitive therapy (MBCT; Segal, Williams, & Teasdale, 2002). These are particularly useful in treating depression, anger, anxiety, and so on in individuals with borderline personality traits.

However, in additional to its use in therapy, mindfulness is also a skill that is useful in developing an awareness of subtle differences in one's emotional experiences (Bishop et al., 2004). The idea of emotional awareness, which is defined as "the extent to which people are aware of emotions in both themselves and others" (Ciarrochi, Caputi, & Mayer, 2003, p. 1478), is not new. Buddhist meditation seeks to improve emotional awareness by teaching its followers to focus attention on specifics of emotional responses (Goleman, 2003; Nielsen & Kaszniak, 2006).

The capacity for mindfulness is associated with emotional intelligence, including emotional clarity and recognition (Baer, Smith, & Allen, 2004; Brown & Ryan, 2003). In order to be mindful, one must view emotions as mental states not demanding an immediate reaction. The reality of psychiatric work, which requires rapid decision-making in time-sensitive situations, rarely allows for emotional self-examination. Yet precisely under these circumstances, inner observation without action is necessary to moderate the urge to preemptively label the experienced emotions. Such rapid labeling may cause clinicians to rely on past emotional experiences instead of recognizing the distinguishing features of the present moment.

The clinician's ability to differentiate similar emotional states is critical to the use of emotions as diagnostic tools for assessing near-term suicide risk. The clinician's negative emotions, such as anxiety and dread, are closer to those targeted by MBCT and DBT (Linehan, 1993a, 1993b; Segal et al., 2002), whereas positive responses, such as unreasonable optimism, have not been targeted. Regardless of the emotion valence, clinicians face additional difficulties admitting to either due to the aforementioned ethical pressures, which result in disapproval of certain emotional responses to patients.

Two examples of "forbidden" emotions are hatred and attraction. Clinicians are likely to use defense mechanisms, such as denial or repression, rather than acknowledge feelings of hate and/or feel sexual attraction toward a patient. Instead of feeling hatred toward patient A, a clinician may acknowledge and recognize a less threatening emotion such as dislike. Similarly, instead of feeling lust toward patient B, a clinician may acknowledge a more acceptable emotion such as feeling concerned.

FROM RESCUE FANTASY TO HELPLESSNESS AND ANGER

Although all patient–clinician encounters are unique, generally in psychotherapy, therapists are likely to respond positively to positive emotions and negatively to negative emotions. This emotional alignment may have many mechanisms, including emotional contagion, which makes one feel depressed around depressed people and happy around happy people (Bartel & Saavedra, 2000; Hatfield, Cacioppo, & Rapson, 1993; Kramer, Guillory, & Hancock, 2014; Sy, Côté, & Saavedra, 2005). As psychotherapy or any other patient–clinician professional encounter progresses, patients' emotions evolve, as do those of their clinicians. An example of an emotional dynamic that may develop between a suicidal patient and a therapist is described next.

Case 43

When the suicidal patient Anne sees a new therapist, Dr. B, for the first time, she hopes that the therapist will be able to relieve her despair and to make her life at least tolerable. In Anne's mind, her new therapist will be able to put a healing balm, so to speak, on her psyche and to cure her emotional pain.

In reality, Dr. B has certain clinical skills in which she has been trained. She will use these to the best of her ability, which is commensurate with her training and talent and is influenced by her personality and temperament, in addition to events taking place in her personal life. Although Dr. B's training allows her to minimize personal factors, they still influence her emotional response to Anne. Whether positive or negative, her emotions are never neutral and include some apprehension.

Initially, Anne likes Dr. B and finds her manner soothing, and Anne's emotional pain begins to ease. Anne starts thinking that she may have finally found a doctor who can help her long-standing struggle with depression, as well as her recent sense that she is sinking into a deep hole of despair from which there is no escape. Feeling better, Anne begins to idealize Dr. B and tells her that she has finally met a doctor who understands her. Flattered, and seeing that Anne's affect is brightening, Dr. B feels relieved and hopeful for her new patient, who she finds likable. "I may actually save this woman," she thinks, not quite realizing that she is experiencing a "rescue fantasy."

Anne's improved mood is short-lived, and her repetitive, ruminating thoughts soon push her back toward the feeling of anguish from which there seems to be no exit. Her suicidal urges return, and the hope she felt after meeting Dr. B dissipates. "She does not care about me," thinks Anne, "She is listening to me because she is getting paid. . . . Does she really care?"

Anne is late for her session with Dr. B, and the first words out of her mouth are "I forgot my checkbook. Do you care or are you only seeing me for the money?" Dr. B is well trained and understands that she is being tested. However, wanting to show Anne that she cares and to develop a therapeutic alliance, Dr. B says something she knows she should not: "It's OK, you will pay me later. . . . You need therapy." She also offers Anne her cell phone number, should she feel particularly down. Anne agrees to continue, and Dr. B breathes a sigh of relief: "I dodged a bullet, I really understand her and I can prevent her suicide." This scenario, in which a patient's testing of the clinician's commitment results in that clinician's overinvolvement, is common.

After 2 weeks, Anne is still despondent. She attends her sessions and calls Dr. B every other day, but her ruminations keep her up at night. "Dr. B is no different from any of my previous therapists. She can't understand what I am going through, and no one can," she thinks, as her idealization of Dr. B turns into disappointment. "I don't know what your experience is with treating depression, but your therapy is not working," Anne tells her. Dr. B starts feeling angry: She thinks, "I am not charging her, she is calling me at all hours, and she is not even grateful." Being a professional, Dr. B tries not to show her anger, but she cannot fully control it. "I have been working in this field for 10 years. I am very experienced," she says, not realizing how defensive she sounds.

Anne is 30 minutes late for her next appointment and does not answer her phone. Dr. B's heart sinks, and she assumes the worst. She leaves an anxious message: "Anne, please call me back as soon as you can, I am worried about you." Anne calls back at 9 p.m.: "I have been having suicidal thoughts," she says, "but I am not going to do anything." Dr. B is relieved but very angry. She dreads the next session. This time, Anne arrives 10 minutes late. "I forgot and fell asleep," she says, "but these sessions are not helping. My bad thoughts are still there. You don't understand what I am going through, and you never will."

Dr. B is livid. "No wonder you have no friends," she thinks, "If this is how you treat people who help you, who could stand being with you?" "We have been making progress," she says out loud, "I have been trying very hard to help you, but if you feel that we are not connecting, I can refer you to one of my colleagues." "Yes, maybe next time," says Anne, sarcastically. "I will find you somebody who is more experienced than I am," says

Dr. B, thinking that she sounds concerned, and not realizing she also comes across as sarcastic. "She can't wait to get rid of me," thinks Anne as she leaves the session.

Dr. B felt relieved: She knew exactly to whom she wanted to refer Anne. However, her relief was short-lived. She could not put the troublesome patient out of her mind. When the phone rang at 5 a.m., Dr. B thought "Anne," and she was right: Anne was in the medical intensive care unit after she had overdosed on Tylenol. She died 2 days later of liver failure.

When discussing Anne's case, the root cause analysis concluded that Dr. B did everything correctly: The patient was not suicidal, she had promised to come to the next appointment, and Dr. B. had no grounds to hospitalize her. Dr. B, however, was very distressed by Anne's suicide and particularly the fact that, in retrospect, she "knew" that the intensity of her initial positive response to Anne was unique, as was the rapidity with which these feelings changed to dread. If/when she has a similar reaction to a patient in the future, she may recognize this as a sign of high imminent suicidal risk.

This vignette describes the evolution of a therapeutic relationship between a suicidal patient and an experienced therapist from hope for a cure on both sides to despair and suicide by the patient and an increasingly intense negative emotional response on the part of the doctor. The doctor initially had the somewhat unrealistic belief that she had unique rapport with Anne, and she felt affection for her new patient. As treatment progressed, that affection changed to increasingly intense anger, anxiety, and dread before meeting with her and unrecognized hostility with resulting rejecting behavior.

There may be many reasons for Dr. B's insensitivity to Anne's increasing despair, which resulted in the deterioration of their therapeutic relationship. Volumes have been written about the psychotherapeutic process and about therapists' emotional responses to their patients (Varghese & Kelly, 1999). Research ties the psychotherapeutic outcome to therapists' ability to recognize and repair ruptures in therapeutic relationships (Eubanks-Carter, Muran, & Safran, 2015; Lombardo, Milne, & Proctor, 2009). The latter in part depends on their ability to assess their own emotions as these change during their work with patients.

Correspondingly, in working with suicidal individuals, clinicians able to distinguish the unique emotions aroused in them by those patients' suicidal narratives and crises are better at assessing their patients' risk for near-term suicide. Both the positive and the negative emotions felt by Dr. B were responses to Anne's feelings of despair and to her suicidal urges. The fact that Anne was her first thought when the phone rang at 5 a.m. shows that Dr. B had some awareness that her reaction to Anne was different from that to other suicidal patients. However, she was not able to identify it as such during their last session.

Dr. B's emotional response to Anne has two distinct phases: the initial positivity and unrealistic expectation of saving Anne and later anxiety, hostility, and dread. In other real-life clinical scenarios, paradoxical hopefulness and dread before seeing the patient can happen in isolation, at the same time, or fluctuate from session to session. However, the previous discussed characteristic mixture of feelings about the suicidal patient is unique and can be recognized and used as a diagnostic tool.

COUNTERTRANSFERENCE LOVE

When clinicians minimize a patient's suicide risk factors or believe that they have a unique relationship with a patient, they allow their affection for the patient to cloud their judgment. This countertransference love, and resulting optimism, is a complex emotional response to the patient's suicidal narrative or suicide crisis and is also a predictor of near-term suicide risk (Maltsberger & Buie, 1974; Marcinko et al., 2008; Nivoli, Nivoli, Nivoli, & Lorettu, 2011). In our retrospective study, optimism was one of the emotions clinicians felt in the last session before a suicide attempt or completed suicide (Yaseen et al., 2013). Prospectively, optimism was, paradoxically, associated with near-term suicidal behavior (Hawes, Yaseen, Briggs, & Galynker, 2017).

The psychological mechanisms underlying countertransference love may involve reaction formation (discussed later). Clinicians who suddenly believe that their suicidal patient is no longer suicidal need to ask themselves if the patient's history supports their sudden optimism. What are the chronic risk factors? Does the patient's life fit into the suicidal narrative? Does the patient have symptoms and signs of a suicidal crisis? An affirmative answer to any of these questions calls for suicide risk reassessment.

If the answer to any of the previous questions is "yes," then a clinician must ask him- or herself whether he or she has a unique understanding of the patient being evaluated and if it can be attributed to a common social or cultural background or to a feeling of being connected for no particular reason. The sense of having a unique bond with a suicidal patient is a sign of unrecognized countertransference love; this calls for rational reassessment of one's emotions.

Case 44

Dr. A, a postgraduate year 2 (PGY-2) resident of Albanian descent, was assigned a suicidal Albanian patient, Edith, because of their common background and language. Dr. A felt like he was put on the spot but also felt flattered that the team trusted his judgment and his clinical skills. He eagerly started working with Edith, a recent 60-year-old immigrant, who reminded him of his mother. Edith was hospitalized twice in Albania with depression. She was living with her son, a building superintendent, and felt like a burden to him. She told Dr. A that she had no friends and no job. Dr. A could relate to this because he remembered his family having a difficult time after their immigration. Hopeful about the patient's future, he spent a lot of time daily helping her understand American society. Edith's mood improved. No longer suicidal, she told Dr. A that he was better than her own son, who was too busy to visit her in the hospital. Dr. A was relieved and thought that the patient could be discharged with a follow-up in one of the local clinics, which had an interpreting service. On the day of discharge, Edith was very disappointed that Dr. A would not be her outpatient doctor. She thanked him profusely, and he felt good about his work with her. She denied suicidal ideation, she but jumped off the roof of her son's building 3 hours after her discharge.

This vignette illustrates unrecognized countertransference love. Because of his own family's immigrant experience, Dr. A overidentifies with Edith and does not fully appreciate her psychopathology and the intensity of her suicidal narrative. Her narrative includes burdensomeness (to her son), alienation (from her past and culture), and entrapment (seeing no good options). Dr. A's "rejection" of her as an outpatient further contributes to her narrative.

In this case, the clinician's belief that he has a special relationship with this patient was unwittingly created by the treatment team, which put an inexperienced doctor in a position of responsibility without supervision by more experienced clinicians. He thus did not properly assess the patient's stresses or the intensity of her suicidal crisis.

COUNTERTRANSFERENCE HATE

Countertransference is a psychoanalytic term that describes therapists' emotional responses to their patients' way of relating to them, or transference. In 1974, Maltsberger and Buie described "countertransference hate"—simultaneous feelings of aversion and malice that suicidal patients invoke in psychotherapists. The authors suggested therapists manage this negative countertransference through full awareness, self-restraint, and appreciation of their own defense mechanisms.

The term countertransference implies knowledge of the exact psychological mechanism of therapists' emotional responses, which have never been proven experimentally. This term is accepted in psychoanalytic literature but not in clinical literature, which is evidence-based. The descriptive term "emotional response" is more suited for clinical work. However, the term "countertransference hate" is so widely known and accepted that it is used interchangeably with "negative emotional response," which does not relay the full emotionality of clinicians' reaction to acutely suicidal individuals.

Of the two components of countertransference hate, aversion is more problematic. Aversion may result in (conscious or unconscious) abandonment of the patient, which in turn may precipitate suicidal action. Malice is less dangerous (although more painful to tolerate) because it is almost always conscious and therefore easier to manage.

Countertransference hate may develop when patients test the clinician's commitment to them in the course of a long-term therapeutic relationship, during an emergency department one-time suicide risk assessment, or prior to discharge from the acute psychiatric unit. Testing of the clinician by suicidal patients often manifests as provocation, such as direct disparagement of the clinician's appearance, occupation, experience, and training—for example, "You are too young to understand," "I would like a female psychiatrist," or "Which medical school did you go to?" The most difficult direct provocations to handle are threats of suicide.

Indirect provocations (e.g., persistent evasiveness, lack of eye contact, and disturbing silences) are more subtle and more difficult to detect. These tend to create a sense of seemingly unfounded unease, discomfort, anger, or irritation directed either at the patient or inward. Other indirect provocations include sudden unexpected cheerfulness, optimism, and minimization of stressors that only minutes ago seemed overwhelming. Finally, there may be continuing expectations of the therapist to "know" what the patient is thinking or to develop a miracle cure. These unreachable expectations can make the clinician feel like a failure.

Regardless of how experienced a clinician may be, he or she will always respond to this testing with some degree of irritation or other negative emotions, which are often too uncomfortable to experience in their raw form. These responses are managed through well-known psychological defenses (i.e., countertransference hate), which reduce discomfort but also obscure its source, creating a possibility that a clinician would unknowingly act out his negative emotion to the patient's detriment. Fortunately, these defenses can be brought into consciousness and used diagnostically to identify patients at imminent suicide risk.

PSYCHOLOGICAL DEFENSES

Identification of the defense mechanisms used to make the "forbidden emotions" of countertransference love and countertransference hate more palatable is a technique to be used when mindfulness is either not possible or ineffective. Maltsberger and Bouie (1974) gave examples of five frequently encountered psychological defenses: reaction formation, denial, turning against self, projection, and repression.

Reaction Formation

Reaction formation is a defense that turns an unacceptable emotion into its exact opposite. This defense is most characteristically used in situations in which a person is trapped with no possibility of escape, and experiencing the unacceptable emotion is life threatening. The most famous example of reaction formation is "Stockholm syndrome," in which a hostage or kidnap victim "falls in love" with his or her captor.

In suicide assessment work, a reaction formation would be attraction or even love toward a high-risk patient, who might otherwise provoke extreme anxiety. The clinician may experience a "rescue fantasy" of him- or herself miraculously curing the patient, projecting eagerness and urgency. Reaction formation often leads to overinvolvement with the patient, which is time-consuming, stressful, and ultimately unsustainable, resulting in physical withdrawal (referring the patient out) or emotional abandonment and disengagement.

Case 45

In July of her PGY-3, Dr. C is given a sign-out by the outgoing resident, who warns him about her most difficult case, Sarah, who is a 38-year-old bipolar woman with several previous suicide attempts. Sarah is known as one of the most challenging patients in the clinic; she has chronic suicidal ideation, no social support, poor boundaries, and poor treatment adherence. Upon meeting the patient, Dr. C is surprised that Sarah is an attractive woman who seems eager to receive help and open to trying new medications. She agrees to take a new selective serotonin reuptake inhibitor (SSRI), and when leaving she gives Dr. C a bright smile. "She can't be so bad," thinks Dr. C, "and I am good at convincing people to take their meds. I will turn her around."

Repression

Repression is an unconscious defense mechanism that prevents disturbing emotions from becoming conscious. In psychiatry and in medicine overall, repression removes from consciousness intense negative feelings directed toward the patient, which are considered shameful and unprofessional. When working with suicidal patients, repression results in the desire to escape from the stress-laden engagement. When brought to consciousness, it is experienced as a thought such as "I don't want this patient in my office." When doctors repress unacceptable feelings, patients see them as aloof and disconnected, and they feel rejected.

Case 46

Arthur is a 50-year-old obese malodorous male with opiate use disorder, substance-induced mood disorder, and a history of near-lethal heroin overdose. Dr. D does not look forward to his sessions with Arthur, which often start late, run short, and are limited to the assessment of Arthur's adherence to treatment, recent stressful life events, and suicidal ideation. Arthur's answers are predictable, which gives Dr. D time during the session to check his e-mail and Facebook postings.

In this example of repression of revulsion, Dr. D perceives himself as being professional, whereas Arthur views him as arrogant and indifferent.

Turning Against the Self

Turning against the self is a defense mechanism in which a person becomes the target of his or her own unacceptable emotions. Turning against the self is a form of the displacement defense mechanism, in which unacceptable emotions are redirected on a substitute target. Typical examples of displacement are kicking the dog out of frustration with superiors at work or hating all members of the opposite sex when having romantic relationship difficulties.

Turning against the self is normally used in reference to hatred, anger, and aggression, and it is the Freudian explanation for feelings of inferiority, guilt, and depression. The idea that "depression is anger turned inwards" has entered mainstream and pop psychology and is accepted by many laypeople.

When faced with a difficult suicidal patient, a clinician may feel incompetent and worthless and think that he or she should refer the patient to somebody else more competent. The danger of the turning against the self defense is that the doctor's actions reflect his or her inner hopelessness, and the patient may feel abandoned and rejected. The sense that their psychiatrist is giving up on them only adds to the suicidal narrative elements of burdensomeness and alienation, as in the following case.

Case 47

Amy, a 55-year-old woman with treatment-resistant bipolar depression and several past suicide attempts, was admitted to an inpatient unit after she was taken off a bridge by the police. The patient's major fear was that she was a burden to her husband and to her doctors, who she feared would collude to send her to a state hospital. Her psychiatrist of many years was feeling like he had run out of options. Seeing the patient was making him depressed, and he felt trapped by his commitment to her. "I have failed her," he thought, "I need to refer her out to more competent clinicians at the NIMH." When he told Amy that he would like to transfer her to the NIMH for a clinical trial for a new antidepressant, Amy said, "This is the end. You are shipping me off."

Projection

Projection is a defense in which a person attributes his or her own undesired emotions to another person. Projection often results from poor insight into one's own motivations and feelings.

In working with suicidal patients, the unacceptable thoughts are hatred for the patients and even violent fantasies ("murder" as per Maltzberger). These thoughts are projected onto the patient, and the clinician believes that it is the patient who hates him or her. The clinician's conscious emotion is fear, which could result in unwarranted aggressiveness and poor judgment, as in the following case.

Case 48

Phoebe, an 18-year-old African American female, was admitted to an inpatient unit after a suicide attempt by drinking methanol. During the interview, she refused to get up and to answer most questions, turning her back on the interviewer. The harried interviewing attending was getting frustrated. He touched the patient's shoulder. The girl looked at her and turned her back again without saying a word. "She hates me," thought the attending, and said, "If you do not talk to us, we'll have security discharge you."

Denial

Denial is the refusal to accept reality, acting as if a painful event, thought, or feeling does not exist. It is considered the most primitive of the defenses because it is the first one to develop in small children, who escape into fantasy to avoid unpleasant reality. People often use denial to avoid dealing with problems in their lives that they do not wish to admit.

For instance, functioning alcoholics often deny they have a drinking problem, pointing to how well they function in their jobs. People often use the denial defense when facing humiliating and potentially catastrophic problems, such as infidelity of spouses, deception by business partners, or emerging serious mental illness in children.

In suicide work, denial usually means that the clinician does "not notice" obvious features of the suicidal narrative or signs of a suicidal crisis. Both countertransference love and countertransference hate may underlie clinicians' denial. A clinician who likes a patient who is at high suicide risk may easily believe the patient's assurances that he or she has no suicidal intent. Strong dislike toward a patient may result in the same outcome. In both scenarios, the suicidal patient may perceive the clinician's acceptance of his or her (false) assurances of safety as rejection.

Case 49

Linda, a 28-year-old disheveled woman with bipolar depression, was being evaluated in an affective disorders clinic. Linda told the evaluating clinician that she had tried all possible treatments, even electroconvulsive therapy, and nothing seemed to help. She told the doctor that she was suicidal and had even thought of the method: suffocation with a plastic bag. "I can help you," said the doctor, thinking about how to avoid such a high-risk case: "You need psychotherapy, let's make an appointment for next week with our therapist. Can you promise me that you will not harm yourself?" The patient committed to safety, but the following morning her parents found her, barely breathing, with a plastic bag over her head.

Rationalization

Rationalization is a defense mechanism in which unacceptable behavior, motives, or feelings are logically justified or made tolerable by plausible means (also known as "making excuses").

In the medical field, rationalization is sometimes seen in the "covering up" of mistakes (Banja, 2004). The following are common excuses:

- "Why disclose the error? The patient was going to die anyway."
- "Telling the family about the error will only make them feel worse."
- "Well, we did our best. These things happen."
- "If we're not too certain the error caused the harm, we don't have to tell."

In suicide risk assessment, rationalization is used primarily to cover countertransference hate and disgust, which manifests as lack of effort to properly assess risk. For example,

- "I am doing my job, aren't I? I can't go 'above and beyond' for every patient I see."
- "Given my workload, I am doing the best I can."
- "People determined to kill themselves will always manage to."
- "We can't predict suicide anyway."
- "This patient's life is miserable; they have nothing to live for."

Case 50

Edward, a 75-year-old-man with a history of Parkinson's disease, was admitted to an inpatient psychiatric unit for suicidal ideation following a massive heart attack. He told the team that his life was over: He was sick, he was alone, and he could no longer do things he used to enjoy. The team was so affected by his despair that it left without doing a thorough evaluation of his suicidal risk. "If I were this sick, I would want to kill myself," one of the doctors said.

CONFLICTED EMOTIONAL RESPONSES MAY PREDICT AN IMMINENT ATTEMPT

The thwarting of the clinician's attempts at connection by a suicidal patient may result in countertransference hate (Maltsberger & Buie, 1974). As discussed previously, such reactions may, in turn, elicit a variety of compensatory defense mechanisms serving to neutralize unacceptable emotional states threatening a positive view of the self (Baumeister et al., 1998; Maltsberger & Buie, 1974). Our recent research shows that these are primarily reaction formation and denial (Hawes, Yaseen, Briggs, & Galynker, 2017; Yaseen, Galynker, Cohen, & Briggs, in press).

Reaction formation may result in hopeful rescue fantasies with anxious urgency to cure (Rycroft, 1995). Likewise, interventions driven by clinicians' reaction formation against countertransference hate may take the form of overinvolvement or inappropriate optimism (Maltsberger & Buie, 1974). Such actions are most problematic during hospital discharge and the unavoidable withdrawal of inpatient care; they may result in patients' feelings of abandonment and despair (Schechter, Goldblatt, Ronningstam, Herbstman, & Maltsberger, 2016), increasing suicide risk.

Alternatively, denial of countertransference hate toward the acutely suicidal patient, in which the clinician is unaware of negative feelings toward that patient, may result in hopelessness and feelings of indifference. Inappropriate clinical responses in such cases are overt rejection and abandonment (Maltsberger & Buie, 1974).

Unconscious defenses against an intense negative reaction to a patient's hostility and to experiencing the patient's strong negative affect may render clinicians both unaware of their countertransference and prone to inappropriate behavioral responses. Although defenses work outside of consciousness, conflict in clinicians' emotional responses along the hopefulness–hopelessness and distress–non-distress dimensions of conscious are more indicative of short-term risk than primary emotions.

Our research is consistent with these theories. For high-risk inpatients, we recently demonstrated that clinicians' conflicting emotion combinations of distress and hope, consistent with a reaction formation defense, and of non-distress and hopelessness, consistent with a denial defense, were predictive of suicide outcomes after discharge. Moreover, these two conflicting emotional responses of clinicians were predictive above and beyond other risk factors, such as depression, entrapment, and suicidal ideation. This result underscores the value and the need for attention to patient–clinician relational factors in work with patients at risk for suicide (Yaseen et al., 2016).

ASSESSING ONE'S OWN EMOTIONAL RESPONSE

To summarize briefly, clinicians working with imminently suicidal patients often feel countertransference love, but more often they feel countertransference hate. Most often, these two emotions are consciously experienced as vague positive or negative feelings, respectively. Because both countertransference love and, particularly, countertransference hate can be viewed as "unprofessional" or unethical, clinicians use common psychological defenses to modify these unacceptable emotional states.

The previously discussed conceptual framework is invaluable in understanding clinicians' interactions with suicidal individuals. Clinicians high in emotional intelligence may use mindfulness to directly assess to what extent they may be experiencing countertransference love and/or hate and to identify the conflicting emotions consistent with various defense mechanisms.

Examining one's own psychological defenses is another technique. Some defense mechanisms, such as rationalization or turning against self, are relatively easy to identify. Others may be more difficult, even for clinicians of high emotional intelligence. Even those skilled in emotional differentiation may not be able to recognize their own denial, repression, and projection.

Clinicians can decipher their emotional responses by identifying the related emotions and behaviors, which are either more acceptable or more obvious. In high-risk inpatients, a number of these have been shown to predict post-discharge suicidal behavior. Clinicians can identify such emotions/behaviors by asking themselves direct questions and giving honest answers. This technique can be used by all; it requires no special talent for emotional differentiation—just internal honesty.

A clinician can use the following five questions to probe reaction formation, in order of increasing emotional intensity:

1. Do I see him/her more frequently, or for longer sessions, than other patients?
2. Does he/she make me feel good about myself?
3. Do I like him/her very much?
4. Do I look forward to seeing him/her all day?
5. Do I feel sexually attracted to him/her?

An affirmative answer to one or more of these questions regarding a high-risk patient suggests the *reaction formation defense*, associated with increased risk for a suicide attempt in the near future. Whereas clinicians are likely to perceive the first two questions as routine, they may be threatened by the fifth question. Although sexual attraction per se is not unethical, any action resulting from it is unethical. Many clinicians would find being attracted to a patient so threatening that they may use every possible defense mechanism to protect themselves from it. In imminent risk assessment, sexual attraction to a patient is a diagnostic sign that needs to be noted and processed rationally. In doing so, being nonjudgmental toward oneself is essential and can be made easier through mindfulness.

The five questions to probe denial, manifested as distancing from the patient, are the following, also in order of increasing emotional intensity:

6. Do I return his/her phone calls less promptly than I should?
7. Does he/she make me feel like my hands are tied?
8. Do I feel dismissed or devalued?

9. Do I wish I had never treated him/her and/or do I dread seeing him/her?
10. Does he/she give me chills or make my skin crawl?

An affirmative answer to one of these questions suggests a *distancing emotional response, consistent with the denial defense* and indicative of increased risk for a suicide attempt in the near future. Countertransference hate is often easier to uncover for clinicians because dislike of a patient is father away from a possible ethical misconduct than sexual attraction and may be easier to admit to oneself. For the same reason, denial may be easier to identify than reaction formation.

When asking the previous questions, it saves time to go in reverse order and to ask the most emotionally loaded question first. If the answer is positive, there is no need to ask the other, less charged questions.

The 11th question, "Do I feel guilty about my feelings toward him/her?" applies to both positive and negative emotional responses. Many clinicians feel guilty when admitting both extremes of feelings. This question should be asked last, as a reality check. Guilt is a diagnostically valuable emotional response. Feeling guilt in the absence of a positive or negative response should indicate that the true response may not have been uncovered and may warrant a re-examination for a defense mechanism other than reaction formation and denial.

Furthermore, feeling positive emotions does not preclude from feeling negative emotions: Both are often felt at the same time, creating a confusion of undifferentiated and unpleasant tension mixing excitement and anxiety. This confused state is exactly when the probing questions are most helpful in teasing out more differentiated and diagnostic emotions. The following case is an example of an internal dialogue probing mixed countertransference:

Case 51

Stanley, a 55-year-old highly accomplished male without a psychiatric history, was admitted to an inpatient unit following a drug overdose. He overdosed after a fight with his wife when she told him that she was filing for divorce. The wife visited the unit and reconciled with the patient, who was then set for discharge. The intern felt intensely anxious about it: "On the negative side, this patient makes my skin crawl," she thought, "He is putting me in an impossible bind: I think that if his wife leaves him, he will kill himself. And yet I need to discharge him because he says he is not suicidal. On the positive side, I think I could help him. I really understand him, and he appreciates me. He makes me feel good about myself. Do I feel a special bond?"

CASE EXAMPLES

Case 52: High Risk for Imminent Suicide–Reaction Formation

Christie was referred to Dr. E by his residency training director, who told him, "She has chronic suicidal ideation and two serious past attempts, one of them very recently.

Wealthy parents who are overinvolved. You are a strong resident, and if anybody can work with her, you can." Dr. E felt put on the spot and became very anxious. "Bad luck" he thought, "I am now under the microscope with a high-risk. This is all I need."

Dr. E was dreading meeting Christie. When he finally did, he was pleasantly surprised. Christie was a very attractive 21-year-old Chinese woman dressed in skin-tight jeans and a T-shirt. She seemed exceptionally bright and motivated to be in treatment. With her she brought a neatly organized folder with pictures and notes. "These are all the men in my life I had relations with and crushes on," she said, "My middle school tennis coach, my high school English teacher, and my college Spanish professor. You need to know everything about me."

The session went very well. Dr. E felt an instant rapport with Christie, as if he had known her for a long time. She was cooperative, open, insightful, and ready to change. "You are very different from my previous therapists," she said at the end of the session, "When is our next session?"

Instead of a weekly visit, Dr. E scheduled Christie for 2 days later. His distress diminished. Moreover, he felt elated and looked forward to their next session so he could implement a strategy he had designed to treat her suicidality, which he was sure would be successful. In supervision, however, the attending alerted him to a discrepancy between his exuberant and hopeful response to Christie and the severity of her illness, as well as her chronic risk for suicide.

Dr. E asked himself the 11 questions probing his emotions and gave the following answers:

Question	Answer
1. Did I (plan to) see her more frequently?	Yes
2. Does she make me feel good about myself?	Yes
3. Do I like her very much?	Yes
4. Do I look forward to seeing her all day?	Don't know
5. Do I feel sexually attracted to her?	Yes
6. Do I return her phone calls less promptly than I do with my other patients?	Don't know
7. Does she make me feel like I was put in an impossible bind?	Yes
8. Do I feel dismissed or devalued?	No
9. Do I wish I had never taken her on as a patient?	Yes
10. Does she give me chills or make my skin crawl?	No/no
11. Do I feel guilty about my feelings toward her?	Yes

When analyzing the answers to the probing questions, Dr. E was able to identify his unusually positive response to Christie, his uncharacteristic scheduling of her, and even his attraction to her. He was then able to identify his developing overinvolvement with Christy. Furthermore, recognizing early distress and subsequent hopefulness in himself made him realize his own reaction formation defense, which reduced the anxiety he initially felt about the case. He then assessed Christie as having elevated risk for imminent suicide.

Case 53: High Risk for Imminent Suicide—Repression and Denial

Leo was admitted to an inpatient psychiatric unit with the chief complaint, "I am desperate, and I need to be admitted to the psychiatric unit, because I do not want to repeat what I did in April." In April, Leo attempted suicide by overdose on benzodiazepines and alcohol and also drank a detergent. Prior to the attempt, he posted a long suicide note on his Facebook page. His suicide attempt was interrupted by the police: Somebody who read the Facebook page had called 911. He was then admitted first to the intensive care unit and later for 2 weeks to an inpatient psychiatric unit. Leo did not follow up with his post-discharge outpatient treatment.

During his assessment, Leo told the resident, Dr. N, that his most recent stressor was a comment at work about his hair loss: It made him think that he was going to become bald like his father, whom he detested. His April attempt followed a comment by his date that she could not understand him because of his accent. Leo was a Bulgarian immigrant who left Bulgaria at age 16 years, and he was very proud of his English.

Dr. N initially liked talkative Leo. However, as the interview dragged on, he became increasingly irritated and angry because Leo was talking only about his hair and his looks, and he was difficult to understand, just like his date had told him. Leo was turning out to be a self-absorbed entitled type. Whatever question he was asked, his response was about either his receding hair or him being overweight, both of which made him feel excluded.

"I am weird," said Leo, "and I like weird girls. But even they don't go out with me. It is my hair. Also I am not athletic, I am overweight, and I am Bulgarian." Dr. N thought that Leo's whining was completely unfounded. He was a tall, attractive, muscular guy, with regular dark hair. "What a wimp," thought Dr. N, "He will never be happy."

Dr. N started Leo on an SSRI for his depression. On the unit, Leo was intrusive, and in groups he continued to perseverate on his appearance. The staff disliked him, and Dr. N always saw him last. On Friday, Leo denied suicidal ideation and plan. Mindful of the need to shorten length of hospital stay, Dr. N discharged him from the unit with a Monday follow-up appointment. He was relieved: Dr. N was very aware that he had disliked Leo, but he thought he had provided good care.

Leo was readmitted on Sunday night after another overdose. A different admitting team decided that Leo was delusional and put him on an antipsychotic. Dr. N realized that he had not recognized Leo's first episode of schizophrenia and felt guilty about his anger at the patient. His answers to the 11 questions would have been as follows:

Question	Answer
1. Do I see him more frequently or for longer sessions than other patients?	No
2. Does he make me feel good about myself?	No
3. Do I like him very much?	No
4. Do I look forward to seeing him all day?	Definitely no

5. Do I feel sexually attracted to him?	No
6. Do I return his phone calls less promptly than I do with my other patients?	N/A
7. Does he make me feel like my hands are tied?	No
8. Do I feel dismissed or devalued?	No
9. Do I wish I had never taken him on as a patient and do I dread seeing him?	Yes/yes
10. Does he give me chills or make my skin crawl?	Yes/yes
11. Do I feel guilty about my feelings toward him?	Yes

Dr. N's emotional response to Leo is fairly characteristic of repression and denial defenses against countertransference hate. He represses his hate toward the patient, and his conscious experience is anger and irritation. He uses denial to distance himself from the patient. As a result, his superficial mental status examination misinterprets Leo's delusional perception of his appearance as self-absorption. In reality, Leo's desperation was a sign of entrapment in his delusional world, with both emotions being symptoms of the suicidal crisis. If Dr. N were to ask himself the countertransference questions, he would have realized that his emotional response to the patient indicates high risk for imminent suicide.

Case 54: Low Risk for Imminent Suicide

Dr. K was asked to assess Rosette, a 23-year-old mother of three and a clinical trial participant, because she was having suicidal thoughts and wanted to be admitted to the hospital for protection, as she was "last time." She had one recent hospitalization after a suicide attempt when she took 18 pills of lorazepam and cut her left wrist because she felt overwhelmed taking care of her children. She agreed to be in the study at that time.

The resident assistant called the study clinician, Dr. K, to assess Rosette's suicide risk. Rosette was a slim, neatly dressed Latina who seemed to be bewildered by Dr. K's sudden appearance. She explained to Dr. K that she was on her way to be admitted to a hospital she was at previously, but she decided to stop at the research office for a follow-up assessment on the way. Her boyfriend was waiting for her outside in the car with their daughters to drive her to the emergency department.

Upon further questioning, Rosette told Dr. K that she had difficulty staying home with her children for long periods of time. Her oldest daughter was oppositional, and the baby was colicky. Rosette was always exhausted, and she had difficulty controlling her anger and thought that she must be a bad mother. Last night, she inflicted superficial cuts on her thighs because seeing blood made her feel good. She said that something needed to change or she would kill herself.

Dr. K had a dilemma: A suicidal patient with a history of a suicidal attempt felt unsafe and wanted to be admitted, but to a different hospital. Should he walk her to his hospital's emergency room or trust her to go to the other emergency room? As the study's principal investigator, he was responsible for her safety. Dr. K felt irritated by the patient's manipulative behavior with regard to her boyfriend. "Manipulative patients do kill themselves," he thought, "particularly those with borderline personality disorder, which she probably has."

"Do you feel trapped in your situation?" he asked and proceeded to assess her for suicidal narrative and suicidal crisis. Neither was present. Dr. K then walked to the patient's car, confirmed that her boyfriend was driving her to the other hospital's emergency department, and instructed him to call him if there was a problem. Although he did not need to ask himself the probing questions, his answers would have been as follows:

Question	Answer
1. Do I see her more frequently or for longer sessions than other patients?	N/A
2. Does she make me feel good about myself?	No
3. Do I like her very much?	No
4. Do I look forward to seeing her all day?	N/A
5. Do I feel sexually attracted to her?	No
6. Do I return her phone calls less promptly than I do with my other patients?	N/A
7. Does she make me feel like my hands are tied or that I am put in an impossible bind?	Yes
8. Do I feel dismissed or devalued?	No
9. Do I wish I had never taken her on as a patient and/or do I dread seeing her?	No
10. Does she give me chills or make my skin crawl?	No
11. Do I feel guilty about my feelings toward her?	No

Despite Rosette's determination to be admitted to a psychiatric unit and her past history of suicidal behavior, Dr. K's emotional response to Rosette indicates low risk for imminent suicide. He diffuses his anger with rationalization and then calmly performs an assessment of her suicide risk. Despite his negative response to Rosette, his walking her down and speaking to the boyfriend is perceived as caring.

CLINICIANS' FEELINGS AND SUICIDAL PATIENTS

Suicide is devastating for the relatives of its victims. Deaths of a spouse, a parent, or a child are at the top of the life stressors severity list (Holmes & Rahe, 1967; Rahe & Arthur, 1978), but their death by suicide is even more dreadful because it is viewed as preventable (Feigelman, Gorman, & Jordan, 2009; Hendin, Lipschitz, Maltsberger, Haas, & Wynecoop, 2000). In addition to grieving, survivors of significant other suicide often blame themselves for missing the warning signs, for being absent in the time of crisis, and for acting in a way that could have pushed their loved one toward suicide.

Psychiatrists who lose their patients to suicide also feel a devastating sense of loss (Hendin et al., 2000). They often second-guess their actions prior to the patient's suicide, identifying signs of the catastrophe that they may have missed. The literature is full of reports describing the anguish and guilt clinicians experience following a patient's suicide (Hendin et al., 2000; Hendin, Haas, et al., 2004; Richards, 2000; Veilleux, 2011). These emotions are compounded by doubts about one's professional skills, perceived treatment mistakes, and fears of lawsuits.

The flood of disturbing emotions that clinicians experience following their patients' suicide is accompanied by the memories of negative or uncomfortable feelings toward these patients prior to their deaths. Prominent among these may be anger, hostility, anxiety, frustration, and helplessness (Hendin et al., 2000; Hendin, Haas, et al., 2004; Richards, 2000; Veilleux, 2011). Also common are negative emotions related to their reluctance to treat such patients, delays in answering their phone calls, or attempts to discharge them prematurely from one's caseload.

Maltzberger and Buie (1974) noted that the dysphoria during an encounter with a suicidal patient may be too intense to be experienced consciously. As discussed previously, clinicians employ unconscious defenses to transform these responses into more acceptable emotions and thoughts, which may be then brought into consciousness. However, clinicians need to be aware that they may still act out their emotional responses either through overinvolvement with patients or through distancing and rejection.

Suicidal patients, who often feel alienated and lonely, are exquisitely sensitive to their clinicians' feelings toward them. During the evaluation or treatment, they try to guess clinicians' "real" emotions. They search for and see the subtle signs of irritation, frustration, or dislike that clinicians may be unaware of. Unfortunately, suicidal patients' perception of their clinicians' dislike may be the final evidence they need to convince themselves that they are a burden to others and that not one person in the world, including their psychiatrist, cares if they live or die. Under these circumstances, a clinician's perceived indifference or dislike may be one of many other factors triggering a suicidal act.

The pressure clinicians feel when deciding whether to discharge or hospitalize suicidal patients weighs heavily on their shoulders. Whether conscious or subconscious, this pressure makes clinicians' emotions even more apparent to those patients—a fact that clinicians are often aware of but powerless to change. A reliable method for assessing imminent suicide risk will both improve the chances of averting a suicide and reduce clinicians' negative responses to suicidal patients.

8

Conducting Short-Term Risk
Assessment Interviews

The preceding chapters discussed the theoretical and historical frameworks for the narrative crisis model of suicidal behavior (Chapters 1 and 2), followed by a detailed discussion of the key constructs used for the assessment of short-term suicide risk (Narrative-Crisis model). This chapter describes several ways to integrate all the constructs into assessment interviews to be used in different clinical settings.

This chapter has five sections. The first section combines all the key constructs of the short-term risk assessment into one comprehensive risk assessment outline according to the narrative crisis model of suicidal behavior. The second section addresses the real-world challenges of risk assessment, limitations of self-reported suicidal ideation and intent, and strategies for minimizing the interview bias. The third section is devoted to the potential advantages and disadvantages of the short-term risk assessment instruments. The fourth section describes three risk assessment interview strategies and gives examples of each. The final section presents the case of "eerie calm" in a patient at imminent risk for suicide.

COMPREHENSIVE ASSESSMENT OUTLINE

The following comprehensive outline summarizes all demographic and clinical information presented previously, which could be used for short-term suicide risk assessments in any clinical setting. The details can be found in the corresponding chapters.

Long-Term Risk Factors

Demographics

- *Age, race, and ethnicity*: In the United States, men and women aged 35–64 years are at highest risk for suicide, but the picture is complex (see Chapter 3). Caucasians and Native Americans have the highest suicide rate.
- *Gender and sexual orientation*: In the United States, suicide rates are higher for men than for women; the highest differential is 5.8 in the 10- to 24-year-old age group. Suicide rates are higher for members of the LGBT community than for heterosexual patients.

Mental Illness and Past Suicide Attempts

- *History of mental illness*: More than 90% of individuals who die by suicide have been diagnosed with a mental illness, most often an affective disorder, schizophrenia, alcohol/drug use disorder, or personality disorder.
- *History of suicide attempt(s)*: Past suicide attempt, however remote, increases lifetime risk of death by suicide 30-fold.

Childhood History

- *Childhood trauma*: Both childhood adversity and childhood trauma are independently associated with increased suicide risk; the highest increase (10–14 times the risk) is seen in adult males who were sexually abused as boys.
- *Parenting style*: Were the patient's parents neglectful, authoritarian, and overbearing, or distant and controlling? Children of mothers with an "affectionless control" parenting style are at higher risk for suicide as adults.
- *Attachment style*: Individuals with insecure and anxious attachment style have increased suicide rates.

Traits

- *Impulsivity*: Impulsivity may be associated with increased short-term suicide risk in crisis-driven suicide attempters (see Chapter 2).
- *Hopelessness and pessimism*: In the United States, although not in some Eastern European cultures, trait hopelessness and pessimism are associated with higher lifetime suicide risk.
- *Perfectionism*: Perfectionism is strongly associated with higher long-term suicide risk and can form a foundation for the first phases of the suicidal narrative.
- *Fearlessness and pain insensitivity (capability)*: Patients who have lower anxiety rates, such as those with externalizing and antisocial traits, are at higher lifetime risk.

Cultural Acceptability

- *Cultural attitudes*: Is suicide accepted or honored in the patient's culture? In certain cultures, suicide is still sanctioned following family dishonor.
- *Immigration status*: Recent immigrants tend to have lower suicide rates, which increase with time and often exceed the suicide rates of those born in the United States.
- *Moral and religious objections*: Faith and strong religious affiliation are two of the strongest protective factors against suicidal behavior.
- *Regional affiliation*: Does the patient live in one of the US "honor" states? Was the patient born in one of those states? Does the patient feel emotional and cultural kinship to one of those states? In the United States, suicide rates are highest in the "honor states" in the western part of the country and Alaska, and they are lowest on the Eastern Seaboard.
- *Suicide in the family*: Mothers' suicides in particular are associated with significant increase in lifetime risk of suicide.
- *Suicide clusters*: Suicides often occur in temporal and geographical clusters, and recent suicides by close others or celebrities increase short-term suicide risk.

- *Suicide exposure and practicing*: Has the patient been discussing suicide in online chat rooms? Has the patient been researching and discussing methods, even when talking about other people? These behaviors signify increased short-term risk.

Stressful Life Events

Work and Career

- *Economic hardship*: Can the patient support him- or herself and his or her family? Is the patient in debt? Has there been recent unemployment or deterioration in socioeconomic status? Economic hardship is one of the two stressful life events (relationship failure is the other) associated most strongly with short-term suicide risk.
- *Business or work failure*: Recent job loss or project termination or failure (particularly if public or humiliating) may feed into the suicidal narrative, increasing short-term risk dramatically.
- *Loss of home*: Recent and particularly impending loss of home increase short-term risk of suicide; foreclosure carries a higher risk than eviction.

Relationship Conflict

- *Romantic rejection*: The recent or impending end of a marriage or long-term relationship, particularly due to infidelity, sharply increases short-term risk for suicide, with most deaths occurring within 24 hours of the event. Recent romantic rejection in adolescents and young adults is also a strong risk factor.
- *Intimate relationship conflict*: Poor relationship quality is a suicide risk factor for women, whereas intimate partner violence is a risk factor for both men and women. Furthermore, men tend to underreport physical abuse due to the shame of appearing "weak."
- *Parents in conflict with children*: In some cultures, being a burden to one's children may feel like a disgrace and may be a short-term risk factor for suicide.
- *Children in conflict with parents*: Conflict with parents, even one that was seemingly trivial, is the most frequent reason for suicide in children and adolescents. Feeling like a burden feeds directly into the suicidal narrative.
- *Ongoing abuse and neglect*: Ongoing sexual, physical or emotional abuse is strongly associated with childhood and adolescent suicide attempts.
- *Bullying*: Bullying is associated with increased suicide risk, particularly in adolescent girls. Workplace bullying by supervisors is more common than is typically acknowledged.

Serious Medical Illness

- *Recent diagnosis*: A diagnosis of a serious medical illness with a poor prognosis significantly reconfigures one's life narrative and can increase suicide risk. In middle-aged adults, short-term risk is highest in the first month after the diagnosis (sixfold increase in risk), and it remains high for the first year.

- *Prolonged and debilitating illness*: Suicide risk is higher for patients while in treatment for cancer or chronic obstructive pulmonary disease, particularly when developing recent comorbid conditions.
- *Acute and chronic pain*: Suicide rates are higher for patients with chronic back pain and chronic headaches. These symptoms also increase the danger of death from unintended opiate overdose.

Serious Mental Illness

- *Recent diagnosis*: In the first 3 months after being given diagnoses of schizophrenia, bipolar disorder, or major depressive disorder (MDD), the suicide risk increases 20-fold for schizophrenia and 10-fold for bipolar disorder and MDD.
- *Recent hospitalization*: In the first week after psychiatric hospitalization, suicide risk is 250 times higher for women and 100 times higher for men compared to that of people never admitted. The risk is 30 times higher in the first month post-discharge.
- *Recent suicide attempts*: Short-term suicide risk is sharply higher in patients with recent suicide attempts, particularly the elderly. Risk is higher in those with multiple attempts, which may indicate rehearsing. Risk is higher with unsuccessful completed attempts (e.g., survival after overdose) compared to aborted attempts (e.g., changing one's mind after ingesting a few pills) or interrupted attempts (e.g., something interfered with pill ingestion).
- *Attempt lethality*: Recent failed attempts by hanging, drowning, or shooting confer a 30–50% risk of death by suicide within the next 6 months. Risk is lowest with failed attempts by cutting.
- *Mental illness exacerbation*: For any diagnosis, an acute episode increases short-term risk by an order of magnitude. The risk is highest for mixed mania (38×), followed by MDD (>20×).
- *Medication changes—initiation, discontinuation, or noncompliance*: Recent treatment initiation with selective serotonin reuptake inhibitors may increase short-term risk by causing anxiety, agitation, irritability, aggressiveness, impulsivity, akathisia, and mixed mania. The same is true in the case of discontinuation or dose reduction of benzodiazepines, antipsychotics, hypnotics, or sedating mood stabilizers and antidepressants. Any changes in medications can contribute to the affective disturbance of suicidal crisis syndrome (SCS).

Recent Substance Misuse

- *Drug/alcohol use disorder*: Suicide rates in patients with alcohol use disorder and substance use disorder are much higher than those in people without these disorders.
- *Acute alcohol intoxication/recent drug use*: One-third to one-half of suicide deaths are preceded by acute use of alcohol and/or drugs.
- *Drug or alcohol withdrawal*: Withdrawal from alcohol and most illicit or prescription drugs of abuse is associated with affective disturbance and changes in arousal, which may exacerbate the suicide crisis.

Suicidal Narrative

Phases of the Narrative

- *Phase 1: Unrealistic life goals*: Life goals that are objectively or perceived as unreachable, given the patient's abilities and background, often form the first phase of the suicidal narrative. Life goals may include realistic or unrealistic career successes or simply having a job and an income. Alternatively, life goals may refer to personal success, such as looks, lifestyle, or relationships.
- *Phase 2: Entitlement to happiness*: Was the patient expecting to be much happier than he or she is currently, and is this due to a belief that the world has failed to deliver on its promise of success and happiness? Was this happiness contingent on an unrealistic goal set in Phase 1?
- *Phase 3: Failure to redirect to more realistic goals*: Is the patient able to appreciate that his or her goals have always been or have become unachievable due to life circumstances? Is the patient able to formulate/accept alternative, more realistic goals when the clinician suggests them? Does the patient continue to insist that only the achievement of the original goal (Phase 1) can bring him or her fulfillment and happiness (Phase 2)?
- *Phase 4: Humiliating defeat*: Has the patient recently suffered, or is he or she about to suffer, a defeat that is perceived as catastrophic, demeaning, or humiliating? Such a defeat, real or imaginary, could involve a loss or impending loss of self, status, or relationship. Typical examples are a terminal medical illness or serious mental illness; a humiliating failure at work or school; real or relative financial hardship or loss of home; and unrequited love, a breakup, or infidelity. Was the humiliation public or was it perceived as public? Has the defeat occurred as a result of failed pursuit of the unrealistic life goal (Phases 1 and 2) and failure to adjust (Phase 3)?
- *Phase 5: Perceived burdensomeness*: Does the patient believe that he or she is a burden to others—particularly parents, children, romantic partners, and close friends—and that these people would be better off if he or she were gone? Does the patient believe he or she is a burden as a result of humiliating failure in Phase 4?
- *Phase 6: Thwarted belongingness*: Does the patient feel alienated, isolated, and lonely? Does the patient's alienation and fear of reaching out stem from the humiliating defeat (Phase 4) and from the guilt and shame after suffering this real or perceived setback? Is the patient's alienation a result of him or her feeling like a burden to others (Phase 5)?
- *Phase 7: Perception of No Future*: Does the patient believe that his or her life situation is unacceptable, intolerable, and inescapable? Can the patient imagine his or her future going forward? Can the patient see any good solutions or good options to find an acceptable alternative? Is the patient capable of communicating a need for help?

Constructing the Suicidal Narrative

- *Suicidal narrative*: Does the patient's life narrative, as described in the course of the assessment, fit the seven phases of the suicide narrative? How good is the fit? In other words, has his or her failure to achieve unrealistic life goals and an inability to adjust to more manageable ones (Phases 1–3) led to a shameful defeat (Phase 4), causing the patient to be a real or perceived burden on others (Phase 5) and to consider him- or herself without a future? If the patient does not volunteer this interpretation, how readily does he or she agree with it?

Suicidal Crisis

Suicidal Ideation, Intent, and Plan

- *(To be assessed last)* Because some patients who intend to die would want to hide their suicidal intent, the early explicit assessment of suicidality may elicit biased responses to the preceding sections of the assessment. For that reason, it is preferable to perform the explicit assessment of suicidal ideation and intent toward the end of the interview.
- *Suicidal ideation*: Does the patient have persistent thoughts of death as a way to escape an unacceptable life situation that is perceived as intolerable and inescapable? Is there an explicit desire to die or be dead? How frequent and painful are these thoughts?
- *Suicidal intent*: Does the patient set conditions to be met as a reason to live or die? For example: "If I get evicted next week, I am not going to survive"; "If my wife gets custody of the kids, I will kill myself"; "I cannot live without her"; and "If I don't get the job, I have no hope." Has the patient "put his affairs in order" and given away any belongings?
- *Suicide plan*: Has the patient chosen a method? Have there been any preparatory actions for suicide? Has the patient researched the method online? Bought the pills? Gone to the bridge or train tracks? Has the patient sent or posted any explicit or cryptic messages revealing his or her suicidal intent?

Entrapment

- *Entrapment*: Does the patient feel trapped in his or her unbearable life situation? Does the patient see no good solutions to relieve the pain his or her pain? Does death appear to be the only solution to the unbearable pain?
- *Desperation*: How urgent is the need to escape an unbearable life situation? Can the patient wait for relief? Does the promise of relief in the future seem irrelevant because the patient can no longer bear it?

Affective Disturbance

- *Emotional pain*: Does the patient feel inner pain that is too much to bear and needs to be stopped? Is the pain severe and relentless?
- *Depressive turmoil*: Has the patient been experiencing extreme and rapid mood swings from anxiety to depression to anger? Are there also aggressiveness, frustration, anger, and irritation? Do these emotions come in waves? Are they too confusing and intense to differentiate?

- *Extreme (frantic) anxiety*: Is the patient experiencing waves of extreme anxiety? Does the patient feel so vulnerable and defenseless that a minor slight is immensely painful? Does he or she feel or appear frenzied, tense, or on edge?
- *Panic–dissociation*: Is the patient having panic attacks? Are there any dissociative symptoms (during or independent of panic attacks)? Do ordinary things look strange or distorted? Does the ground feel solid or rubbery? Does the patient feel strange sensations in his or her body or skin? Does the patient experience burning on the skin, feeling blood rushing in his or her veins, eyelids burning, or ears ringing?
- *Fear of dying*: During a panic attack, is the patient afraid of suddenly dying or being killed? (This fear is not of death itself but of the suddenness of it.)
- *Acute anhedonia*: Does the patient express an inability to experience, remember, or imagine experiencing things as enjoyable?

Loss of Cognitive Control

- *Ruminations*: Does the patient have persistent ruminations about his or her own distress and its possible causes and consequences? About the life events and actions that brought on the distress? Does he or she ruminate about possible solutions to these problems (reflective pondering)?
- *Cognitive rigidity*: Can the patient deviate from or offer alternatives to his or her repetitive negative pattern of thought (cognitive flexibility)? Can the patient accept alternative explanations offered by the clinician? Is there any flexibility in thinking with regard to any subject?
- *Ruminative flooding*: Does the patient feel that he or she has lost control over his or her thinking and that changing these thoughts is impossible even with extreme mental effort? Does the patient experience pain or pressure in the head from having only negative thoughts? Does the patient feel that his or her head may explode from all the negative thinking?
- *Thought suppression*: What happens when the patient tries to suppress repetitive negative or disturbing thoughts? Are these efforts successful, or do the unpleasant thoughts, including those about suicide, return with even more intensity?

Disturbance in Arousal

- *Agitation*: Is the patient agitated, restless, or hypervigilant during the assessment? Have the patient's significant others noticed him or her to be unusually irritable or anxious? Does the patient feel agitated inside? Is he or she aware of increased irritability or lower frustration tolerance?
- *Global insomnia*: Is the patient having difficulty falling asleep, particularly because of ruminative thinking? Does he or she wake up repeatedly at night? Is the patient bothered by dreams, nightmares, or night terrors? Does the patient feel exhausted in the morning?

Preliminary Risk Assessment

- In the preliminary risk assessment, the clinician integrates all the clinical material obtained with the exception of the clinician's emotional response component, which is assessed separately.

Clinician's Emotional Response

- *Reaction formation of countertransference hate*: Does the clinician have an unusually positive emotional response to the patient? Does he or she feel compelled to see the patient more frequently or for longer sessions than other patients? What are the answers to the following questions: Does the patient make me feel good about myself? Do I like the patient very much? Do I look forward to seeing the patient all day? Do I feel sexually attracted to the patient? Positive answers to these questions, particularly when the clinician's feelings are otherwise distressing, conflicted, or induce guilt, indicate reaction formation defense. The use of this defense suggests increased short-term suicide risk.
- *Denial of countertransference hate*: Does the clinician have an unusually negative emotional response to the patient? Does the case seem hopeless? Does the clinician postpone seeing the patient until the very end of the day or return phone calls less promptly than usual? What are the answers to the following questions: Does the patient make me feel like my hands are tied? Do I feel dismissed or devalued by the patient? Do I wish I had never met the patient and/or do I dread seeing the patient? Does the patient give me chills or make my skin crawl? Positive answers to these questions, particularly when the clinician's feelings are conflicted, indicate the use of the denial defense to "countertransference hate." Like reaction formation, this indicates higher short-term suicide risk.

Final Risk Assessment

- In the final risk assessment, the clinician integrates the preliminary risk assessment with the information obtained through the analysis of his or her emotional responses and corrects for the potential biases due to either "reaction formation" or "denial."

SUICIDAL IDEATION AND INTENT: SELF-REPORT AND ITS LIMITATIONS

The leading sentence in the proposed *Diagnostic and Statistical Manual of Mental Disorders* (American Psychiatric Association, 2013) criteria for the suicide crisis syndrome describes

> persistent thoughts of wanting to die or kill oneself as a way to escape an unacceptable life situation, which is perceived as simultaneously painfully intolerable and inescapable. Typical situations include a loss or impending loss of self-worth, status, or attachment, such as terminal illness, humiliating failure at work, or rejection by a romantic partner, respectively.

Therefore, one of the key items of short-term suicide risk is the assessment of the intensity of the suicidal ideation and suicide intent.

Predominantly, it is mental health professionals who conduct suicide risk assessments of patients. Sixty-five percent of them ask these questions during routine visits, compared to 13% of primary care doctors and 10% of medical specialists (Smith et al., 2013). Traditionally, in such assessments, clinicians overwhelmingly rely on suicidal patients' truthful reporting of their suicidal ideation, intent, and plan, using three direct questions:

1. Have you been thinking about suicide?
2. Do you have an intention to commit suicide?
3. What is your plan?

Unfortunately, patients' self-report of these factors during the risk assessment interview is a poor predictor of imminent suicidal behavior. The main reasons for poor predictive validity of self-reporting in explicit suicide risk assessment are the patient hiding his or her suicidal intent, lack of conscious awareness of suicidal intent, inability to communicate a need for help, and the fleeting nature of the suicidal crisis.

Many acutely suicidal individuals who are thinking about ending their lives will deny or minimize their suicidal ideation and will hide their intent and the plan. Even patients who have made up their mind to end their lives may not tell the truth to the evaluating clinicians. Suicidal people determined to die are aware that their admission of having a suicidal plan may result in involuntary hospitalization. Of patients who die by suicide, 85% deny suicidal ideation when assessed, and three-fourths do so within 7 days of their suicide. They know how the game is played, so to speak.

There may be other, unconscious reasons for the high denial rates. Some patients are unable to recognize their own suicidal feelings and thoughts due to poor emotional differentiation or the use of psychological defenses. Moreover, inability to ask for help by communicating despair and suicidal thoughts to close others is associated with increased suicide risk (Gvion et al., 2014; Levi-Belz et al., 2014). Thus, low self-disclosure in and of itself may be a risk factor for suicide. Moreover, whereas mental pain and depression predict suicidal behavior, difficulties with self-disclosure are related to its lethality and seriousness (Gvion et al., 2014; Levi-Belz et al., 2014).

It appears that a combination of intense mental pain with an inability to communicate this pain to others enhances the risk of more lethal suicidal behaviors (Levi-Belz et al., 2014). Interestingly, aggression and impulsivity in lethal and nonlethal attempters appear to be similar (Gvion et al., 2014). Thus, inability to share feelings is an important risk factor for suicide, above and beyond the contribution of psychiatric illness and mental pain (Busch, Fawcett, & Jacobs, 2003; Horesh, Zalsman, & Apter, 2004; Levi et al., 2008).

Another complicating factor is that patients' suicidal intent or their awareness of it can change sharply over a short period of time. The duration of conscious suicidal thinking could be as short as 10 minutes for half of the suicide attempters (Deisenhammer et al., 2009). Patients with longer conscious suicidality have a higher suicidal intent; impulsivity is not associated with the duration of the suicidal process. The short time window for identifying suicidal intent may explain why these patients do not communicate their suicidal feelings to others despite being in close contact with them.

Self-report of past and current suicidal behavior can be equally unreliable. Some suicidal individuals may hide their past attempts because they understand that revealing the existence of these past attempts may result in their involuntary hospitalization. Others may be deeply ashamed of their past attempts either because they failed or because they attempted them in the first place. Moreover, others may simply "forget" that they attempted suicide (e.g., "I just took some pills. It was a long time ago").

In summary, although patients' suicidal ideation, intent, and plan are central to the suicidal process, the accurate assessment of these factors is challenging and unreliable. Specifically, patients' denials should be considered in the context of their other SCS symptoms and in relation to the strength of their suicidal narrative.

SUICIDE RISK ASSESSMENT INSTRUMENTS

Short-Term Risk Assessment Instruments and the SAD PERSONS Scales

Under the ideal circumstances, clinicians using the previously described comprehensive assessment outline would obtain all the necessary information to make the best clinical decisions regarding their patients' short-term suicide risk. Yet, due to limited time and resources, or due to explicit administrative policies, most clinicians will have to make their decisions based on short interviews and on concise risk assessment questionnaires. Although the use of these interviews and questionnaires may make clinicians feel secure about their assessment, this security is not supported by research.

To date, more than 20 suicide risk assessment tools have been developed for prediction of future suicidal behavior (Roos, Sareen, & Bolton, 2013). Surprisingly, predictive validity for future suicide attempts for some of these tools has never been tested, whereas other tools, such as the Beck Depression Inventory, the Beck Hopelessness Scale, and the Scale for Suicidal Ideation, are only effective at predicting long-term suicidal behavior. The most well known among them is the SAD PERSONS scale (SPS), which was developed in 1983 based on 10 risk factors, taken from published literature reports (Patterson, Dohn, Bird, & Patterson, 1983).

SAD PERSONS is an acronym based on the following suicide risk factors :

S: male sex
A: old age
D: Depression
P: Previous attempt
E: Excess alcohol or substance use
R: Rational thinking loss
S: Social support lacking
O: Organized plan
N: No spouse
S: Sickness

Each affirmative answer to these risk factors is given 1 point, and the total score is then mapped onto a risk assessment scale as follows:

- 0–4: Low
- 5–6: Medium
- 7–10: High

Remarkably, the SAD PERSONS scale has been widely used for years without ever being tested if it can predict suicidal behavior prospectively. A prospective study was conducted only relatively recently among a large group of general psychiatric referrals ($N = 4019$) (Bolton et al., 2013), and the full scale had no predictive value. Only individual items from the scale, such as alcohol abuse and suicidal ideation with intent, were associated with near-term suicide attempts.

In 1996, the scale was modified into the Modified SAD PERSONS scale (MSPS), which has a similar acronym but slightly different risk factors. The yes/no answers to whether these risk factors are present are weighted either 1 or 2, as follows:

S: Male sex → 1
A: Age 15–25 or 59+ years → 1
D: Depression or hopelessness → 2
P: Previous suicidal attempts or psychiatric care → 1
E: Excessive ethanol or drug use → 1
R: Rational thinking loss (psychotic or organic illness) → 2
S: Single, widowed, or divorced → 1
O: Organized or serious attempt → 2
N: No social support → 1
S: Stated future intent (determined to repeat or ambivalent) → 2

Similar to the original version, the total score is then mapped onto a risk assessment scale, also modified, as follows:

- 0–5: May be safe to discharge
- 6–8: Probably requires psychiatric consultation
- >8: Probably requires hospital admission

As the parent scale, the MSPS was implemented without its validity assessed to predict future suicidal behavior in prospective studies. When such testing was done, the MSPS proved not to be predictive of future suicidal behavior. Recently, the SPS proved less effective in predicting suicide attempts over 6 months than the clinician's "best guess" mapped onto a 10-point Likert scale (Wang et al., 2015).

Other assessment scales (Lecrubier et al., 1997; Oquendo, 2015) are no better at predicting suicide attempts or completed suicide short-term than the SPS and the MSPS. Thus, although having a score-producing algorithm that would allow clinicians to act (and relieve them of the burden of legal responsibility for consequences of their action) would be comforting, no such scale is currently available. The skepticism with regard to the short risk assessment scales is underscored by British guidelines for suicide risk assessment (Harding, 2016):

> Assessing the risk of suicide in a person expressing suicidal thoughts, or presenting with self-harm or a suicide attempt is crucial in attempting to prevent deaths. There are a number of risk-predicting score systems for determining suicidal intent. However, none have good predictive ability, and National Institute for Health and Care Excellence (NICE) guidelines advise these should *not* be used. Instead a comprehensive clinical interview should be used for assessment.

The Modular Assessment of Risk for Imminent Suicide Clinical Tool

Aiming to design a theoretically sound, practical tool for prospective assessment of short-term suicide risk, we recently developed the Modular Assessment of Risk for Imminent Suicide (MARIS). As shown by De Los Reyes and others, having more than one informant improves the diagnostic accuracy of psychiatric assessment, including that of a suicide risk (De Los Reyes et al., 2015). Accordingly, MARIS utilizes the clinician's emotional responses as a diagnostic tool, making the evaluating clinician the second informant.

MARIS is a two-part, two-informant assessment measure that takes less than 5 minutes to administer. Because MARIS was designed to be a practical tool for use by frontline clinicians everywhere, the scale includes only selected aspects of the previously presented comprehensive interview outline. In high-risk psychiatric inpatients, MARIS was predictive of suicidal behavior during the initial 4–8 weeks after discharge, with an odds ratio = 19 (Hawes et al., 2017).

Part 1 of MARIS contains two self-report patient modules that assess the SCS intensity and acceptability of suicide as a solution to life's problems. Part 2 consists of two clinician-rated modules that assess the explicit suicide intent and attempt history and the clinician's emotional response to the patient. Thus, MARIS is focused on the crisis aspect of the short-term risk assessment.

Currently, MARIS is strictly a research tool. More studies with diverse patient populations and clinical settings are needed to establish a validated scoring system with clear cut-off scores to guide clinical decision-making. Until such time, clinicians may use MARIS as an efficient tool for obtaining clinical material on suicide and on their own emotional response to patients.

MARIS

Part 1: Self-Report

Name or Pt. ID # _____   Date _____

Module 1: Suicide Crisis Syndrome—Short Form

Please rate how much each of the following applies to you by writing the appropriate number on the line following each question. Follow the scale below:

> 0 – Not at all
> 1 – A little
> 2 – Somewhat
> 3 – Quite a bit
> 4 – Extremely

In the past couple of days, when you felt your worst . . .

1. Did you become afraid that you would die? _____
2. Did you think something, like a heart attack or accident, would suddenly kill you? _____
3. Did you feel your thoughts are confused? _____
4. Did you feel there is no exit? _____
5. Did you feel that your head could explode from too many thoughts? _____
6. Did you feel bothered by thoughts that did not make sense? _____
7. Did you feel trapped? _____
8. Did you feel like you were getting a headache from too many thoughts in your head? _____

Subtotal 1: _____

Module 2: Suicide Opinion Questionnaire—Short Form

Please rate your general opinion on the following statements about suicide by writing the appropriate number on the line following each question. Follow the scale below:

> 0 – Strongly disagree
> 1 – Disagree
> 2 – Undecided
> 3 – Agree
> 4 – Strongly agree

1. The method used in a given suicide probably reflects whether the action was impulsive or carefully and rationally planned. _____
2. Most people who commit suicide do not believe in an afterlife. _____
3. In general, suicide is an evil act. _____

4. Sometimes suicide is the only escape from life's problems. _____
5. A suicide attempt is essentially a "cry for help." _____
6. Usually, relatives of a suicide victim had no idea of what was about to happen. _____
7. Long-term self-destructive behaviors, such as alcoholism, may represent unconscious suicide attempts. _____
8. Suicide occurs only in civilized societies. _____

Subtotal 2: _____

Part 2: Clinician Assessment

Pt. Name or ID # _____   Date _____

Module 3: The Short Clinical Assessment of Risk for Suicide

Please answer the following questions with regard to your patient.

1. Previous suicide attempt (action taken with at least some intent to die as a result of that action)?   Yes (2)/No (0)
2. Previous attempt by hanging, asphyxiation (e.g., carbon monoxide), or firearm? Yes (2)/No (0)
3. Alcohol or drug abuse present?   Yes (1)/No (0)
4. Recent relapse or escalation in drug/alcohol use?   Yes (1)/No (0)
5. Indicates intent to end own life at some point?   Yes (1)/No (0)
6. Age 19–45 years?   Yes (1)/No (0)
7. Able to think rationally?   Yes (2)/No (0)

Subtotal 3: _____

Module 4: Clinicians Emotional Response

Rate how much each of the following is true regarding how you felt with/about this patient by writing the appropriate number on the line following each item. Follow the scale below:

0 – Not at all
1 – A little
2 – Somewhat
3 – Quite a bit
4 – Extremely

1. S/he made me feel good about myself. _____
2. I liked him/her very much. _____
3. I felt like my hands were tied or that I was put in an impossible bind. _____
4. I felt dismissed or devalued. _____
5. I felt guilty about my feelings toward him/her. _____

6. I thought life really might not be worth living for him/her. _____
7. This patient gave me chills. _____
8. I had to force myself to connect with him/her. _____
9. I feel confident in my ability to help him/her. _____
10. We trust one another. _____

Subtotal 4: _____
Grand total: _____

Note: Copyright by Zimri Yaseen and Igor Galynker. Reproduced with permission.

RISK ASSESSMENT INTERVIEW STRATEGIES

The comprehensive short-term risk assessment outline delineates all the information needed to make an assessment of the suicide risk and to formulate the clinical plan. Three interviewing strategies to obtain this clinical material are suggested next. The strategy choice depends primarily on the amount of time a clinician has for the assessment, the patient's awareness of the suicidal intent, and the patient's willingness to be forthcoming with the interview.

The interview strategies described differ in their duration and in the question order, but all are conversational interviews rather than fixed checklists. In a conversational interview, the clinician takes questions from the list but asks them in an order guided in part by the patient's answers. Although ultimately all the questions are asked, the patient has some control over the interview, which feels like a dialogue rather than an interrogation.

The comprehensive risk assessment interview covers many subjects, which may be confusing to the patient and to the interviewing clinician. To maintain conceptual clarity, we recommend conducting the interview in modules reflecting the components of the narrative crisis model, as delineated in the interview outline. These modules are Trait Vulnerability, Stressful Life Events, Suicidal Narrative, Suicide Crisis Syndrome, and Clinician's Emotional Response.

The three interview strategies are the comprehensive interview, the MARIS interview, and the expanded MARIS interview. Their main features and intended use are as follows:

- The comprehensive interview largely follows the comprehensive assessment outline and is best used in outpatient screenings, when time is not a factor. The comprehensive interview differs from the outline in that all of the explicit suicide-related questions—that is, those regarding acceptability, family history and suicide clusters, recent attempt history, suicidal ideation, intent, and plan—are asked at the end. Estimated assessment time is 90 minutes.
- The MARIS interview works best in emergency room setting, when time is a factor. The MARIS interview has just four modules: Suicide Crisis Syndrome, Acceptability of Suicide, Explicit Risk Assessment, and Clinician's Emotional Response. The interview should take 20 minutes if the suicide risk is present and obvious. If no clinical judgment can be made after the MARIS interview, it must be expanded to the extended MARIS interview.

- The extended MARIS interview includes the MARIS interview with additional Stressful Life Events and Suicidal Narrative modules. It is almost always an extension of the concise MARIS interview when more information is required. The extended MARIS interview takes 30–40 minutes.

Comprehensive Interview

The comprehensive interview strategy is based on the comprehensive assessment outline with one exception: All the explicit suicide-related questions—that is, those regarding acceptability, family history and suicide clusters, attempt history, recent attempt history, suicidal ideation, intent, and plan—are asked at the end. This adjustment is made to improve the reliability of the patient's self-report.

Suicidal individuals who have decided to die and who know that they are being assessed for suicide risk have reasons to deny or minimize their current and past suicidal ideation and behavior. Consequently, an interviewer who asks explicit questions about a patient's suicidality runs the risk of being misled by denials and nonreport of psychopathology by the patient who is trying to minimize his or her risk of hospitalization. However, for patients who do want clinicians' help with staying alive, which are the majority, this is the most important part of the assessment. Moreover, a suicidal patient may perceive lack of explicit assessment as callous, adding this to the experience of the suicidal narrative.

One possible solution to this clinical dilemma is for the clinician to begin the assessment interview with less obvious aspects of the imminent risk evaluation. Questions about history and symptoms are rarely perceived as threatening. They may help the clinician build rapport unaffected by the patient's possible desire to conceal his or her suicidal intent. The bulk of the assessment thus consists of a conversational interview about the patient's life narrative. The interview starts by asking about the long-term factors, followed by the evaluation of the patient's more recent stressors and then the assessment of the signs and symptoms of SCS other than suicidal ideation. The explicit direct and detailed questions about the patient's past and present suicidal behavior are not asked until the very end.

The Comprehensive Interview Strategy (Figure 8.1)

- The clinician starts the interview by establishing rapport. If the patient brings up suicide, the clinician acknowledges it but then indicates that he or she will return to the issue later in the interview.
- The first module of the interview focuses on long-term factors, such as perfectionism, impulsivity, fearlessness, and childhood trauma. Questions about past attempts, family history of suicide, or suicide clusters are saved for the fifth module.
- The second module consists of the conversational interview about the patient's life events and possible recent stressors.
- The third module assesses the patient's perception of his or her life stressors in terms of the phases of the suicidal narrative. The clinician should attempt to construct the suicidal narrative and obtain the patient's feedback on it.

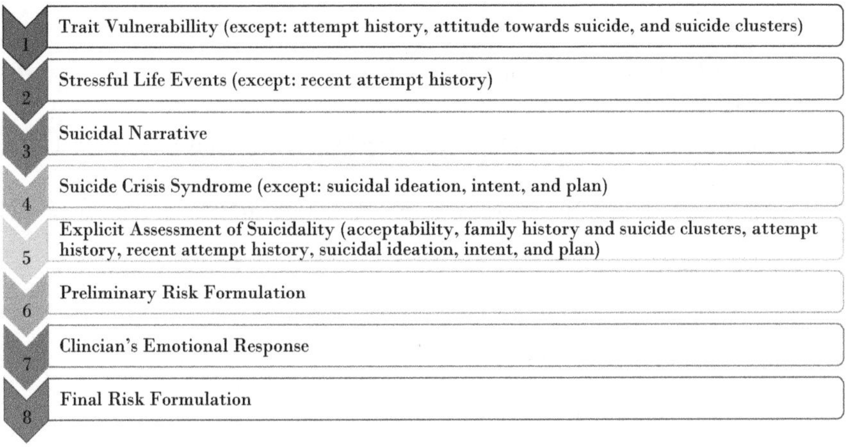

1. Trait Vulnerabillity (except: attempt history, attitude towards suicide, and suicide clusters)

2. Stressful Life Events (except: recent attempt history)

3. Suicidal Narrative

4. Suicide Crisis Syndrome (except: suicidal ideation, intent, and plan)

5. Explicit Assessment of Suicidality (acceptability, family history and suicide clusters, attempt history, recent attempt history, suicidal ideation, intent, and plan)

6. Preliminary Risk Formulation

7. Clinician's Emotional Response

8. Final Risk Formulation

Figure 8.1 Comprehensive short-term risk assessment interview.

- The fourth module is the mental status assessment aimed at eliciting symptoms of SCS, such as entrapment, affective disturbance, and ruminative flooding. No questions about suicidal ideation are asked at this stage.
- The fifth module is a direct assessment of the suicide-related clinical material listed in the comprehensive assessment, including family history of suicide, suicide clusters, attitudes toward suicide, recent and remote past suicidal behavior and current ideation, intent, and plan.
- The sixth module is the clinician's preliminary formulation of short-term risk based on the obtained objective clinical material.
- The seventh module involves the clinician's assessment of his or her emotional response to the patient, with emphasis on possible reaction formation or denial defenses to "countertransference hate."
- The eighth and the final module involves the reassessment of the preliminary formulation, which takes into account the clinician's emotional response.

Case 55: Comprehensive Short-Term Risk Assessment Interview Example

Location: Outpatient office.

Patient: Hans is a 30-year-old man with a history of bipolar disorder and alcohol use.

Circumstances/chief complaint: Patient was brought in by his parents for an assessment because he said he was going to kill himself.

History of present illness: Hans was still living with his parents on their full financial support. They recently refused to help him start a marijuana-growing business.

Building Rapport

DR: Hello Hans, how are you feeling today?

HANS: Fine.

DR: I understand that you may need help with your bipolar disorder. Is that so?

HANS: Yes.

DR: Let's start then. You know, my interview may be a little longer than usual, but bear with me. OK?

HANS: OK.

Trait Vulnerability

DR: How old are you?

HANS: 30.

DR: You came here with your parents; what's your relationship like with them?

HANS: You don't fool around ... go straight to the point. ... The relationship is not good.

DR: Sorry to hear that. Why?

HANS: They always criticize me. I can't win.

DR: Are you close with them?

HANS: Closer than I want to be.

DR: Sounds like your relationship with them is too close for your comfort. Are they strict?

HANS: I told you I can't seem to do anything right.

DR: Are they abusive?

HANS: I guess you can call this emotional abuse.

DR: Any physical or sexual abuse?

HANS: No.

DR: Any history of mental illness in the family?

HANS: My grandfather. He killed himself when I was little.

DR: I am sorry to hear that. I will return to that later if you do not mind. Did you have any traumatic experiences as a child?

HANS: I was bullied in middle school.

DR: It must have been really painful, if you to bring it up now. Why were you bullied?

HANS: I was fat and I was not athletic.

DR: Is this when you first saw a psychiatrist?

HANS: No, that was in elementary school for ADHD. I was on Ritalin and Seroquel and other stuff.

DR: Did you have friends in elementary school?

HANS: Yeah.

DR: And in high school?

HANS: I had a few.

DR: Girlfriends?

HANS: Not really ...

DR: What is your sexual orientation?

HANS: I am very straight.

DR: I see. Do you have a girlfriend now?

HANS: Yeah! But don't tell my parents. They don't approve.

DR: It seems that your care about your parents' approval. . . . Are you a sensitive person?

HANS: I am pretty thin-skinned. Things get to me.

DR: When things get to you, do you try to avoid the conflict?

HANS: It depends. I fight with my parents a lot.

DR: How about street fights? Did you get into fights as a kid?

HANS: Not really. I am pretty laid back.

DR: Is it fair to say that you are not a perfectionist?

HANS: Yeah.

DR: Some more questions about you as a person: Do you generally see a glass as half full or half empty? Are you an optimist or a pessimist?

HANS: A pessimist. Definitely.

DR: OK. Finally, are you a spontaneous person or a planner?

HANS: Mmmm . . . not a planner. I can be pretty impulsive.

Trait Vulnerability Summary

Hans is a 30-year-old male with a long history of mood disorder and anxiety disorder, and he also has a history of childhood bullying. His attachment style appears to be anxious and fearful. Hans acknowledges his own impulsivity and lack of perfectionism and has dependent traits.

Stressful Life Events

DR: Are you working?

HANS: No. . . . I want to start a business.

DR: Want kind of business?

HANS: Growing medical marijuana.

DR: Do you have a plan?

HANS: No, but I have a friend who does. I just need my parents to put up some money.

DR: Are they willing?

HANS: No. That's why we've been fighting.

DR: How does the fighting make you feel?

HANS: I feel that they owe me. I have had a mental illness since I was little. I graduated from high school. I finished college. I worked before. I have been trying to be productive. Now that I have an opportunity "to grow up" (their words) and to be independent, they are not helping. I am not asking for much, and they can afford it.

DR: I see. When they want you "to grow up," do they threaten to kick you out of the house?

HANS: No. I can live in the basement forever.

DR: What's "growing up" then?

HANS: Get a job and find my own place. Even if I flip hamburgers.

DR: When was your last job, and what was it?

HANS: Two years ago. I worked for my dad.

DR: And?

HANS: I left because I was mistreated. My brother, "the manager," is only 2 years older than me! They wanted me to make copies.

DR: Do you think that your parents are unfair to you?

HANS: Always. Since I can remember.

DR: What does your girlfriend think about this?

HANS: She thinks I am crazy . . . and she thinks they should be more supportive.

DR: Why do your parents dislike her?

HANS: Because she drinks and does drugs. They also think she is not smart.

DR: Does she use drugs? Is she smart?

HANS: She smokes pot and she drinks, like everybody else. And hangs out with crazy me. And she laughs at my jokes.

DR: Things are OK with your girlfriend, it seems. Is this long term?

HANS: No (smiles), but she does not know it.

DR: Noted (smiles). . . . How does all this affect your depression?

HANS: Makes it worse . . . I have been drinking more. I am 30 years old, living with my parents, and my life is not going anywhere. I, finally, could succeed at something, and they are not supportive.

DR: Is your depression worse than usual?

HANS: Yes but I can work! I just need the money to start my business.

DR: What medications are you taking?

HANS: I have been taking the same meds for years: Seroquel, Lamictal, Lexapro, and Adderall.

DR: Have the doses been changed recently?

HANS: No. Same old, same old.

DR: How much have you been drinking?

HANS: Two or three beers a day.

DR: What about on weekends?

HANS: Mmmm, more on weekends, with my buddies . . . maybe five beers.

DR: Do you black out?

HANS: Occasionally (smiles).

DR: How much worse is your drinking than, say, last year?

HANS: Well . . . about the same, now that you asked.

Stressful Life Events Summary

Hans reports no recent relationship or health-related stressors and no recent increase in alcohol use. He reports an ongoing conflict with his parents and a possible upcoming change in his financial status, depending on how the current conflict is resolved. He exhibits externalizing traits (narcissistic and antisocial).)

Suicidal Narrative

DR: So, Hans, if I may: What are your life goals?

HANS: A big question. . . . What does everybody wants? I want to be happy. I would like to have a business, a family, and a house with a backyard. The American Dream.

DR: Are your goals realistic? You are 30, depressed, living with your parents . . . and I presume that your parents are paying for this appointment.

HANS: Are you telling me that I am a failure?

DR: No, I didn't mean to . . . I have just repeated what you said earlier. Do you think your goals are achievable?

HANS: Yes they are. I want to start this business with my friend!

DR: OK. Let's say the business does not happen. Will you be able to modify your life goals? Maybe scale down a little? A job, maybe, a smaller house?

HANS: I am not giving up yet. I do not work well in the corporate environment.

DR: Has life been fair to you? Are you getting the share of happiness you deserve given what you have been through?

HANS: Nobody understands how hard life has been for me. I have been always struggling. And I have been trying. I have been looking for opportunities. The medical marijuana business is a once-in-a-lifetime opportunity. The window will close soon.

DR: Let me ask you another question. Say your parents will not finance your MJ adventure. What would you feel?

HANS: Really angry. I won't have another opportunity like this!

DR: Would this feel like a defeat for you?

HANS: Yeah . . . it would take a while to get over it. . . . My depression will get worse.

DR: Will you be able to get over it?

HANS: I have doctors . . . friends . . . I hope so.

DR: What if your parents stop supporting you altogether?

HANS: What do you mean? They can't just cut me off. They won't . . . they never mentioned it.

DR: Do they make you feel like you burden them, financially or emotionally?

HANS: No. They tell me I am not using my talents, but they promised to support me until I find something that makes me happy.

DR: Earlier you said that you were bullied in school . . . for being different, really. Do you still feel like that? That you are different and that you don't belong?

HANS: I don't. I am not good at political games. I found out when I worked for my father.

DR: Do you want to belong? Maybe giving it another try if the MJ business does not work out?

HANS: That's just too painful. I don't think I can.

DR: So, you future hinges on the marijuana business. Can you see your future without it?

HANS: Mmmmm ... maybe another business. I want this one though.

DR: (Constructing suicidal narrative) Let's see if I understand: It sounds like your life goal is to be like everybody else, but your mental illness makes you a misfit in a corporate environment. The marijuana business is an opportunity but there may be other options. It seems that although your parents are supportive, they also do not understand you. Given how hard your life is, it is only fair that they support you until you find happiness. Is this a reasonable summary?

HANS: Yes, except, if they don't fund my business, I am going to kill myself.

Suicidal Narrative Summary

Hans's perception of his past, present, and future is not consistent with a compelling suicidal narrative. His goals are achievable, he can redirect to lesser goals, he feels entitled rather than burdensome, and he feels connected. Hans has a sense of a future.

Suicide Crisis Syndrome

DR: Hans, I will ask you about your suicidal thoughts very shortly. But first, please tell me more about your current thoughts. Do you feel trapped in your life situation?

HANS: What do you mean?

DR: I mean: Is your life unbearable and do you want to escape it?

HANS: No, I feel mistreated by my parents, but I want to work on it.

DR: Are you patient enough for this type of work?

HANS: Well, the sooner it resolves the better.

DR: Is the your situation causing you emotional pain?

HANS: Of course.

DR: Is the pain there all the time? How intense is it?

HANS: Very. It comes and goes, but I want it to stop. Enough is enough.

DR: Have you had intense mood swings lately? When you feel so bad it's hard to tell what you are feeling?

HANS: Sometimes, but mostly I know what I am feeling.

DR: You told me that you have anxiety. Have you been feeling vulnerable and defenseless, that even a minor slight is immensely painful? Like your parents' criticism?

HANS: It's not minor, doc. They know which buttons to push.

DR: Do you ever feel strange sensations in your body and skin?

HANS: No, that's weird.

DR: Are you enjoying things you usually enjoy? Like food, sex, watching TV?

HANS: Not as much as I wish.

DR: Do you often think about what led to all your problems?

HANS: Are you kidding me? I am 30, living in my parents basement. I think about this all the time.

DR: Do you obsess about possible solutions to your problems?

HANS: Yeah, I need to start a business!

DR: Is your thinking circular, always coming back to the same thing?

HANS: Always the same thing.

DR: Can you change your thoughts with a lot of effort? Can you shut down the unwanted thoughts?

HANS: I can't.

DR: What happens when you try? Do your bad thoughts become even more intense?

HANS: Yes they do.

DR: How do you sleep?

HANS: Not well. Too many things to think about.

Suicide Crisis Syndrome Summary

Although Hans complains of severe emotional pain and some anhedonia, he does not acknowledge entrapment. He reports ruminations, thought suppression, and some cognitive rigidity, which add up to significant loss of cognitive control. His insomnia reveals disturbance in arousal.

Explicit Suicide Risk Assessment

DR: Now, to the main reason you are here. . . . I understand that when your parents told you they would not give you money, you said you would kill yourself.

HANS: And I meant it.

DR: Your grandfather killed himself. Do you remember him?

HANS: I do. We were buddies. I was seven when he died. He was a drinker and he shot himself.

DR: Did you know it at the time?

HANS: No, I only learned when I was in high school. It was a blow. Made me think.

DR: What do you mean?

HANS: Think about suicide. Taking your own life.

DR: What are your thoughts about suicide.

HANS: It's an option. When things get really tough.

DR: In your mind, can a suicide be a solution to life's problems?

HANS: If the pain is too strong.

DR: Did you know other people who had died by suicide?

HANS: Two of my friends died from a heroin overdose.

DR: Were those suicides?

HANS: They did not leave notes or anything. . . . Robin Williams killed himself.

DR: What did his suicide mean to you?

HANS: He was bipolar or something. If nobody could help him, then some cases are just beyond hope. Maybe my grandfather was one of those.

DR: And can you be helped?

HANS: I simply need that money for my business.

DR: But what if your parents refuse to fund your business?

HANS: Then I will kill myself.

DR: How?

HANS: With a gun, like my grandfather.

DR: Do you have a gun?

HANS: I know how to get one.

DR: How?

HANS: Friends. I am not going to tell you.

DR: Have you attempted suicide before?

HANS: I tried once.

DR: What did you do?

HANS: I took pills when I was in high school.

DR: And what happened?

HANS: Just went to sleep.

DR: And?

HANS: Woke up the next day and decided to go on.

DR: Do you remember what pills?

HANS: No, it was 15 years ago.

DR: Are you planning to end your life now?

HANS: If my parents don't support me . . .

DR: What would be your plan?

HANS: I told you I would shoot myself.

DR: I hope it won't come to that. I hope that your depression improves and that you will either negotiate your business plans with your parents or find an alternative. Can I speak to them?

HANS: Yeah, that's OK. Keep me posted.

Explicit Suicide Risk Assessment Summary

Hans reveals remote history of one suicide attempt, acceptance of suicide as a solution to life's problems and no moral objections to it, as well as awareness of a celebrity suicide. He has suicidal ideation and conditional intent with a high-lethality plan.

Preliminary Risk Formulation

Hans is a 30-year-old single white male with mood disorder and likely severe personality disorder with dependent, narcissistic, antisocial, and borderline features who is being assessed because he had threatened suicide. His trait vulnerability is primarily due to his lack of moral objection to suicide, his anxious attachment style, his grandfather's suicide, and his past low-lethality impulsive suicide attempt. His stressful life events are his parents' refusal to fund his unrealistic business plans and their frustration with his dependency on them. Hans's perception of his life is inconsistent with the suicidal narrative. Hans reports some symptoms of SCS, which include suicidal ideation, intent, and plan of high lethality, emotional pain, mild anhedonia, some loss of cognitive control, and insomnia. To summarize, Hans' indirect assessment indicates low risk but is contradicted by the high-risk self-report of explicit intent. The doctor's opinion was that Hans's self-report was both dramatic and vague, casting doubt on his sincerity. Because of the presumed better reliability of the information obtained indirectly, the doctor's preliminary formulation was that Hans was at low risk for short-term suicidal behavior.

Doctor's Emotional Response

The doctor's self-examination of his emotional response revealed anger and disdain for the patient. The doctor became aware of this early in the course of the interview, when Hans responded to his disdain in the following exchange:

> DR: Are your goals realistic? You are 30, depressed, living with your parents . . . and I presume that your parents are paying for this appointment.
> HANS: Are you trying to tell me that I am a failure?

The doctor judged Hans to be entitled and exploitative toward his parents. He thought Hans was manipulating the interview by exaggerating his suicidal risk. The doctor felt guilty about his negative emotional response to the patient affecting his behavior in a way that would minimize his further involvement in this troubling case. The doctor then realized that he was experiencing "countertransference hate" and using denial defense mechanism to minimize his discomfort. He then factored this conclusion into his revised final risk assessment.

Final Risk Formulation

Hans is a 30-year-old male with a history of mood disorder, alcohol use disorder, and suicide attempt who was brought in by his parents for suicidal threat. Hans' trait vulnerability is due to his age, race, history of mental illness, history of suicide attempt, his acceptability of suicide as a solution to life's problems, his anxious and fearful attachment style, and his impulsivity. His stressful life events include potential personal defeat (if his parents refuse to support his marijuana business), which could become crushing with the threat of loss of his parents' financial support and home. His suicidal narrative is fragmented and noted primarily for entitlement to happiness but can become coherent with the loss of parents' financial support and home. His SCS includes suicidal ideation and plan, emotional pain, and loss of cognitive control. The revised overall risk formulation was that, at the time of the assessment, despite significant SCS, Hans was at low risk for short-term suicidal behavior because of his lack of the suicide narrative. However, the doctor thought that the risk could increase sharply with the threat of loss of home and financial support, and he scheduled a family meeting.

The previous comprehensive interview is typical of a short-term risk assessment performed during consultations in outpatient psychiatric clinics. The interview illustrates how modular assessment based on the narrative crisis model of suicidal behavior can bring conceptual clarity to the complex clinical material. The interview also demonstrates how delaying the explicit risk assessment until the end allows most of the interview to be unaffected by self-report bias. Finally, the interview illustrates how a denial defense against "countertransference hate" toward a manipulative patient can both bias the assessment and be factored into adjustment of risk by a shrewd clinician. The revised risk formulation correctly identified potential high risk in the near future and included the family meeting into the treatment plan.

The MARIS Interview

The MARIS interview is a concise interview based on the MARIS instrument to be used primarily in ongoing inpatient or emergency department assessments. Because MARIS is a self-report questionnaire, its items are worded differently from the language used during a face-to-face conversational interview. However, the MARIS structure provides a useful framework for an abbreviated assessment of short-term suicide risk. MARIS modules provide a useful algorithm for a focused bare-bones interview when the clinician is either short on time or already knows the patient making, thus the comprehensive interview unnecessary (Figure 8.2).

The MARIS Interview Strategy

- As in the comprehensive interview, the clinician first builds rapport. He or she then quickly transitions to the first SCS module—the mental status examination aimed at eliciting symptoms of entrapment, affective disturbance, and loss of cognitive control. As in the comprehensive interview, no questions about suicidal ideation or intent are asked until the end.
- The second module assesses the patient's attitudes toward suicide as a solution to life's problems. Both morally and culturally permissive and prohibitive attitudes should be assessed. Although this module does not question about the patient's suicidality directly, its purpose as a suicide risk assessment tool is more transparent than that of the first module.

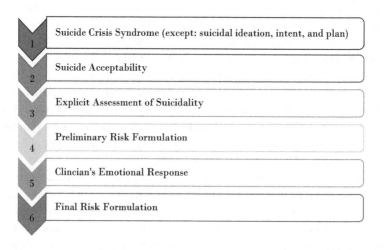

1. Suicide Crisis Syndrome (except: suicidal ideation, intent, and plan)
2. Suicide Acceptability
3. Explicit Assessment of Suicidality
4. Preliminary Risk Formulation
5. Clincian's Emotional Response
6. Final Risk Formulation

Figure 8.2 MARIS interview.

- The third module is an abbreviated explicit assessment of suicide-related clinical material similar to the comprehensive assessment, including family history of suicide, suicide clusters, and suicidal behavior, ideation and plan, with the emphasis on current and recent.
- In the fourth module, the clinician makes the preliminary assessment of the short-term risk and makes preliminary clinical decisions regarding the immediate treatment, disposition, and follow-up.
- The fifth module involves the clinician's assessment of his or her emotional reaction to the patient, with an emphasis on possible "countertransference love" and "countertransference hate" to be factored into the final decision-making process.
- The sixth and final module involves the synthesis of all the clinical material into the final formulation of risk and the decision regarding treatment, disposition, and follow-up.

Case 56: MARIS Interview Example

Location: Inpatient psychiatric unit.

Patient: Karen is an attractive 37-year-old woman with a history of MDD and generalized anxiety disorder who is being assessed prior to her planned discharge from an inpatient unit.

Circumstances/chief complaint: Karen was admitted after a suicide attempt by asphyxiation using a plastic bag after her boyfriend told her he wanted to break-up.

Hospital course: The patient's depression and anxiety appeared to have improved somewhat with antidepressant treatment. Her boyfriend had agreed to start couples counseling. Karen's affect had brightened. She was attending groups, making future plans (with and without her boyfriend), and waiting impatiently for discharge.

Suicide Crisis Syndrome

DR: How are you feeling today?

KAREN: Better . . . much calmer than before.

DR: Very good, what's on your mind?

KAREN: A lot. . . . Why does Alex want to break up? Why I did what I did. Why was I feeling so bad? How can I avoid feeling this bad again?

DR: Sounds like you still have too many thoughts in your head . . .

KAREN: Yes, but differently . . . these thoughts are positive and constructive.

DR: Do you still feel pressure in your head from thinking too much?

KAREN: Sometimes . . . but it's OK, I need to think.

DR: Do you feel pain in your head from having too many thoughts?

KAREN: Maybe just once.

DR: Are your thoughts confused?

KAREN: A little. . . . He was leaving then he was staying, than he was leaving again. The couples sessions make you think. . . . But it's all good.

DR: Are you scared that something bad may happen?

KAREN: Not as much as before.

DR: Is your fear coming in waves?

KAREN: Yes, it's hard to know how you are going to feel the next moment.

DR: Are you able to enjoy things?

KAREN: On the unit? . . . Frankly, it feels like jail, but maybe when I leave.

DR: Do you feel trapped?

KAREN: Being locked up does not help.

DR: Do you feel like there is an exit from your life situation?

KAREN: I don't see any yet, but I will work on them with the therapist after the discharge. When will that be?

Suicide Crisis Syndrome Summary

Karen has some symptoms of SCS, such as entrapment, ruminative flooding, and anhedonia, but her thinking is more positive than on admission.

Acceptability

DR: Do you feel that suicide is a possible solution to one's problems?

KAREN: It can end the suffering for some people. I thought it would end mine, but I was wrong

DR: Is suicide immoral?

KAREN: I don't think it's immoral. My attempt was premature. I can see the future now.

DR: And from a religious point of view?

KAREN: I am not religious.

DR: What about how it affects others?

KAREN: I don't want to hurt anybody. But I was a burden to Alex, and maybe I still am. I hope not.

Acceptability Summary

The patient continues to accept suicide as a solution to life's problems.

Explicit Assessment

DR: And in your case?

KAREN: Alex says he loves me. I would never hurt him again.

DR: But you did hurt him the first time . . .

KAREN: I thought I was a burden and I would always be a burden. Time heals.

DR: Are you still thinking about suicide?

KAREN: Not really. . . . Therapy helps, and the antidepressants. I am looking forward to seeing Alex. He is coming in the evening.

DR: Are you planning to kill yourself?

KAREN: Not anymore. Even if things with Alex do not work out. I should be strong enough to be on my own. The therapy is helping me figure things out.

DR: What do you mean?

KAREN: I am feeling better. I am not in the dark place I was in before. I am working on my problems.

DR: And what will you do if you are in a dark place as before?

KAREN: I will call my therapist, my parents; I will go to the ER.

DR: How many times have you attempted suicide?

KAREN: Two. But the first time was long ago.

DR: How?

KAREN: When I was young I took pills.

DR: And recently?

KAREN: I put a bag over my head.

DR: And what happened?

KAREN: Alex found me unconscious and called the police.

DR: If you feel bad, would you attempt suicide on the unit?

KAREN: How? Everybody is watching you all the time.

DR: I see. I hope you feel better. I will talk to the team.

Explicit Assessment Summary

Karen has had two attempts of increasing lethality but currently denies suicidal intent and commits to safety.

Preliminary Risk Formulation

Karen is a 37-year-old woman with chronic mental illness and two suicide attempts. The last attempt was by asphyxiation when she was experiencing severe symptoms of SCS. Her lack of moral prohibitions against suicide puts her at a higher risk. However, at present, her SCS has resolved. She has no suicidal ideation or intent, does not feel entrapment, and has future plans. Her mood symptoms have improved with treatment. The preliminary conclusion is that Karen is at a low short-term suicide risk and could be discharged.

Doctor's Emotional Response

The doctor's self-assessment of his emotions revealed that he liked Karen, felt empathy for her, and was somewhat attracted to her. The doctor noted that he was looking forward to seeing Karen and that her neediness made him feel powerful and confident. He also felt proud that she improved under his care and was no longer suicidal. The doctor noted that he felt slightly guilty about his attraction to Karen and concluded that he was using the reaction formation defense to a suicidal patient. Knowing that denial may have biased his risk assessment toward lower risk, the doctor has revised the formulation.

Karen is a 37-year-old woman with a history of chronic mental illness, two suicide attempts, and recent high-lethality attempt by asphyxiation. Despite denying suicidal intent, she reports significant SCS symptoms, both affective disturbance (depressive turmoil and anhedonia) and loss of cognitive control (ruminations, reflective pondering, and ruminative flooding). Her sense of entrapment has lessened, but the future she can picture is contingent on her keeping Alex. She has no moral prohibitions against suicide, and her commitment to safety on the unit is actually due to means restriction and being watched. Given the intense residual SCS symptoms, and uncertainty of her future with Alex, she is at high risk for suicide if discharged. Moreover, she is at high risk on the unit, subject to Alex's intention to stay or to leave. The doctor's revised conclusion was that Karen is at high short-term risk for suicide.

(Following his assessment, the doctor ordered a room search, which discovered a plastic bag under Karen's mattress. Karen admitted to a conditional plan to use the bag to end her life if Alex decides to leave. She was placed on close observation, and a meeting with Alex was scheduled.)

The previous MARIS interview was focused but sufficiently detailed to reveal Karen's continuing suicidal crisis and acceptability of suicide. The clinician's use of the reaction formation defense indicated higher risk that the patient would be otherwise. No additional interviewing was necessary to make the correct clinical decision to do a search, which revealed Karen's preparatory actions for suicide on the unit, and to place her on close observation afterwards.

Karen's case illustrates a frequent clinical situation in which a recently suicidal patient denies suicidality, wanting to convince the clinical team that the patient is safe for discharge. In Karen's case, both the residual SCS symptoms and the intense emotional response allowed the clinician to diagnose high suicide risk with relative ease. For another, more difficult diagnostic dilemma, see the section "The Case of Eerie Calm" later in this chapter.

Expanded MARIS Interview

Due to its intended use as a brief assessment and screening tool, MARIS focuses primarily on SCS, as does the MARIS interview. The MARIS format allows clinicians to detect the suicidal crisis and to identify individuals with no moral prohibitions against suicide and with high trait vulnerability due to past history. Furthermore, the MARIS interview gives clinicians an opportunity to factor in their strong emotional responses into clinical decision-making.

The MARIS interview is well suited for detection of suicide crisis and crisis-driven short-term suicide risk, but it is less sensitive to the high risk due to strong suicidal narrative. For that reason, in cases in which no SCS is elicited during the MARIS interview, the clinician would need to continue the interview using the expanded MARIS interview format, which adds the modules that target recent life stressors and the suicidal narrative.

After completing the additional modules, the clinician would need to reassess his or her emotional response to the patient, which may change as a result of the new information. Overall, the expanded MARIS interview is the comprehensive assessment differently organized, with the explicit part of the assessment moved to the beginning of the interview (Figure 8.3).

Case 57: Expanded MARIS Interview Example

Location: Emergency department.

Patient: Ellen is a 47-year-old woman with a long history of depression.

Circumstances/chief complaint: Ellen's husband brought her in for an evaluation of her depression.

History of present illness: The patient's husband was worried that Ellen's new antidepressant was making her worse. He has never seen her so depressed.

Suicide Crisis Syndrome

DR: Good evening Ellen, How are you feeling?

ELLEN: I feel depressed.

DR: What is making you depressed?

ELLEN: I have been having problems at work.

DR: I promise, we'll talk about your work a little later, but for now, can we talk about how these problems make you feel and think?

ELLEN: If you say so.

DR: OK. . . . Do you feel trapped in your work situation?

ELLEN: Well, I can't see a way out of it . . .

DR: Do you think about your problems, and being trapped, all the time?

ELLEN: Most of the time.

DR: Can you stop these thoughts when you try?

ELLEN: Sometimes . . . and sometimes I can't.

DR: Do these thoughts give you headaches?

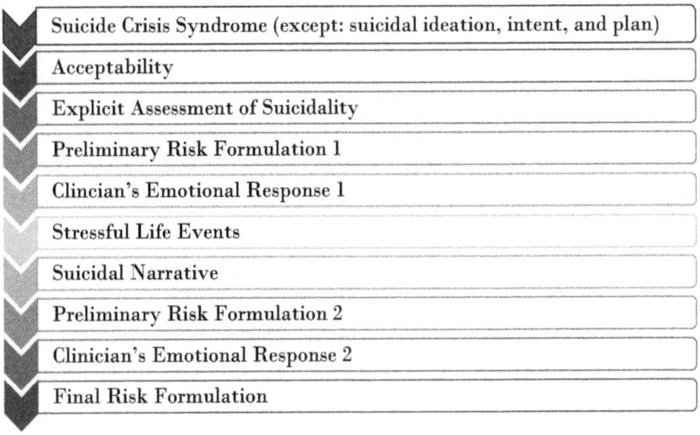

Suicide Crisis Syndrome (except: suicidal ideation, intent, and plan)
Acceptability
Explicit Assessment of Suicidality
Preliminary Risk Formulation 1
Clincian's Emotional Response 1
Stressful Life Events
Suicidal Narrative
Preliminary Risk Formulation 2
Clinician's Emotional Response 2
Final Risk Formulation

Figure 8.3 Expanded MARIS interview.

ELLEN: Sometimes.

DR: Do these thoughts make you feel pressure in your head?

ELLEN: (Smiles) Not right now.

DR: It sounds that sometimes they do, though. When you feel your worst, are you afraid that something horrible may happen, like a heart attack, and—kill you?

ELLEN: No.

DR: Have you been feeling mental pain?

ELLEN: Yes, it has been terrible.

DR: Does this pain come in waves?

ELLEN: More like in shocks.

Suicide Crisis Syndrome Summary

Ellen has a strong sense of entrapment, significant loss of cognitive control, and affective disturbance.

Acceptability

DR: Some people believe than when things are really bad in life, suicide may be the only escape.

ELLEN: I would agree. Sometimes, life may just be too painful to bear.

DR: Do you think other people can tell when somebody is suicidal?

ELLEN: Not if the person keeps the plans secret.

DR: Are you religious?

ELLEN: I am Jewish, but I am not observant.

Acceptability Summary

Ellen accepts suicide as a solution to life's problems and pains.

Explicit Assessment

DR: Is suicide a possible solution for you?

ELLEN: You said this is not about me. I am depressed.

DR: Have you ever attempted suicide before?

ELLEN: No, but I thought about it.

DR: Recently?

ELLEN: No. . . . Years back when I was having a rough time.

DR: Worse than now?

ELLEN: Now is actually tougher.

DR: At the time, did you have a plan?

ELLEN: Kind of.

DR: What was it?

ELLEN: I would jump off something high . . . no chance of surviving and becoming a vegetable.

DR: You seem very clear-headed about this. Do you still have this plan?

ELLEN: No . . . it was in the past.

DR: Any thoughts about suicide now?

ELLEN: I am depressed but not suicidal.

DR: If discharged and feeling suicidal, will you ask for help?

ELLEN: Yes, I am here aren't I?

Explicit Assessment Summary

Ellen denies suicidal ideation and intent, and she commits to safety.

Preliminary Risk Formulation

Ellen is a 47-year-old woman with a history of depression and past high-lethality suicide plan she did not enact. She currently has significant SCS, and she accepts suicide as a solution to problems. She denies suicidal ideation and intent, and she commits to safety. The information is contradictory. Although both Ellen and her husband state that this is her worst depression, she is less suicidal than during the previous, less severe episode. Moreover, her self-report of no ideation contradicts her high-intensity SCS. The preliminary formulation is that no conclusion regarding risk can be made, necessitating the expanded interview.

Doctor's Emotional Response 1

The doctor's self-assessment of her emotional responses revealed sympathy and liking for Ellen, as well as her confidence in her ability to help her. The doctor also felt unease about not having a clear understanding of her suicide risk. The doctor concluded that she felt no "countertransference hate" to the suicidal patient and that she was using neither the reaction formation nor the denial defenses; she then proceeded with the expanded MARIS interview.

Stressful Life Events

DR: Now let's talk about your work. Why do you feel trapped at work?

ELLEN: I don't think I am getting my grant renewed.

DR: What does that mean for you?

ELLEN: This means I cannot continue my research. I have had this grant for 15 years. This may be the end of my academic career.

DR: Will you lose your job?

ELLEN: Almost certainly. There won' be enough bridge money to write another grant, and I don't have tenure. Nobody has tenure anymore. You are expected to bring in your own research money.

DR: And if you can't?

ELLEN: I will tell my researchers to look for jobs and look for one myself.

DR: What jobs would you look for?

ELLEN: I can work in the pharmaceutical industry. . . . I never thought that would happen to me.

DR: What is wrong with the pharma?

ELLEN: Everything. It's all about profit. I worked there before I got my PhD. I hated it.

DR: Are there other options?

ELLEN: I can teach in some community college. (Laughs sarcastically)

DR: How are things financially?

ELLEN: My husband has a good job. Finances are not the issue.

DR: Are things OK with your husband?

ELLEN: As OK as they will ever be. He is limited.

DR: What are his limitations?

ELLEN: He is in construction. He never understood science.

DR: How is your health?

ELLEN: I am fine.

DR: Are things OK with your children?

ELLEN: They are in college. They are fine.

Stressful Life Events Summary

Ellen is facing a job loss, which could be career-ending. She also feels chronically isolated and misunderstood at home.

Suicidal Narrative

DR: It sounds like you have high standards. . . . Are you a perfectionist?

ELLEN: How can one be an imperfect scientist?

DR: Do you set high goals for yourself?

ELLEN: You can't be in medicine otherwise. It takes 5 years to accomplish anything, and it better be consequential. I wanted to find a cure for cancer. And our results are incredible!

DR: Hmm. Are you an overachiever?

ELLEN: I am a hard worker and I don't cut corners.

DR: Were you expecting to be happier at this stage in your life? Has life treated you fairly?

ELLEN: Ha! I brought in $15 million of grant money and $10 million in overhead that *all* went to the school. Don't you think I deserve better?

DR: I certainly do, and sounds like you did amazing work. But I am not the decider, unfortunately. If you do not get the bridge money, will you be able to change to plan B? Maybe, indeed, in industry, or . . . teaching?

ELLEN: I can't even think about this. . . . This would be so humiliating. What will I tell my colleagues? I will be too ashamed to attend the meetings! I will have nothing to present . . .

DR: Do you know other scientists who did not get their grants renewed?

ELLEN: Yes . . . and they are pitied or avoided.

DR: Are you afraid that you will become one of them?

ELLEN: For sure. . . . I will be too humiliated to look people in the eye. I will not leave my apartment.

DR: But life is unpredictable. People understand. Life rarely turns out the way you have imagined. Can you imagine a different future? As project leader in industry, or star teacher?

ELLEN: I can't. According to you, I am a failure.

DR: Absolutely not, but is this how you see yourself? A failure?

ELLEN: (Nods)

DR: Now I understand why you feel trapped. That time, when you were suicidal and you thought of jumping, was it also related to work?

ELLEN: Yes, somebody could not reproduce my results and questioned my scientific integrity. It was political.

DR: And what happened?

ELLEN: My mentor stepped in and they backed off.

DR: I see. . . . Let me stop for now. Can I speak to your husband if you do not mind?

Suicidal Narrative Summary

Ellen's perception of her life includes all phases of the suicidal narrative: perfectionism, failure to disengage from an unreachable goal (continuing her research), humiliating failure, alienation, and a sense of no future. Her suicidal narrative is so clear that the doctor does not even reprise it for the patient.

Preliminary Risk Formulation 2

Ellen is a 47-year-old woman with history of depression and of past high-lethality plan during a *less severe* episode. She lacks moral prohibitions against suicide. Her stress due to the perception of imminent career-ending job loss is overwhelming. Currently, Ellen sees herself in an unacceptable life situation due to humiliating work failure. She cannot imagine a future and sees her situation as simultaneously painfully intolerable and inescapable—that is, she perceives her life as clear suicidal narrative. Ellen has many symptoms of SCS, and other than her superficial denial of suicidal intent, all other clinical information suggests very high short-term risk.

Clinician's Emotional Response 2

The doctor's second self-assessment of her emotional responses was less sympathetic toward the patient than her first, and she felt irritated at Ellen's lack of flexibility. The doctor still felt deep concern for the patient. Her initial unease about not understanding her suicide risk changed to a concern that, if discharged, Ellen may kill herself by jumping off a building. The doctor concluded that she was not experiencing "countertransference hate" to the suicidal patient, nor was she using the reaction formation or the denial defenses. She felt no need to revise her diagnostic formulation and called the husband regarding possible hospitalization.

Final Risk Formulation

The final risk formulation is the same as preliminary risk formulation 2.

THE CASE OF EERIE CALM

The criteria for SCS, which precedes suicide, describe entrapment dominated by urgency to escape an unbearable life situation when escape is perceived as impossible. Thus, death appears as the only achievable solution to unbearable pain. SCS also involves at least one symptom of affective disturbance, loss of cognitive control, and hyperarousal. Many patients with SCS project a feeling of unnerving intensity, which could make a clinician feel uncomfortable. Yet some individuals prior to their suicide appear calm, composed, and even placid.

There are a number of reasons why suicidal individuals may appear calm and content in the hours or minutes preceding suicide. First, the symptoms of SCS (e.g., entrapment or ruminations) describe subjective inner experiences that are not always visible to an outside observer, particularly if the patient does not reveal his or her inner state. Agitation and insomnia are readily observable, but agitation may be intermittent, whereas insomnia is not specific to suicidal individuals. Thus, even patients with severe SCS may appear calm outwardly.

Second, SCS severity may be lower for narrative-driven suicides than for crisis-driven suicides. For example, an elderly person with advancing malignancy and poor pain control may be more distressed by the pain and the prospect of imminent death than by SCS symptoms. For individuals in this type of situation, death as the only perceived solution to the unbearable pain may seem a respite, and after they had already planned the suicide, they may suddenly appear calm.

Third, in some individuals SCS may be of sudden onset and last only hours or even minutes (Deisenhammer et al., 2009). When assessed prior to their suicide crises, these individuals may not feel entrapped and may experience no symptoms of affective disturbance or loss of cognitive control. They may also appear calm or, if not, they may look and behave like their usual selves to outsiders.

Clinicians can encounter either of the previously discussed scenarios when treating recently suicidal individuals. The calm, the upbeat mood, and even elation exhibited by those who were desperate just recently can have an eerie unreal quality, which makes clinicians feel a deep sense of unease. The abrupt change in affect could also be confusing for their loved ones. The eeriness and confusion derive from the difficulty in reconciling the patient's sudden change in mental state and his or her unchanged or almost unchanged life narrative, which had just recently brought on the patient's suicide attempt.

On the one hand, the patient's relatives and clinicians feel relieved at the patient's change; they want to believe that the patient is no longer suicidal and views life differently.

They want the patient discharged from the hospital. On the other hand, the sudden incongruent "exemplary" mental state of somebody who has just survived a suicide attempt and who was recently finding no reason to live makes clinicians anxious and insecure.

Clinicians most frequently experience this unease when treating psychiatric inpatients admitted because of their explicit suicidal intent or after a suicide attempt. Some may have already planned their next and more lethal suicide attempt and want to be discharged so they can accomplish their goal. Others may be so deeply embarrassed by their attempt failure, their subsequent hospitalization, and their new "sick role" that they are in denial that the circumstances that brought on their suicide attempt have not changed. In either case, such patients explicitly deny suicidal intent, follow the unit routine, and promise to comply with any discharge treatment plan.

Because outwardly these patients are not suicidal, exhibit "insight" into their behavior, and agree to the outpatient follow-up, their psychiatrists can no longer justify their hospitalization to the bed utilization review or the managed care companies. Some of these patients leaving the hospital with family members, with a follow-up plan and after "warm hand-off" to outpatient clinicians with a safety plan, may go on to kill themselves, sometimes within hours of discharge.

The first post-discharge week carries the highest risk of suicide death, which in comparison with those never hospitalized is 252:1 for women and 108:1 for men. A prospective study (Yaseen et al., 2014) showed that both ultra-high and ultra-low scorers on the Suicide Trigger Scale (STS-3) risk assessment scale were likely to attempt suicide within the first 2 months after discharge. In fact, the majority were the ultra-low scorers, who very quickly after their admission denied having any symptoms of the STS that brought them to the hospital in the first place.

How can the clinician justify continuing hospitalization of a patient who has exhibited insight into his or her behavior, has agreed to treatment follow-up, and has "committed" to safety when the clinician's intuition and inner discomfort tell him or her that the patient is at acute risk? One option is to forcefully explore the patient's abrupt changes in mood and the possibility of the patient viewing his or her life as suicidal narrative or feeling SCS symptoms:

You seem so calm. Is this how you feel inside?
Are you able to see your future clearly now? What are your options?
Your mood change is a little unexpected. You wanted to die just last week. What changed?
You felt so trapped last week. What happened to those feelings?
Please tell me, how is your thinking? What were your thoughts like last night?

Answers revealing that the patient's continuing perception of having no good options for the future or continuing SCS symptoms would indicate high short-term risk for suicide. These answers would need to be carefully documented in the chart followed by a conclusion that the patient requires further inpatient hospital stay for safety and treatment. Vague answers should raise concern about the genuineness of the patient's insight, which also should be documented as a justification for the extended hospital stay.

The following case is representative of an eerie calm exhibited by a patient after high-lethality suicidal behavior.

Case 58

Michael, a 55-year-old single man, was transferred to an inpatient unit from the hospital intensive care unit after a failed suicide attempt by hanging on a door handle. He was found unconscious and, as result of his attempt, suffered a subclavian steal syndrome but no anoxic brain injury. Prior to his suicide attempt, Michael, who was gay, worked as a manager in a rug store owned by his friend John, with whom he may have been involved in a long-term love affair. One month prior to Michael's suicide attempt, John, who was married, suddenly told Michael that was retiring and moving to Florida. He then left town and delegated Michael to close the store and let go of the long-term employees who were like a family to Michael. Feeling betrayed and devastated, Michael did as he was told, but the night after the last person left and he closed the store for good, he tried to hang himself. He passed out and would have died, but the handle to which he had tied the rope broke off.

After a week-long stay in the medical intensive care unit, Michael was transferred to an inpatient psychiatric unit, where he was given an antidepressant. Michael was withdrawn and quiet at first. However, on the second day his affect brightened, and on the third day Michael was seen smiling and even joking. In sessions with his doctor, he was remorseful about his attempt, which he called stupid. He participated in all groups and activities, where he exhibited superficial insight and avoided questions about his personal life. His general plan after the discharge was to take medications and get some therapy to "sort things out" and "to figure out how I could be so stupid." Michael's affect was bright, and he denied suicidal intent. However, Michael's improvement made the staff feel uneasy. His change in mood seemed sudden and unjustified. He did not want to discuss John and his anger at him for leaving for Florida and making him do the dirty work of laying people off and closing the store.

Still, after a week-long hospital stay, Michael maintained his bright affect and the team discussed the patient's progress and discharge plans. Some staff members felt uneasy about discharging him because his progress was "too good to be true" and nobody really knew what was "inside his head." However, his longer hospital stay could not be justified because Michael was "saying and doing all the right things."

The next day, Michael was given an outpatient appointment with a psychiatrist, and he was discharged to the care of a friend. When leaving, Michael said good-bye and thanked the nurses for taking good care of him. The friend picked him up, drove Michael home and left him in his 18th-floor apartment. He and Michael agreed to meet for lunch the next day and do something afterwards. However, tragically, 2 hours later, Michael jumped to his death off his apartment balcony.

Michael's case is an illustration of the patient's eerie calm after a high-lethality attempt, which made clinicians feel anxious and uneasy because the changes in mood and affect were not justified by the changes in the patient's life narrative and stressors. At least two scenarios are possible. The first scenario is that on the unit Michael sincerely believed that his attempt was in the past and that the future looked brighter with medications and therapy. However, something did not go as planned when he got home: For instance, John refused to talk to him. Such a refusal might have precipitated his second suicidal crisis and his suicide. The second scenario is that Michael planned his suicide all along and was actively hiding his intent. In either case, the sudden change in mood and the lack of detail in the patient's description of his mental state to justify such a change gave his calm affect an eerie quality and made the staff feel uneasy.

9

Interventions

With Raquel Rose and Nicolette Molina

INTRODUCTION

Currently, there are no US Food and Drug Administration-approved treatments for suicidal behavior despite suicide being one of the leading causes of death in the United States. In 1999, "The Surgeon General's Call to Action to Prevent Suicide" (US Public Health Service, 1999) emphasized the need for empirically supported suicide prevention and treatment strategies, particularly for adolescents. Although there is no gold standard for suicide treatments, there are available interventions that provide potentially effective treatment. Many of these have psychosocial frameworks for intervention during an acute suicidal episode, including assessing for risks and resources, creating a safe haven (through crisis intervention, emergency department visit, and means restriction), stabilizing symptoms, and trying to limit side effects (Gunnell et al., 2013). Other treatments include biological therapeutics and virtual tools.

MEDICATIONS AND BIOLOGICAL INTERVENTIONS

Past drug treatments have shown some effectiveness with suicidal patients. However, this was likely due to the treatment of an underlying diagnosis that has high comorbidity with suicidal behavior (e.g., bipolar disorder and depression) because 90% of those who die from suicide have another underlying mental disorder (Chang, Gitlin, & Patel, 2011). Although the literature is sparse on a direct connection between biological therapeutics and suicide prevention, the mitigating effects of some drug treatments warrant further scrutiny.

Clozapine (Antipsychotics)

Clozapine, an atypical antipsychotic, is used to treat schizophrenia when more conventional medicines have been ineffective. Due to clozapine's ability to act on multiple neurotransmitter systems, it has many side effects, some of which are significant (Foster, 2013). However, in a randomized, controlled, multicenter InterSept study that compared clozapine to a more widely prescribed antipsychotic (olanzapine) with regard to their ability to reduce suicidal outcomes, clozapine showed a significantly higher reduction in suicide attempts (Thomas, Jiang, & McCombs, 2015).

Lithium

Lithium is a widely used and well-studied medication. The data on the anti-suicidal action of lithium are conflicting (Tondo, Hennen, & Baldessarini, 2001). However, Cipriani and colleagues (2005) found that suicidal behavior and mortality decreased significantly in patients who received lithium treatment. A follow-up study found that lithium was statistically more effective than a placebo and a comparable drug in decreasing suicide deaths (Cipriani, Hawton, Stockton, & Geddes, 2013). Although the mechanism is not fully understood, it is hypothesized that lithium mitigates suicide by diminishing impulsivity (Müller-Oerlinghausen & Lewitzka, 2010). A concern with ongoing use of lithium is its toxicity profile, particularly when used long term. Potential long-term side effects include diabetes insipidus, thyroid dysfunction, kidney dysfunction, and neurotoxicity (Gonzalez, Bernstein, & Suppes, 2008).

Ketamine (Anesthetic Agents)

Anesthetic agents are garnering attention as therapeutics for suicide patients. Generally used by pediatricians and veterinarians, ketamine has been used effectively in emergency procedures and for treatment of chronic pain. Recent evidence indicates that ketamine at low levels may also demonstrate antidepressant properties, which can last 3–7 days, in as quickly as 40 minutes after an intravenous infusion (Murrough et al., 2013). Early data suggest that ketamine may result in transient or even sustained reduction in suicidal ideation (Al Jurdi, Swann, & Mathew, 2015). More evidence is needed to establish the scope and efficacy of ketamine treatment of suicidal ideation and behavior. In the interim, Lee et al. (2016) proposed that the antidepressant and anti-suicidal effects reported with ketamine administration are mediated, in part, by targeting neural circuits that subserve cognitive processing relevant to executive function and cognitive–emotional processing.

The major concern regarding ketamine and ketamine-like compounds is their potential for abuse and their current classification as controlled substances (Newport, Schatzberg, & Nemeroff, 2016). However, given that ketamine is fast-acting, it may respond to a specialized need for those in a crisis or waiting for traditional medication to take effect. With further research, ketamine may become an acute intervention to mitigate immediate suicide concerns (Newport et al., 2015).

PSYCHOSOCIAL INTERVENTIONS

Psychosocial interventions have long been used to treat various mental illnesses, and some have been tailored to work with suicidal patients with varying levels of success.

Dialectical Behavior Therapy

Originally created to treat individuals with borderline personality disorder (BPD), dialectical behavior therapy (DBT) is a multicomponent intervention that has strong experimental support for its ability to decrease suicidal and self-injurious behaviors. The two core principles that inform DBT are that individuals with BPD lack important interpersonal, self-regulation (including emotional regulation), and distress tolerance skills and that personal and environmental factors often block and/or inhibit the use of behavioral skills that these patients do have and reinforce dysfunctional behaviors.

To address these two factors, DBT immerses the patient in individual therapy, group skills training, and between-session telephone coaching, and it provides the patient with a therapist consultation team. In 1993, Linehan, Heard, and Armstrong found that participants randomized to the DBT treatment condition exhibited significantly less parasuicidal behavior and anger and better self-reported social adjustment during the 6-month follow-up period. DBT is also an attractive intervention due to its effectiveness even when separated into its components. With limited funding, heavy caseloads, time restrictions, and the unique severity of each suicidal patient, an intervention such as DBT can be a good treatment option (Linehan et al., 2015).

Cognitive–Behavioral Therapy for Suicidal Patients

In their manualized cognitive–behavioral therapy for suicidal patients (CBT-SP), Drs. Barbara Stanley and Gregory Brown sought to reduce risk and prevent relapse into a suicidal state while tailoring treatment to the needs of adolescents. CBT-SP focuses on developing cognitive, behavioral, and interaction skills with the hope that these skills will help adolescents resist suicidal thoughts and behaviors by modifying reactions to stressors. In a 2009 study, CBT-SP was shown to be a viable treatment to administer to suicidal adolescents, but further testing in randomized controlled trials was recommended (Stanley et al., 2009).

Collaborative Assessment and Management of Suicidality

Developed by Dr. David A. Jobes, the Collaborative Assessment and Management of Suicidality (CAMS) is an evidence-based intervention that emphasizes collaborative assessment and intervention planning between patient and clinician. Pivotal to CAMS is the utilization of the Suicide Status Form (SSF), a multipurpose tool to plan, track, and conceptualize patient outcomes.

CAMS is a therapeutic framework for clinicians' engagement with and treatment of suicidal individuals (Jobes & Shneidman, 2006). Typically, CAMS is initiated with the collaborative completion of the SSF, which is then used to guide the treatment planning and tracking of suicide risk and also the outcome of care. The clinician and the patient then collaboratively develop the Crisis Response Plan, a suicide-specific, problem-focused treatment plan aiming to stabilize the patient. The treatment targets conceptualize the "drivers" of suicidality, which are the specifics that make the patient suicidal.

CAMS also aims to help a suicidal patient develop an existential purpose—a life worth living (Jobes, Comtois, Brenner, & Gutierrez, 2011). CAMS is thus a philosophical as well as a clinical instrument, which specifies a series of steps that are guided by the SSF tool. Its goal is to build a strong clinical alliance and increase patient motivation and engagement in care.

All interventions in CAMS are designed to either reduce or eliminate the impact of suicidal drivers and design alternatives to suicidality. Problem-focused interventions for suicidal drivers in CAMS may include treatments of hopelessness, emotional dysregulation, interpersonal isolation, impulsivity, or difficulties in planning for the future. CAMS-based care can and should be concomitant with psychopharmacology, substance abuse treatment, treatment of health care issues, or vocational counseling.

CAMS is not a new psychotherapy but, rather, an organizational clinical framework for maintaining a collaborative focus on the elimination of suicidal ideation and behavior as a means of coping. In CAMS, a clinician is free to use his or her own expertise to select and implement effective clinical interventions.

The acceptance of CAMS has been growing during the past decade. CAMS is now used in multiple settings in the United States (Ellis, Allen, Woodson, Frueh, & Jobes, 2009) and abroad (Nielsen, Alberdi, & Rosenbaum, 2011). The psychometric assessment properties of the SSF have been established and replicated (Conrad et al., 2009; Jobes, Jacoby, Cimbolic, & Hustead, 1997), with good support for the qualitative assessment of the SSF (Jobes & Mann, 1999; Jobes et al., 2004). Several studies support the feasibility of CAMS and the SSF with suicidal outpatients (Jobes, Wong, Conrad, Drozd, & Neal-Walden, 2005; Nielsen et al., 2011).

Attachment-Based Family Therapy

Attachment-based family therapy (ABFT) turns its scope to examine family interaction and function. Research supports that negative family function is a risk factor for youth suicide and depression. Conflicts with family precede 20% of suicide deaths and 50% of nonfatal suicidal acts by adolescents (Diamond et al., 2010). Although several family studies have shown promising results in treating suicidal youth, ABFT is one of the first manualized family therapies tailored to address severely depressed and suicidal populations (Ewing, Diamond, & Levy, 2015; Shpigel & Diamond, 2012). ABFT focuses on increasing family cohesion and parent–adolescent attachment bonds to create a safe "nest" for the adolescent to mature.

Safety Planning Intervention

One particularly promising intervention is the creation of a personalized safety plan. Identified as a best practice by the Suicide Prevention Resource Center, the Safety Planning Intervention (SPI) was created by Drs. Barbara Stanley and Gregory Brown and intended to be administered as a stand-alone intervention in emergency departments and other acute settings. Although not a treatment, it is meant to be multifaceted in addressing different aspects of safety and is written as a prioritized list of coping strategies and support sources a person can quickly consult. A safety plan in its simplest state is an actionable plan for managing suicidal behavior that is collaborative, documented, and accessible (Currier et al., 2015).

A safety plan (SP) is most effective when developed as a combined effort between patient and clinician early in the course of treatment. The plan is a strategy for the patient to use if a suicidal crisis arises. Although the structure of the treatment derives from the clinical judgment of the clinician, the plan itself is personalized by and for the patient to suit his or her level of suicidality.

An effective SP is composed of the following:

- Recognition of warning signs. Patients will ask themselves "What situations make me feel like I want to kill myself?" as well as contextual details such as "What happens before, who am I with, what am I doing, how do I feel, what am I thinking?"
- Internal coping strategies, where patients are asked what they think they can do to reduce suicidal urges both acutely and long term.
- Socializations to distract from a suicidal crisis and obtain support. The patient will compile a list of healthy people and activities that can serve as distractions. The patient can also compile a list of people or activities that magnify the suicidal crisis.
- Social contacts (family or friends) who may offer help to resolve the crisis if urges become too overwhelming to manage alone.
- Professionals and agencies that are trained to help resolve a suicidal crisis.

Lethal means restriction is a common goal in psychosocial interventions and critical for creating an effective safety plan. Caregivers focus on the reduction of lethal means and eventually eliminate potential methods for self-harm. Many empirical studies have shown that means restriction is effective (Barber & Miller, 2014; Glasgow, 2011). Generally, clinicians ask patients which means they would use during a suicidal crisis and collaboratively identify ways to limit or remove access. Although lethal means restriction is not a guaranteed barrier to a suicide attempt, the added obstacle may act as a delay or deterrent until proper coping strategies can be implemented or social supports contacted.

ALTERNATIVE AND DIGITAL INTERVENTIONS

Treatment adherence can make the most effective interventions difficult, providing a critical niche for nontraditional and Internet/application (app)-based treatments. Apps can serve as vital connectors between treatment of acute episodes and long-term maintenance. With the explosion of mobile phone usage, an app could be considered more accessible than standard care. Even current Internet powerhouses Facebook and Twitter have multiple pages dedicated to suicide support groups, both officially monitored and community made. Particularly for the adolescent population, app and Internet-based interventions could prove more "interesting" and accessible.

Mindfulness Meditation

Mindfulness meditation has been utilized in nonclinical settings of a multitude of cultures for centuries and is gaining traction as a useful addition to empirically supported treatments. According to Hanh and Kotler (1996), mindfulness meditation focuses on keeping one's consciousness alive to the present reality. Mindfulness training aims to teach people a new way of paying attention to the present to deal more skillfully with what happens rather than going on "autopilot" or wishing that reality differed from its current state. For patients who are caught in a suicide crisis and can only see their circumstance through a narrowed tunnel of despair, altering this perception of circumstances may decrease ruminating on future "catastrophes" and focus on current thought processes and physiological alarms.

Apps and Internet Tools

Applications and Internet tools offer a proactive preventative supplement to traditional treatments due to their wide availability and customizability. Virtual versions of concepts such as the "hope box" or "automatic thought record" can provide easily available coping mechanisms. Virtual hope boxes contain items such as letters, poetry, and virtual coping cards, selected with the help of a therapist, that serve as pleasant memories and distractions from a stressor or acute crisis ("Virtual Hope Box," n.d.). Another resource is podcasts, which can serve as useful tools in developing a suicide prevention strategy. Currently, the Centers for Disease Control and Prevention has five podcasts on the topic of suicide, providing information on warning signs, coping strategies, and resources.

Although useful, the research affirming the effectiveness of app-based interventions is still in its infancy. Another major challenge is that confidentiality and security, such as HIPAA, are not yet required of mobile applications, which may create confidentiality and security conflicts. However, the current body of literature has supported the potential of these treatments. Further research is needed.

MISSING THE BIGGER PICTURE

Suicide, even in modern psychiatry and psychology, still has many uncharted territories, and despite the best efforts of a dedicated clinician and care team, a patient can still carry out a successful suicide attempt. Many clinicians/caregivers will retrospectively ask themselves, "Was there sufficient evidence to suggest that a patient's suicide could have been anticipated?"

Risk Assessment and Self-Care

The previous question has given increased importance to proper risk assessment and documentation. Risk assessment collects data regarding the presence versus the absence of suicide risk factors and protective factors. These factors can provide a clearer picture of the state of the patient and aid more accurate diagnoses.

Self-care can be a process that begins before a first attempt. Physically, individuals should focus on sleep, nutrition, and exercise. Emotionally, patients should focus on mood, spirit, and self-examination (Hirsch, 2006). In addition, a robust social network has been shown to be a protective factor against suicide. In 2012, Fassberg and colleagues found that increased social interactions, particularly for older men, decreased suicide ideation and number of suicide attempts.

SUMMARY

Current biological and psychosocial interventions, although having varying degrees of effectiveness, now span the entire timeline of the suicide crisis. Whether aiming to prevent suicidal crises with self-care and support or redirecting a decompensating patient by restricting means, research has made strides in providing tailored treatments that may prevent suicidal crises. Among the available medications, clozapine and lithium stand out as the best psychopharmacological options, and among the behavioral treatment options, DBT and CAMS have the most experimental support.

Conclusion
Being Vigilant

The Suicidal Crisis: Clinical Guide to the Assessment of Imminent Suicide Risk was conceived in 2014 to be the first text devoted to the assessment of imminent risk for suicide. In 2017, it is still true that no such book is available on the market. During this time period, changing suicide patterns worldwide have made this guide even more essential for clinicians than when it was first conceptualized.

During the past several years, the suicide rates in the United States and the United Kingdom have remained at peak highs. Moreover, during this time, the US rate has continued to steadily climb. According to a 2015 report by the Centers for Disease Control and Prevention, 42,773 people died by suicide in 2014 compared to 29,199 in 1999; the overall suicide rate has risen 24% from 1999 to 2014 (American Foundation for Suicide Prevention, 2016; Tavernise, 2016). Overall, in every age group except older adults, suicide in the United States is at its highest levels in nearly 30 years.

A recent Danish population-based study underscored that patients with mental illness and recent suicidal behavior are at high risk for suicide. It came as no surprise that of all individuals first presenting to an emergency department after attempted suicide between 1996 and 2011, those most prone to repeated attempts and suicide deaths were individuals with recent psychiatric treatment and recent psychiatric hospitalizations for their first attempt.

In response to the urgent need to stem the rise in suicide, rates fueled in part by high suicide rates in the mentally ill during transition of care, the National Institute of Mental Health has prioritized research into risk detection, engagement, and continuity of care during known periods of heightened risk, such as care transfers between systems (e.g., handoffs between emergency departments and inpatient psychiatric or substance abuse units, and transitions between outpatient mental health/substance abuse programs and primary care settings) ("RFA-MH-16-800: Applied Research Toward Zero Suicide Healthcare Systems (R01)," 2016). This new focus underscores the need for a teaching and clinical manual to help frontline clinicians identify and treat those at imminent risk for suicide in emergency departments and during other high-vulnerability time periods.

I wrote *The Suicide Narrative* with that exact purpose in mind. It is intended explicitly for use by frontline clinicians and clinical institutions assessing high-risk suicidal patients, as well as for medical and graduate schools training clinicians to perform such assessments. The foundational belief of Zero Suicide ("Zero Suicide," 2015) is that suicide deaths by individuals under care within health and behavioral health systems are preventable. My sincere hope is that this guide will help clinicians and organizations practice the Zero Suicide approach, prevent suicides, and save lives.

Appendix

Answers to Test Cases

Test Case 1: Lenny's Suicide Implicit Factors Assessment Table

Component	Risk Level				
	Minimal	Low	Moderate	High	Severe
Attitudes				X	
Moral religious prohibitions/permissiveness				X	
Capability—trait	X				
Capability—practicing	X				
Family or friend suicide				X	
Suicide clusters					X
Total				X	

Lenny is alienated from his family and has no moral objections to suicide. He believes that suicide is justifiable if one is in too much pain. These two factors put him at high risk. He is fearful of pain and timid, decreasing his risk. However, he had a strong and personal reaction to his friend's suicide, increasing his risk. Overall, Lenny is at high risk for imminent suicide.

Test Case 2: Zhang's Suicide Implicit Factors Assessment Table

Component	Risk Level				
	Minimal	Low	Moderate	High	Severe
Perfectionism				X	
Entitlement to happiness				X	
Failure to disengage				X	
Social defeat				X	
Thwarted belongingness				X	
Perceived burdensomeness				X	
Entrapment				X	
Total				X	

Zhang's whole life may be seen as one evolving suicidal narrative. Perfectionist since childhood, devoted to the goal of becoming a doctor to uphold the honor of his family, he does not have the mental aptitude to achieve his goal, nor does he have the flexibility to disengage from it. Abandoning a medical career will signify disgrace for his family and ostracism in his community. He is not even in a position to seek support from his family or friends, which leaves him isolated, internally humiliated and defeated, without any chance for support from others. His failure is about to become public, and he is at a very high risk of ending his life, either to avoid the pain of admitting his failure to his parents or after facing their inevitable extreme disappointment.

Test Case 3: Jackie's Suicide Crisis Syndrome Intensity Assessment Table

Symptom	Symptom Intensity				
	Minimal	Low	Moderate	High	Severe
Part A					
Suicidal ideation					X
Suicide intent and plan					X
Entrapment					X
Desperation				X	
Part A summary					X
Part B					
Affective disturbance					
Emotional pain			X		
Depressive turmoil		X			
Frantic anxiety	X				
Panic–dissociation		X			
Fear of dying					X
Anhedonia	X				
Affective disturbance summary		X			
Loss of cognitive control					
Ruminations		X			
Rigidity			X		
Thought suppression	X				
Ruminative flooding	X				
Loss of cognitive control summary		X			
Overarousal					
Agitation		X			
Insomnia		X			
Part B summary		X			
Overall summary			X		

Jackie's mother's death by suicide increases her suicide risk long term, whereas her recent overdose increases her suicide risk both long term and short term. Her Part A SCS assessment shows clear and intense suicidal ideation and intent with a moderate lethality plan, as well as entrapment, which, however, is conditional on external circumstances. In contrast, her Part B assessment shows only minimal and low-intensity symptoms of affective disturbance, loss of cognitive control, and overarousal. Thus, Jackie's overall short-term risk is moderate. The divergent Part A and Part B symptom levels illustrate both the inconsistent relationship between the self-reported suicidal ideation and suicide risk and the usefulness of the full SCS assessment for short-term risk determination.

References

Abramowitz, J. S., Tolin, D. F., & Street, G. P. (2001). Paradoxical effects of thought suppression: A meta-analysis of controlled studies. *Clinical Psychology Review, 21*(5), 683–703.

Adam, K. S., Keller, A., West, M., Larose, S., & Goszer, L. B. (1994). Parental representation in suicidal adolescents: A controlled study. *Australian and New Zealand Journal of Psychiatry, 28*, 418–425. doi:10.3109/00048679409075868

Adam, K. S., Lohrenz, J. G., Harper, D., & Streiner, D. (1982). Early parental loss and suicidal ideation in university students. *Canadian Journal of Psychiatry, 27*(4), 275–281.

Ægisdóttir, S., White, M., Spengler, P., Maugherman, A., Anderson, L., Cook, R., . . . Rush, J. (2006). The meta-analysis of clinical judgment project: Fifty-six years of accumulated research on clinical versus statistical prediction. *The Counseling Psychologist, 34*(3), 341–382. doi:10.1177/001100000528587

Affrunti, N. W., & Ginsburg, G. S. (2012). Maternal overcontrol and child anxiety: The mediating role of perceived competence. *Child Psychiatry & Human Development, 43*(1), 102–112. doi:10.1007/s10578-011-0248-z

Afifi, T. O., Enns, M. W., Cox, B. J., Asmundson, G. J., Stein, M. B., & Sareen, J. (2008). Population attributable fractions of psychiatric disorders and suicide ideation and attempts associated with adverse childhood experiences. *American Journal of Public Health, 98*(5), 946–952. doi:10.2105/ajph.2007.120253

Aguirre, R. T. P., McCoy, M. K., & Roan, M. (2013). Development guidelines from a study of suicide prevention mobile applications. *Journal of Technology in Human Services, 31*(3), 269–293. doi:10.1080/15228835.2013.814750

Ahlm, K., Lindqvist, P., Saveman, B. I., & Björnstig, U. (2015). Suicidal drowning deaths in northern Sweden 1992–2009: The role of mental disorder and intoxication. *Journal of Forensic and Legal Medicine, 34*, 168–172. doi:10.1016/j.jflm.2015.06.002

Ajdacic-Gross, V. (2008). Methods of suicide: International suicide patterns derived from the WHO mortality database. *Bulletin of the World Health Organization, 86*(9), 726–732. doi:10.2471/blt.07.043489

Akiskal, H. S., & Benazzi, F. (2005). Psychopathologic correlates of suicidal ideation in major depressive outpatients: Is it all due to unrecognized (bipolar) depressive mixed states? *Psychopathology, 38*(5), 273–280.

Akiskal, H. S., & Benazzi, F. (2006). The DSM-IV and ICD-10 categories of recurrent [major] depressive and bipolar II disorders: Evidence that they lie on a dimensional spectrum. *Journal of Affective Disorders, 92*(1), 45–54.

Akiskal, H. S., Benazzi, F., Perugi, G., & Rihmer, Z. (2005). Agitated "unipolar" depression re-conceptualized as a depressive mixed state: Implications for the antidepressant–suicide controversy. *Journal of Affective Disorders, 85*(3), 245–258.

Al Jurdi, R. K., Swann, A., & Mathew, S. J. (2015). Psychopharmacological agents and suicide risk reduction: Ketamine and other approaches. *Current Psychiatry Reports, 17*(10), 81. doi:10.1007/s11920-015-0614-9

Aliverdinia, A., & Pridemore, W. A. (2009). Women's fatalistic suicide in Iran: A partial test of Durkheim in an Islamic republic. *Violence Against Women*, 15(3), 307–320. doi:10.1177/1077801208330434

American Foundation for Suicide Prevention. (2016). *Suicide statistics*. Retrieved from https://afsp.org/about-suicide/suicide-statistics

American Psychiatric Association. (2013). *Diagnostic and statistical manual of mental disorders* (5th ed.). Arlington, VA: American Psychiatric Publishing.

Andreassen, C. S., Griffiths, M. D., Sinha, R., Hetland, J., & Pallesen, S. (2016). The relationships between Workaholism and symptoms of psychiatric disorders: A large-scale cross-sectional study. *PLOS ONE*, 11(5), e0152978. doi:10.1371/journal.pone.0152978

Anestis, M. D., & Joiner, T. E. (2011). Examining the role of emotion in suicidality: Negative urgency as an amplifier of the relationship between components of the interpersonal-psychological theory of suicidal behavior and lifetime number of suicide attempts. *Journal of Affective Disorders*, 129(1-3), 261–269. doi:10.1016/j.jad.2010.08.006

Angst, J., Angst, F., & Stassen, H. H. (1999). Suicide risk in patients with major depressive disorder. *Journal of Clinical Psychiatry*, 60, 57–62; discussion 75–76, 113–116.

Appleby, L., Kapur, N., Shaw, J., Hunt, I. M., Flynn, S., & Rahman, M. S.; University of Manchester Centre for Mental Health and Risk. (2012). *The national confidential inquiry into suicide and homicide by people with mental illness: Annual report*. Retrieved from http://research.bmh.manchester.ac.uk/cmhs/research/centreforsuicideprevention/nci

Apter, A., Kotler, M., Sevy, S., Plutchik, R., Brown, S., Foster, H., . . . van Praag, H. (1991). Correlates of risk of suicide in violent and nonviolent psychiatric patients. *American Journal of Psychiatry*, 148(7), 883–887. doi:10.1176/ajp.148.7.883

Apter, A., Plutchik, R., & van Praag, H. M. (1993). Anxiety, impulsivity and depressed mood in relation to suicidal and violent behavior. *Acta Psychiatrica Scandinavica*, 87(1), 1–5. doi:10.1111/j.1600-0447.1993.tb03321.x

Baca-Garcia, E., Diaz-Sastre, C., Garcia Resa, E., Blasco, H., Braquehais Conesa, D., Oquendo, M. A., . . . de Leon, J. (2005). Suicide attempts and impulsivity. *European Archives of Psychiatry and Clinical Neuroscience*, 255, 152–156.

Baca-Garcia, E., Perez-Rodriguez, M. M., Man, J. J., & Oquendo, M. (2008). Suicidal behavior in young women. *Psychiatric Clinics of North America*, 31(2), 317–331. doi:10.1016/j.psc.2008.01.002

Baer, R. A., Hopkins, J., Krietemeyer, J., Smith, G. T., & Toney, L. (2006). Using self-report assessment methods to explore facets of mindfulness. *Assessment*, 13(1), 27–45. doi:10.1177/1073191105283504

Baer, R. A., Smith, G. T., & Allen, K. B. (2004). Assessment of mindfulness by self-report: The Kentucky Inventory of Mindfulness Skills. *Assessment*, 11(3), 191–206. doi:10.1177/1073191104268029

Bagge, C. L., Glenn, C. R., & Lee, H. J. (2013). Quantifying the impact of recent negative life events on suicide attempts. *Journal of Abnormal Psychology*, 122(2), 359–368. doi:10.1037/a0030371

Bagge, C. L., Lee, H. J., Schumacher, J. A., Gratz, K. L., Krull, J. L., & Holloman, G. (2013). Alcohol as an acute risk factor for recent suicide attempts: A case–crossover analysis. *Journal of Studies on Alcohol and Drugs*, 74(4), 552–558. doi:10.15288/jsad.2013.74.552

Bagge, C. L., & Sher, K. J. (2008). Adolescent alcohol involvement and suicide attempts: Toward the development of a conceptual framework. *Clinical Psychology Review*, 28(8), 1283–1296.

Bagley, C., Bolitho, F., & Bertrand, L. (1995). Mental health profiles, suicidal behavior, and community sexual assault in 2112 Canadian adolescents. *Journal of Crisis Intervention and Suicide Prevention*, 16(3), 126–131. doi:10.1027/0227-5910.16.3.126

Baldwin, D. S., Montgomery, S. A., Nil, R., & Lader, M. (2007). Discontinuation symptoms in depression and anxiety disorders. *International Journal of Neuropsychopharmacology*, 10(01), 73–84.

Ballard, E. D., Vande Voort, J. L., Luckenbaugh, D. A., Machado-Vieira, R., Tohen, M., & Zarate, C. A. (2016). Acute risk factors for suicide attempts and death: Prospective findings from the STEP-BD study. *Bipolar Disorders*, 18(4), 363–372.

Banja, J. (2004). *Medical errors and medical narcissism*. Sudbury, MA: Jones & Bartlett.

Barber, C. W., & Miller, M. J. (2014). Reducing a suicidal person's access to lethal means of suicide. *American Journal of Preventive Medicine*, 47(3), S264–S272. doi:10.1016/j.amepre.2014.05.028

Barrett, L. F., Gross, J., Christensen, T. C., & Benvenuto, M. (2001). Knowing what you're feeling and knowing what to do about it: Mapping the relation between emotion differentiation and emotion regulation. *Cognition & Emotion*, 15(6), 713–724. doi:10.1080/02699930143000239

Bartel, C. A., & Saavedra, R. (2000). The collective construction of work group moods. *Administrative Science Quarterly*, 45(2), 197. doi:10.2307/2667070

Barzilay, S., & Apter, A. (2014). Psychological models of suicide. *Archives of Suicide Research*, 18(4), 295–312. doi:10.1080/13811118.2013.824825

Battauz, M., Bellio, R., & Gori, E. (2007). Reducing measurement error in student achievement estimation. *Psychometrika*, 73(2), 289–302. doi:10.1007/s11336-007-9050-z

Baumeister, R. F. (1990). Suicide as escape from self. *Psychological Review*, 97(1), 90–113. doi:10.1037/0033-295x.97.1.90

Baumeister, R. F., & Leary, M. R. (1995). The need to belong: Desire for interpersonal attachments as a fundamental human motivation. *Psychological Bulletin*, 117(3), 497.

Baumeister, R. F., & Scher, S. J. (1988). Self-defeating behavior patterns among normal individuals: Review and analysis of common self-destructive tendencies. *Psychological Bulletin*, 104(1), 3–22. doi:10.1037/0033-2909.104.1.3

Beautrais, A. L., Joyce, P. R., & Mulder, R. T. (1997). Precipitating factors and live events in serious suicide attempts among youths aged 13 through 24 year. *Journal of American Child Adolescent Psychiatry*, 36(11), 1543–1551. doi:10.1016/S0890-8567(09)66563-1

Beck, A. T. (1996). Beyond belief: A theory of modes, personality and psychopathology. In P. M. Salkovaskis (Ed.), *Frontiers of cognitive therapy* (pp. 1–25). New York, NY: Guilford.

Beck, A. T. (2005). The current state of cognitive therapy. *Archives of General Psychiatry*, 62(9), 953. doi:10.1001/archpsyc.62.9.953

Beck, A. T., Brown, G., & Steer, R. A. (1989). Prediction of eventual suicide in psychiatric inpatients by clinical ratings of hopelessness. *Journal of Consulting and Clinical Psychology*, 57(2), 309–310. doi:10.1037/0022-006x.57.2.309

Beck, A. T., Kovacs, M., & Weissman, A. (1975). Hopelessness and suicidal behavior: An overview. *Journal of the American Medical Association*, 234(11), 1146–1149.

Beck, A. T., Schuyler, D., & Herman, J. (1974). Development of suicidal intent scales. In A. Beck, H. Resnik, & D. J. Lettieri (Eds.), *The prediction of suicide* (pp. 45–56). Bowie, MD: Charles.

Beck, A. T., Steer, R. A., Kovacs, M., & Garrison, B. (1985). Hopelessness and eventual suicide: A 10-year prospective study of patients hospitalized with suicidal ideation. *American Journal of Psychiatry*, 142(5), 559–563. doi:10.1176/ajp.142.5.559

Becker, E. S., Strohbach, D., & Rinck, M. (1999). A specific attentional bias in suicide attempt-ers. *Journal of Nervous and Mental Disease, 187*, 730–735.

Benazzi, F. (2007). Bipolar disorder—Focus on bipolar II disorder and mixed depression. *Lancet, 369*(9565), 935–945.

Benazzi, F., & Akiskal, H. S. (2001). Delineating bipolar II mixed states in the Ravenna–San Diego collaborative study: The relative prevalence and diagnostic significance of hypo-manic features during major depressive episodes. *Journal of Affective Disorders, 6*, 115–122.

Bertolote, J. M., & Fleischmann, A. (2015). A global perspective in the epidemiology of sui-cide. *Suicidologi, 7*(2), 6–8. doi:10.5617/suicidologi.2330

Birchwood, M., Trower, P., Brunet, K., Gilbert, P., Iqbal, Z., & Jackson, C. (2007). Social anx-iety and the shame of psychosis: A study in first episode psychosis. *Behavioral Research Therapy, 45*(5), 1025–1037. doi:10.1016/j.brat.2006.07.011

Bishop, S. R., Lau, M., Shapiro, S., Carlson, L., Anderson, N. D., Carmody, J., . . . Gerald, D. (2004). Mindfulness: A proposed operational definition. *Clinical Psychology: Science and Practice, 11*(3), 230–241. doi:10.1093/clipsy/bph077

Blonigen, D. M., Hicks, B. M., Krueger, R. F., Patrick, C. J., & Iacono, W. G. (2005). Psychopathic personality traits: Heritability and genetic overlap with internalizing and externalizing psychopathology. *Psychological Medicine, 35*(5), 637–648. doi:10.1017/s0033291704004180

Bolton, J. M., Spiwak, R., & Sareen, J. (2012). Predicting suicide attempts with the SAD PERSONS scale. *The Journal of Clinical Psychiatry, 73*(06), e735–e741. doi:10.4088/jcp.11m07362

Borges, G., & Loera, C. R. (2010). Alcohol and drug use in suicidal behavior. *Current Opinion in Psychiatry, 23*(3), 195–204.

Borges, G., Orozco, R., Rafful, C., Miller, E., & Breslau, J. (2011). Suicidality, ethnicity and immigration in the USA. *Psychological Medicine, 42*(06), 1175–1184. doi:10.1017/s0033291711002340

Borges, G., & Rosovsky, H. (1996). Suicide attempts and alcohol consumption in an emer-gency room sample. *Journal of Studies on Alcohol, 57*(5), 543–548.

Bowlby, J. (1969). *Attachment and loss: Vol. 1. Loss.* New York, NY: Basic Books.

Bowlby, J. (1980). *Attachment and loss: Vol. 3. Loss: Sadness and depression.* London, England: Hogarth.

Brent, D. A., Kerr, M. M., Goldstein, C., Bozigar, J., Wartella, M., & Allan, M. J. (1989). An out-break of suicide and suicidal behavior in a high school. *Journal of the American Academy of Child & Adolescent Psychiatry, 28*(6), 918–924. doi:10.1097/00004583-198911000-00017

Brent, D. A., & Mann, J. J. (2005). Family genetic studies, suicide, and suicidal behavior. *American Journal of Medical Genetics Part C: Seminars in Medical Genetics, 133C*(1), 13–24. doi:10.1002/ajmg.c.30042

Brent, D. A., & Mann, J. J. (2006). Familial pathways to suicidal behavior—Understanding and preventing suicide among adolescents. *New England Journal of Medicine, 355*, 2719–2721.

Brent, D. A., Perper, J. A., Moritz, G., Allman, C., Friend, A., Roth, C., . . . Baugher, M. (1993). Psychiatric risk factors for adolescent suicide: A case–control study. *Journal of the American Academy of Child & Adolescent Psychiatry, 32*(3), 521–529. doi:10.1097/00004583-199305000-00006

Bridge, J. A. (2008). Suicide trends among youths aged 10 to 19 years in the United States, 1996–2005. *Journal of the American Medical Association, 300*(9), 1025. doi:10.1001/jama.300.9.1025

Bridge, J. A., Asti, L., Horowitz, L.M., Greenhouse, J.B., Fontanella, C.A., Sheftall, A. H., ... Campo, J. V. (2015). Suicide trends among elementary school-aged children in the United States from 1993–2012. *Journal of the American Medical Association Pediatrics, 169*(7), 673–677. doi:10.1001/jamapediatrics.2015.0465

Brooks, D. (2015, June 12). How adulthood happens. *The New York Times.* Retrieved from http://www.nytimes.com/2015/06/12/opinion/david-brooks-how-adulthood-happens.html?_r=0

Brown, G. K., Henriques, G. R., Sosdjan, D., & Beck, A. T. (2004). Suicide intent and accurate expectations of lethality: Predictors of medical lethality of suicide attempts. *Journal of Consulting and Clinical Psychology, 72*(6), 1170–1174. doi:10.1037/0022-006X.72.6.1170

Brown, G. W., Harris, T. O., & Hepworth, C. (1995). Loss, humiliation and entrapment among women developing depression: A patient and non-patient comparison. *Psychological Medicine, 25*(1), 7–21.

Brown, J., Cohen, P., Johnson, J. G., & Smailes, E. M. (1999). Childhood abuse and neglect: Specificity of effects on adolescent and young adult depression and suicide. *Journal of the American Academy of Child and Adolescent Psychiatry, 38*(2), 1490–1496. doi:10.1097/00004583-199912000-00009

Brown, K. W., & Ryan, R. M. (2003). The benefits of being present: Mindfulness and its role in psychological well-being. *Journal of Personality and Social Psychology, 84*(4), 822–848. doi:10.1037/0022-3514.84.4.822

Bruck, E., Winston, A., Aderholt, S., & Muran, J. (2006). Predictive validity of patient and therapist attachment and introject styles. *American Journal of Psychotherapy, 60*, 393–406.

Bruwer, B., Govender, R., Bishop, M., Williams, D. R., Stein, D. J., & Seedat, S. (2014). Association between childhood adversities and long-term suicidality among South Africans from the results of the South African Stress and Health study: A cross-sectional study. *BMJ Open, 4*(6). doi:10.1136/bmjopen-2013-004644

Bryan, C. J., Hernandez, A. M., Allison, S., & Clemans, T. (2012). Combat exposure and suicide risk in two samples of military personnel. *Journal of Clinical Psychology, 69*(1), 64–77. doi:10.1002/jclp.21932

Bryan, C. J., Hitschfeld, M. J., Palmer, B. A., Schak, K. M., Roberge, E. M., & Lineberry, T. W. (2014). Gender differences in the association of agitation and suicide attempts among psychiatric inpatients. *General Hospital Psychiatry, 36*(6), 726–731.

Busch, K. A., Fawcett, J., & Jacobs, D. G. (2003). Clinical correlates of inpatient suicide. *Journal of Clinical Psychiatry, 64*, 14–19.

Cacioppo, J. T., & Patrick, W. (2008). *Loneliness: Human nature and the need for social connection.* New York, NY: Norton.

Caetano, R., Kaplan, M. S., Huguet, N., McFarland, B. H., Conner, K., Giesbrecht, N., & Nolte, K. B. (2013). Acute alcohol intoxication and suicide among United States ethnic/racial groups: Findings from the National Violent Death Reporting System. *Alcoholism: Clinical and Experimental Research, 37*(5), 839–846.

Campos, R. C., Besser, A., & Blatt, S. J. (2010). The mediating role of self-criticism and dependency in the association between perceptions of maternal caring and depressive symptoms. *Depression and Anxiety, 27*(12), 1149–1157. doi:10.1002/da.20763

Cantor, C. H., & Slater, P. J. (1995). Marital breakdown, parenthood and suicide. *Journal of Family Studies, 1*(2), 91–102. doi:10.5172/jfs.1.2.91

Carver, C. S., & Scheier, M. F. (1998). *On the self-regulation of behavior.* New York, NY: Cambridge University Press.

Cash, S. J., & Bridge, J. A. (2009). Epidemiology of youth suicide and suicidal behavior. *Current Opinion in Pediatrics, 21*(5), 613–619. doi:10.1097/mop.0b013e32833063e1

Catechism of the Catholic Church. (n.d.). Retrieved from http://www.scborromeo.org/ccc/p3s2c2a5.htm

Centers for Disease Control and Prevention. (2014). *10 leading causes of death by age group, United States.* Retrieved from https://www.cdc.gov/injury/images/lc-charts/leading_causes_of_death_age_group_2014_1050w760h.gif

Centers for Disease Control and Prevention. (2015a). *Suicide facts at a glance.* Retrieved from https://www.cdc.gov/violenceprevention/pdf/suicide-datasheet-a.PDF

Centers for Disease Control and Prevention. (2015b). *Suicide prevention.* Retrieved from http://www.cdc.gov/violenceprevention/suicide/youth_suicide.html

Cha, C. B., Najmi, S., Park, J. M., Finn, C. T., & Nock, M. K. (2010). Attentional bias toward suicide-related stimuli predicts suicidal behavior. *Journal of Abnormal Psychology, 119*(3), 616–622. doi:10.1037/a0019710

Chambers, A. (2010, August 3). Japan: Ending the culture of the "honourable" suicide. *The Guardian.*

Chang, B., Gitlin, D., & Patel, R. (2011). The depressed patient and suicidal patient in the emergency department: Evidence-based management and treatment strategies. *Emergency Medicine Practice, 13*(9), 1–23.

Chang, S., Stuckler, D., Yip, P., & Gunnell, D. (2013). Impact of 2008 global economic crisis on suicide: Time trend study in 54 countries. *BMJ, 347*(1). doi:10.1136/bmj.f5239

Cheatle, M. D. (2011). Depression, chronic pain, and suicide by overdose: On the edge. *Pain Medicine, 12*(Suppl. 2), S43–S48. doi:10.1111/j.1526-4637.2011.01131.x

Chen, Y. Y., Wu, K. C., Yousuf, S., & Yip, P. S. (2012). Suicide in Asia: Opportunities and challenges. *Epidemiological Reviews, 34*(1), 129–144. doi:10.1093/epirev/mxr025

Cheng, A. T. A., Chen, T. H. H., Chen, C. C., & Jenkins, R. (2000). Psychosocial and psychiatric risk factors for suicide: Case–control psychological autopsy study. *British Journal of Psychiatry, 177*(4), 360–365.

Cherpitel, C. J., Borges, G. L., & Wilcox, H. C. (2004). Acute alcohol use and suicidal behavior: A review of the literature. *Alcoholism: Clinical and Experimental Research, 28*(s1), 18S–28S.

Cheung, G., Merry, S., & Sundram, F. (2015a). Late-life suicide: Insight on motives and contributors derived from suicide notes. *Journal of Affective Disorders, 185,* 17–23. doi:10.1016/j.jad.2015.06.035

Cheung, G., Merry, S., & Sundram, F. (2015b). Medical examiner and coroner reports: Uses and limitations in the epidemiology and prevention of late-life suicide. *International Journal of Geriatric Psychiatry, 30*(8), 781–792. doi:10.1002/gps.4294

Ciarrochi, J., Caputi, P., & Mayer, J. D. (2003). The distinctiveness and utility of a measure of trait emotional awareness. *Personality and Individual Differences, 34*(8), 1477–1490. doi:10.1016/s0191-8869(02)00129-0

Cipriani, A., Hawton, K., Stockton, S., & Geddes, J. R. (2013). Lithium in the prevention of suicide in mood disorders: Updated systematic review and meta-analysis. *BMJ, 346.* doi:10.1136/bmj.f3646

Cipriani, A., Pretty, H., Hawton, K., & Geddes, J. R. (2005). Lithium in the prevention of suicidal behavior and all-cause mortality in patients with mood disorders: A systematic review of Randomized trials. *American Journal of Psychiatry, 162*(10), 1805–1819. doi:10.1176/appi.ajp.162.10.1805

Claassen, C. A., Harvilchuck-Laurenson, J. D., & Fawcett, J. (2014). Prognostic models to detect and monitor the near-term risk of suicide. *American Journal of Preventive Medicine, 47*(3). doi:10.1016/j.amepre.2014.06.003

Clark, C. B., Li, Y., & Cropsey, K. L. (2016). Family dysfunction and suicide risk in a community corrections sample. *Crisis, 37*(6), 454–460. doi:10.1027/0227-5910/a000406

Cohen, L. J. (1994). Psychiatric hospitalization as an experience of trauma. *Archives of Psychiatric Nursing, 8*(2), 78–81. doi:10.1016/0883-9417(94)90037-x

Čoklo, M., Stemberga, V., Cuculić, D., Šoša, I., Jerković, R., & Bosnar, A. (2008). The methods of committing and alcohol intoxication of suicides in southwestern Croatia from 1996 to 2005. *Collegium Antropologicum, 32*(2), 123–125.

Conner, K. R., Beautrais, A. L., & Conwell, Y. (2003). Risk factors for suicide and medically serious suicide attempts among alcoholics: Analyses of Canterbury Suicide Project data. *Journal of Studies on Alcohol, 64*(4), 551–554.

Conner, K. R., Huguet, N., Caetano, R., Giesbrecht, N., McFarland, B. H., Nolte, K. B., & Kaplan, M. S. (2014). Acute use of alcohol and methods of suicide in a US national sample. *American Journal of Public Health, 104*(1), 171–178.

Conrad, A. K., Jacoby, A. M., Jobes, D. A., Lineberry, T. W., Shea, C. E., Arnold Ewing, T. D., . . . Kung, S. (2009). A psychometric investigation of the suicide status form II with a psychiatric inpatient sample. *Suicide and Life-Threatening Behavior, 39*(3), 307–320. doi:10.1521/suli.2009.39.3.307

Consoli, A., Payre, H., Speranza, M., Hassler, C., Falissard, B., Touchette, E., . . . Revah-Levy, A. (2013). Suicidal behaviors in depressed adolescents: Role of perceived relationships in the family. *Child Adolescent Psychiatry and Mental Health, 7*(1), 1. doi:10.1186/1753-2000-7-8

Cook, C. R., Williams, K. R., Guerra, N. G., Kim, T. E., & Sadek, S. (2010). Predictors of bullying and victimization in childhood and adolescence: A meta-analytic investigation. *School Psychology Quarterly, 25*(2), 65–83. doi:10.1037/a0020149

Cornette, M. M., Deroon-Cassini, T. A., Fosco, G. M., Holloway, R. L., Clark, D. C., & Joiner, T. E. (2009). Application of an interpersonal–psychological model of suicidal behavior to physicians and medical trainees. *Archives of Suicide Research, 13*(1), 1–14. doi:10.1080/13811110802571801

Cosgrove, V. E., Rhee, S. H., Gelhorn, H. L., Boeldt, D., Corley, R. C., Ehringer, M. A., . . . Hewitt, J. K. (2011). Structure and etiology of co-occurring internalizing and externalizing disorders in adolescents. *Journal of Abnormal Child Psychology, 39*(1), 109–123. doi:10.1007/s10802-010-9444-8

Crowell, S. E., Beauchaine, T. P., & Linehan, M. M. (2009). A biosocial developmental model of borderline personality: Elaborating and extending Linehan's theory. *Psychological Bulletin, 135*(3), 495–510. doi:10.1037/a0015616

Culpepper, L., Davidson, J. R., Dietrich, A. J., Goodman, W. K., & Schwenk, T. L. (2004). Suicidality as a possible side effect of antidepressant treatment. *Journal of Clinical Psychiatry, 65*(6), 742–749.

Currier, G. W., Brown, G. K., Brenner, L. A., Chesin, M., Knox, K. L., Ghahramanlou-Holloway, M., & Stanley, B. (2015). Rationale and study protocol for a two-part intervention: Safety planning and structured follow-up among veterans at risk for suicide and discharged from the emergency department. *Contemporary Clinical Trials, 43*, 179–184. doi:10.1016/j.cct.2015.05.003

Curtin, S., Warner, M., & Hedegaard, H. (2016). *Increase in suicide in the United States, 1999–2014* (NCHS data brief No. 241). Hyattsville, MD: National Center for Health Statistics. Retrieved from https://www.cdc.gov/nchs/products/databriefs/db241.htm

De Los Reyes, A., Augenstein, T. M., Wang, M., Thomas, S. A., Drabick, D. A. G., Burgers, D. E., & Rabinowitz, J. (2015). The validity of the multi-informant approach to assessing child and adolescent mental health. *Psychological Bulletin, 141*(4), 858–900. doi:10.1037/a0038498

Deisenhammer, E. A., Ing, C. M., Strauss, R., Kemmler, G., Hinterhuber, H., & Weiss, E. M. (2009). The duration of the suicidal process: How much time is left for intervention between consideration and accomplishment of a suicide attempt? *Journal of Clinical Psychiatry, 70*, 19–24. doi:10.4088/jcp.07m03904

Dervic, K., Carballo, J. J., Baca-Garcia, E., Galfalvy, H. C., Mann, J. J., Brent, D. A., & Oquendo, M. A. (2011). Moral or religious objections to suicide may protect against suicidal behavior in bipolar disorder. *Journal of Clinical Psychiatry, 72*(10), 1390–1396. doi:10.4088/jcp.09m05910gre

DeWall, C. N., Baumeister, R. F., & Vohs, K. D. (2008). Satiated with belongingness? Effects of acceptance, rejection, and task framing on self-regulatory performance. *Journal of Personality and Social Psychology, 95*(6), 1367–1382. doi:10.1037/a0012632

Dhingra, K., Boduszek, D., & O'Connor, R. C. (2016). A structural test of the integrated motivational–volitional model of suicidal behavior. *Psychiatry Research, 239*, 169–178. doi:10.1016/j.psychres.2016.03.023

Diamond, G. S., Wintersteen, M. B., Brown, G. K., Gallop, R., Shelef, K., & Levy, S. (2010). Attachment-based family therapy for adolescents with suicidal ideation: A randomized controlled trial. *Journal of the American Academy of Child & Adolescent Psychiatry, 49*(2), 122–131. doi:10.1097/00004583-201002000-00006

Dilillo, D., Mauri, S., Mantegazza, C., Fabiano, V., Mameli, C., & Zuccotti, G. V. (2015). Suicide in pediatrics: Epidemiology, risk factors, warning signs and the role of the pediatrician in detecting them. *Italian Journal of Pediatrics, 41*(1), 49. doi:10.1186/s13052-015-0153-3

Dilsaver, S. C., Benazzi, F., Akiskal, H., & Akiskal, K. (2007). Post-traumatic stress disorder among adolescents with bipolar disorder and its relationship to suicidality. *Bipolar Disorders, 9*, 649–655.

Donath, C., Graessel, E., Baier, D., Bleich, S., & Hillemacher, T. (2014). Is parenting style a predictor of suicide attempts in a representative sample of adolescents? *BMC Pediatrics, 14*(1), 1–13. doi:10.1186/1471-2431-14-113

Dougall, N., Lambert, P., Maxwell, M., Dawson, A., Sinnott, R., McCafferty, S., . . . Springbett, A. (2014). Deaths by suicide and their relationship with general and psychiatric hospital discharge: 30-Year record linkage study. *British Journal of Psychiatry, 204*(4), 267–273. doi:10.1192/bjp.bp.112.122374

Dublin, L. I. (1963). *Suicide: A sociological and statistical study.* New York, NY: Ronald.

Dufort, M., Stenbacka, M., & Gumpert, C. H. (2015). Physical domestic violence exposure is highly associated with suicidal attempts in both women and men. Results from the National Public Health Survey in Sweden. *European Journal of Public Health, 25*(3), 413–418. doi:10.1093/eurpub/cku198

Dufrasne, S., Roy, M., Galvez, M., & Rosenblatt, D. S. (2011). Experience over fifteen years with a protocol for predictive testing for Huntington disease. *Molecular Genetics and Metabolism, 102*(4), 494–504. doi:10.1016/j.ymgme.2010.12.001

Ehring, T., & Watkins, E. (2008). Repetitive negative thinking as a transdiagnostic process. *International Journal of Cognitive Therapy, 1*, 192–205.

Ellis, T. (2001). Psychotherapy with suicidal patients. In D. Lester (Ed.), *Suicide prevention: Resources for the millennium* (pp. 129–151). Philadelphia, PA: Brunner-Routledge.

Ellis, T. E., Allen, J. G., Woodson, H., Frueh, B. C., & Jobes, D. A. (2009). Implementing an evidence-based approach to working with suicidal inpatients. *Bulletin of the Menninger Clinic, 73*(4), 339–354. doi:10.1521/bumc.2009.73.4.339

Elman, I., Borsook, D., & Volkow, N. D. (2013). Pain and suicidality: Insights from reward and addiction neuroscience. *Progress in Neurobiology, 109*, 1–27.

Erlangsen, A., Stenager, E., & Conwell, Y. (2015). Physical diseases as predictors of suicide in older adults: A nationwide, register-based cohort study. *Social Psychiatry and Psychiatric Epidemiology, 50*(9), 1427–1439. doi:10.1007/s00127-015-1051-0

Esposito, C. L., & Clum, G. A. (2002a). Psychiatric symptoms and their relationship to suicidal ideation in a high-risk adolescent community sample. *Journal of the American Academy of Child and Adolescent Psychiatry, 41*(1), 44–51. doi:10.1097/00004583-200201000-00010

Esposito, C. L., & Clum, G. A. (2002b). Social support and problem-solving as moderators of the relationship between childhood abuse and suicidality: Applications to a delinquent population. *Journal of Traumatic Stress, 15*(2), 137–146. doi:10.1023/a:1014860024980

Eubanks-Carter, C., Muran, J. C., & Safran, J. D. (2015). Alliance-focused training. *Psychotherapy, 52*(2), 169–173. doi:10.1037/a0037596

Ewing, E. S. K., Diamond, G., & Levy, S. (2015). Attachment-based family therapy for depressed and suicidal adolescents: Theory, clinical model and empirical support. *Attachment & Human Development, 17*(2), 136–156. doi:10.1080/14616734.2015.1006384

Fang, F., Fall, K., Mittleman, M. A., Sparén, P., Ye, W., Adami, H., & Valdimarsdóttir, U. (2012). Suicide and cardiovascular death after a cancer diagnosis. *New England Journal of Medicine, 367*(3), 276–277. doi:10.1056/nejmc1205927

Farmer, A. S., & Kashdan, T. B. (2013). Affective and self-esteem instability in the daily lives of people with generalized social anxiety disorder. *Clinical Psychological Science, 2*(2), 187–201. doi:10.1177/2167702613495200

Fässberg, M. M., Van Orden, K. A., Duberstein, P., Erlangsen, A., Lapierre, S., Bodner, E., . . . Waern, M. (2012). A systematic review of social factors and suicidal behavior in older adulthood. *International Journal of Environmental Research and Public Health, 9*(12), 722–745. doi:10.3390/ijerph9030722

Fawcett, J. (1988). Predictors of early suicide: Identification and appropriate intervention. *Journal of Clinical Psychiatry, 49*, 7–8.

Fawcett, J. (2006). Depressive disorders. In R. I. Simon & R. E. Hales (Eds.), *Textbook of suicide assessment and management* (pp. 1–24). New York, NY: American Psychiatric Publishing.

Fawcett, J., Busch, K. A., Jacobs, D., Kravitz, H. M., & Fogg, L. (1997). Suicide: A four-pathway clinical–biochemical model. *Annals of the New York Academy of Science, 836*, 288–301.

Fawcett, J., Scheftner, W., & Clark, D. (1987). Clinical predictors of suicide in patients with major affective disorders: A controlled prospective study. *American Journal of Psychiatry, 144*(1), 35–40. doi:10.1176/ajp.144.1.35

Fawcett, J., Scheftner, W. A., Fogg, L., Clark, D. C., Young, M. A., Hedeker, D., & Gibbons, R. (1990). Time-related predictors of suicide in major affective disorder. *American Journal of Psychiatry, 147*(9), 1189–1194.

Feigelman, W., Gorman, B. S., & Jordan, J. R. (2009). Stigmatization and suicide bereavement. *Death Studies, 33*(7), 591–608. doi:10.1080/07481180902979973

Fergusson, D. M., Beautrais, A. L., & Horwood, L. J. (2003). Vulnerability and resiliency to suicidal behaviours in young people. *Psychological Medicine, 33*(1), 61–73. doi:10.1017/s0033291702006748

Fergusson, D. M., Horwood, L. J., & Lynskey, M. T. (1996). Childhood sexual abuse and psychiatric disorder in young adulthood: II. Psychiatric outcomes of childhood sexual abuse. *Journal of the American Academy of Child & Adolescent Psychiatry, 35*(10), 1365–1374. doi:10.1097/00004583-199610000-00024

Fergusson, D. M., Woodward, L. J., & Horwood, L. J. (2000). Risk factors and life processes associated with the onset of suicidal behavior during adolescence and early adulthood. *Psychological Medicine, 30*(1), 23–39.

Ferlatte, O., Dulai, J., Hottes, T. S., Trussler, T., & Marchand, R. (2015). Suicide related ideation and behavior among Canadian gay and bisexual men: A syndemic analysis. *BMC Public Health, 15*(1), 597. doi:10.1186/s12889-015-1961-5

Feuer, A. (2008, March 7). Four charged with running online prostitution ring. *The New York Times*. Retrieved from http://www.nytimes.com/2008/03/07/nyregion/07prostitution.html?_r=0

Fiedorowicz, J. G., Leon, A. C., Keller, M. B., Solomon, D. A., Rice, J. P., & Coryell, W. H. (2009). Do risk factors for suicidal behavior differ by affective disorder polarity? *Psychological Medicine, 39*(05), 763–771.

Flowers, K. C., Walker, R. L., Thompson, M. P., & Kaslow, N. J. (2014). Associations between reasons for living and diminished suicide intent among African-American female suicide attempters. *Journal of Nervous and Mental Disease, 202*(8), 569–575. doi:10.1097/nmd.0000000000000170

Foster, T. (2011). Adverse life events proximal to adult suicide: A synthesis of findings from psychological autopsy studies. *Archives of Suicide Research, 15*(1), 1–15. doi:10.1080/13811118.2011.5402213

Foster, T. J. (2013). Suicide prevention as a prerequisite for recovery from severe mental illness. *International Journal of Psychiatry in Medicine, 46*(1), 15–25. doi:10.2190/pm.46.1.b

Fowler, J. C. (2012). Suicide risk assessment in clinical practice: Pragmatic guidelines for imperfect assessments. *Psychotherapy, 49*(1), 81–90. doi:10.1037/a0026148

Fowler, K. A., Gladden, M., Vagi, K. J., Barnes, J., & Frazier, L. (2015). Increase in suicides associated with home eviction and foreclosure during the US housing crisis: From 16 national violent death reporting system states, 2005–2010. *Research and Practice, 105*(312), 311–316. doi:10.2105/AJPH.2014.301945

Fowles, D. C. (2007). The three arousal model: Implications of Gray's two-factor learning theory for heart rate, electrodermal activity, and psychopathy. *Psychophysiology, 17*(2), 87–104.

Freud, S. (1922). *Beyond the pleasure principle*. London, England: International Psycho-Analytical Press.

Friedman, R. A., & Leon, A. C. (2007). Expanding the black box—Depression, antidepressants, and the risk of suicide. *New England Journal of Medicine, 356*(23), 2343–2346.

Freuchen, A., Kjelsberg, E., Lundervold, A. J., & Groholt, B. (2012). Differences between children and adolescents who commit suicide and their peers: A psychological autopsy of suicide victims compared to accident victims and a community sample. *Child and Adolescent Psychiatry Mental Health, 6*(1), 1–12. doi:10.1186/1753-2000-6-1

Fudalej, S., Ilgen, M., Fudalej, M., Wojnar, M., Matsumoto, H., Barry, K. L., . . . Blow, F. C. (2009). Clinical and genetic risk factors for suicide under the influence of alcohol in a Polish sample. *Alcohol and Alcoholism, 44*(5), 437–442.

Gabbay, V., Ely, B. A., Babb, J., & Liebes, L. (2012). The possible role of the kynurenine pathway in anhedonia in adolescents. *Journal of Neural Transmission, 119*(2), 253–260.

Galdas, P. M., Cheater, F., & Marshall, P. (2005). Men and health help-seeking behaviour: Literature review. *Journal of Advanced Nursing, 49*(6), 616–623. doi:10.1111/j.1365-2648.2004.03331.x

Galynker, I. I., Yaseen, Z. S., Briggs, J., & Hayashi, F. (2015). Attitudes of acceptability and lack of condemnation toward suicide may be predictive of post-discharge suicide attempts. *BMC Psychiatry, 15*(1), 87. doi:10.1186/s12888-015-0462-5

Galynker, I., Yaseen, Z. S., Cohen, A., Benhamou, O., Hawes, M., & Briggs, J. (2016). Prediction of suicidal behavior in high risk psychiatric patients using an assessment of acute suicidal state: The suicide crisis inventory. *Depression and Anxiety, 34*(2), 147–158. doi:10.1002/da.22559

Germer, C. K., Siegel, R. D., & Fulton, P. R. (2005). *Mindfulness and psychotherapy*. New York, NY: Guilford.

Geulayov, G., Gunnell, D., Holmen, T. L., & Metcalfe, C. (2012). The association of parental fatal and non-fatal suicidal behaviour with offspring suicidal behaviour and depression: A systematic review and meta-analysis. *Psychological Medicine, 42*, 1567–1580.

Gilbert, P., & Allan, S. (1998). The role of defeat and entrapment (arrested flight) in depression: An exploration of an evolutionary view. *Psychological Medicine, 28*(3), 585–598. doi:10.1017/s0033291798006710

Gilbert, P., & Gilbert, J. (2003). Entrapment and arrested fight and flight in depression: An exploration using focus groups. *Psychology and Psychotherapy: Theory, Research and Practice, 76*(2), 173–188. doi:10.1348/147608303765951203

Gilbert, P., Gilbert, J., & Irons, C. (2004). Life events, entrapments, and arrested anger in depression. *Journal of Affective Disorders, 79*(1-3), 149–160.

Glasgow, G. (2011). Do local landmark bridges increase the suicide rate? An alternative test of the likely effect of means restriction at suicide-jumping sites. *Social Science & Medicine, 72*(6), 884–889. doi:10.1016/j.socscimed.2011.01.001

Glowinski, A. L., Bucholz, K. K., Nelson, E. C., Fu, Q., Madden, P. A., Reich, W., & Heath, A. C. (2001). Suicide attempts in an adolescent female twin sample. *Journal of the American Academy of Child & Adolescent Psychiatry, 40*(11), 1300–1307. doi:10.1097/00004583-200111000-00010

Gold, M. S., Pottash, A. L. C., Sweeney, D. R., & Kleber, H. D. (1980). Efficacy of clonidine in opiate withdrawal: A study of thirty patients. *Drug and Alcohol Dependence, 6*(4), 201–208.

Goldsmith, S. K., Pellmar, T. C., Kleinman, A. M., & Bunney, W. E. (2002). *Reducing suicide: A national imperative*. Washington, DC: National Academies Press.

Goldston, D. B., Reboussin, B. A., & Daniel, S. S. (2006). Predictors of suicide attempts: State and trait components. *Journal of Abnormal Psychology, 115*, 842–849.

Goleman, D. (2003). Maxed emotions. *Business Strategy Review, 14*(2), 26–32. doi:10.1111/1467-8616.00256

Gonzalez, R., Bernstein, I., & Suppes, T. (2008). An investigation of water lithium concentrations and rates of violent acts in 11 Texas counties. *Journal of Clinical Psychiatry, 69*(2), 325–326. doi:10.4088/jcp.v69n0221a

Goschin, S., Briggs, J., Blanco-Luten, S., Cohen, L. J., & Galynker, I. (2013). Parental affectionless control and suicidality. *Journal of Affective Disorders, 151*(1), 1–6. doi:10.1016/j.jad.2013.05.096

Gould, M. S. (1996). Psychosocial risk factors of child and adolescent completed suicide. *Archives of General Psychiatry, 53*(12), 1155. doi:10.1001/archpsyc.1996.01830120095016

Gould, M. S., Wallenstein, S., Kleinman, M. H., O'Carroll, P., & Mercy, J. (1990). Suicide clusters: An examination of age-specific effects. *American Journal of Public Health, 80*(2), 211–212. doi:10.2105/ajph.80.2.211

Griffin, D., & Bartholomew, K. (1994). Models of the self and other: Fundamental dimensions underlying measures of adult attachment. *Journal of Personality and Social Psychology, 67*, 430–445. doi:10.1037/0022-3514.67.3.430

Griffith, J. (2012). Suicide and war: The mediating effects of negative mood, posttraumatic stress disorder symptoms, and social support among Army National Guard soldiers. *Suicide and Life-Threatening Behavior, 42*(4), 453–469. doi:10.1111/j.1943-278x.2012.00104.x

Groenewoud, J. H., van der Maas, P. J., van der Wal, G., Hengeveld, M. W., Tholen, A. J., Schudel, W. J., & van der Heide, A. (1997). Physician-assisted death in psychiatric practice in the Netherlands. *New England Journal of Medicine, 336*(25), 1795–1801. doi:10.1056/nejm199706193362506

Groholt, B., Ekeberg, O., Wichstrom, L., & Haldorsen, T. (1998). Suicide among children and younger and older adolescents in Norway: A comparative study. *Journal of the American Academy of Child and Adolescent Psychiatry, 37*(5), 473–481. doi:10.1097/00004583-199805000-00008

Guintivano, J., Brown, T., & Newcomer, A. (2014). Identification and replication of a combined epigenetic and genetic biomarker predicting suicide and suicidal behaviors. *American Journal of Psychiatry, 171*(12), 1287–1296. doi:10.1176/appi.ajp.2014.14010008

Gunnell, D., Brooks, J., & Peters, T. J. (1996). Epidemiology and patterns of hospital use after parasuicide in the south west of England. *Journal of Epidemiology & Community Health, 50*(1), 24–29. doi:10.1136/jech.50.1.24

Gunnell, D., Eddleston, M., Phillips, M. R., & Konradsen, F. (2007). The global distribution of fatal pesticide self-poisoning: Systematic review. *BMC Public Health, 7*(1), 357. doi:10.1186/1471-2458-7-357

Gunnell, D., & Frankel, S. (1994). Prevention of suicide: Aspirations and evidence. *BMJ, 308*(6938), 1227–1233. doi:10.1136/bmj.308.6938.1227

Gunnell, D., Hawton, K., Bennewith, O., Cooper, J., Simkin, S., Donovan, J., . . . Kapur, N. (2013). A multicentre programme of clinical and public health research in support of the national suicide prevention strategy for England. *Programme Grants for Applied Research, 1*(1), 1–216. doi:10.3310/pgfar01010

Gureje, O., Oladeji, B., Hwang, I., Chiu, W. T., Kessler, R. C., Sampson, N. A., . . . Nock, M. K. (2010). Parental psychopathology and the risk of suicidal behavior in their offspring: Results from the World Mental Health surveys. *Molecular Psychiatry, 16*(12), 1221–1233. doi:10.1038/mp.2010.111

Gururaj, G., Isaac, M. K., Subbakrishna, D. K., & Ranjani, R. (2004). Risk factors for completed suicides: A case–control study from Bangalore, India. *Injury Control and Safety Promotion, 11*(3), 183–191. doi:10.1080/156609704/233/289706

Gvion, Y., Horresh, N., Levi-Belz, Y., Fischel, T., Treves, I., Weiser, M., . . . Apter, A. (2014). Aggression–impulsivity, mental pain, and communication difficulties in medically serious and medically non-serious suicide attempters. *Comprehensive Psychiatry, 55*(1), 40–50. doi:10.1016/j.comppsych.2013.09.003

Hajar, R. (2016). Framingham contribution to cardiovascular disease. *Heart Views, 17*(2), 78. doi:10.4103/1995-705x.185130

Halari, R., Premkumar, P., Farguharson, L., Fannon, D., Kuipers, E., & Kumari, V. (2009). Rumination and negative symptoms in schizophrenia. *Journal of Nervous and Mental Disease, 197*(9), 703–706.

Hanh, T. N., & Kotler, A. (1996). *Peace is every step: The path of mindfulness in everyday life.* New York, NY: Random House.

Harding, M. (2016, August 1). *Suicide risk assessment and threats of suicide.* Retrieved from http://patient.info/doctor/suicide-risk-assessment-and-threats-of-suicide

Harper, S., Charters, T. J., Strumpf, E. C., Galea, S., & Nandi, A. (2015). Economic downturns and suicide mortality in the USA, 1980–2010: Observational study. *International Journal of Epidemiology, 44*(3), 956–966. doi:10.1093/ije/dyv009

Harriss, L., & Hawton, K. (2005). Suicidal intent in deliberate self-harm and the risk of suicide: The predictive power of the Suicide Intent Scale. *Journal of Affective Disorders, 86*(2-3), 225–233. doi:10.1016/j.jad.2005.02.009

Hasin, D. S., Keyes, K. M., Alderson, D., Wang, S., Aharonovich, E., & Grant, B. F. (2008). Cannabis withdrawal in the United States: A general population study. *Journal of Clinical Psychiatry, 69*(9), 1354.

Hatcher, S., & Stubberfield, O. (2013). Sense of belonging and suicide: A systematic review. *Canadian Journal of Psychiatry, 57*(7), 432–436.

Hatfield, E., Cacioppo, J., & Rapson, R. (1993). Emotional contagion. *Current Directions in Psychological Sciences, 2*, 96–99. doi:10.1111/1467-8721.ep10770953.

Haw, C. (1994). A cluster of suicides at a London psychiatric unit. *Suicide and Life-Threatening Behavior, 24*, 256–266.

Haw, C., Hawton, K., Houston, K., & Townsend, E. (2003). Correlates of relative lethality and suicidal intent among deliberate self-harm patients. *Suicide and Life-Threatening Behavior, 33*(4), 353–364. doi:10.1521/suli.33.4.353.25232

Haw, C., Hawton, K., Niedzwiedz, C., & Platt, S. (2013). Suicide clusters: A review of risk factors and mechanisms. *Suicide and Life-Threatening Behavior, 43*(1), 97–108. doi:10.1111/j.1943-278x.2012.00130.x

Hawes, M., Yaseen, Z., Briggs, J., & Galynker, I. (2017). The modular assessment of risk for imminent suicide (MARIS): A proof of concept for a multi-informant tool for evaluation of short-term suicide risk. *Comprehensive Psychiatry, 72*, 88–96. doi:10.1016/j.comppsych.2016.10.002

Hawton, K., Fagg, J., & McKeown, S. P. (1989). Alcoholism, Alcohol and Attempted Suicide. *Alcohol and Alcoholism, 24*(1), 3–9. doi:10.1093/oxfordjournals.alcalc.a044864

Hawton, K., & Van Heeringen, K. (2009). Suicide. *Lancet, 373*(9672), 1372–1381. doi:10.1016/S0140-6736(09)60372-x

Hawton, K., Zahl, D., & Weatherall, R. (2003). Suicide following deliberate self-harm: Long-term follow-up of patients who presented to a general hospital. *British Journal of Psychiatry, 182*(6), 537–542. doi:10.1192/bjp.182.6.537

Heckhausen, J., Wrosch, C., & Schulz, R. (2010). A motivational theory of life-span development. *Psychological Review, 117*, 32–60. doi:10.1037/a0017668

Heikkinen, M., Aro, H., & Lönnqvist, J. (1992). The partners' views on precipitant stressors in suicide. *Acta Psychiatrica Scandinavica, 85*(5), 380–384. doi:10.1111/j.16000447.1992.tb10323.x

Heikkinen, M., Aro, H., & Lönnqvist, J. (1994). Recent life events, social support and suicide. *Acta Psychiatrica Scandinavica, 89*(s377), 65–72.

Hendin, H., Al Jurdi, R. K., Houck, P. R., Hughes, S., & Turner, J. B. (2010). Role of intense affects in predicting short-term risk for suicidal behavior. *The Journal of Nervous and Mental Disease, 198*(3), 220–225. doi:10.1097/nmd.0b013e3181d13d14

Hendin, H., Haas, A. P., Maltsberger, J. T., Koestner, B., & Szanto, K. (2006). Problems in psychotherapy with suicidal patients. *American Journal of Psychiatry, 163*(1), 67–72.

Hendin, H., Haas, A. P., Maltsberger, J. T., Szanto, K., & Rabinowicz, H. (2004). Factors contributing to therapists' distress after the suicide of a patient. *American Journal of Psychiatry, 161*(8), 1442–1446. doi:10.1176/appi.ajp.161.8.1442

Hendin, H., Lipschitz, A., Maltsberger, J. T., Haas, A. P., & Wynecoop, S. (2000). Therapists' reactions to patients suicides. *American Journal of Psychiatry, 157*(12), 2022–2027. doi:10.1176/appi.ajp.157.12.2022

Hendin, H., Maltsberger, J. T., Lipschitz, A., Haas, A. P., & Kyle, J. (2001). Recognizing and responding to a suicide crisis. *Suicide and Life-Threatening Behavior, 31*(2), 115–128. doi:10.1521/suli.31.2.115.21515

Hendin, H., Maltsberger, J. T., Haas, A. P., Szanto, K., & Rabinowicz, H. (2004). Desperation and other affective states in suicidal patients. *Suicide and Life-Threatening Behavior, 34*(4), 386–394. doi:10.1521/suli.34.4.386.53734

Hendin, H., Maltsberger, J. T., & Szanto, K. (2007). The role of intense affective states in signaling a suicide crisis. *Journal of Nervous and Mental Disease, 195*(5), 363–369.

Henry, C., & Demotes-Mainard, J. (2006). SSRIs, suicide and violent behavior: Is there a need for better definition of the depressive state? *Current Drug Safety, 1*, 59–62.

Herszenhorn, D. M. (2013, March 23). Russian oligarch and sharp critic of Putin dies in London. *The New York Times*. Retrieved from http://www.nytimes.com/2013/03/24/world/europe/boris-a-berezovsky-a-putin-critic-dies-at-67.html

Hewitt, P. L., Flett, G. L., Sherry, S. B., & Caelian, C. (2006). Trait perfectionism and suicide behavior. In T. Ellis (Ed.), *Cognition and suicide: Theory, research, and practice*. Washington, DC: American Psychological Association.

Hill, C. L., & Updegraff, J. A. (2012). Mindfulness and its relationship to emotional regulation. *Emotion, 12*(1), 81–90. doi:10.1037/a0026355

Hirsch, J. K. (2006). A review of the literature on rural suicide: Risk and protective factors, incidence, and prevention. *Crisis, 21*(4), 188–199. doi:10.1027/0227-5910.27.4.189

Hochard, K. D., Heym, N., & Townsend, E. (2016). Investigating the interaction between sleep symptoms of arousal and acquired capability in predicting Suicidality. *Suicide and Life-Threatening Behavior*. doi:10.1111/sltb.12285

Hoertel, N., Franco, S., Wall, M. M., Oquendo, M. A., Kerridge, B. T., Limosin, F., & Blanco, C. (2015). Mental disorders and risk of suicide attempt: A national prospective study. *Molecular Psychiatry, 20*(6), 718–726. doi:10.1038/mp.2015.19

Holland, N. (1977). *Literary suicide: A question of style*. Retrieved from http://users.clas.ufl.edu/nholland/suicide.htm

Holmes, T. H., & Rahe, R. H. (1967). The social readjustment rating scale. *Journal of Psychosomatic Research, 11*(2), 213–218. doi:10.1016/0022-3999(67)90010-4

Horesh, N. (2001). Self-report vs. computerized measures of impulsivity as a correlate of suicidal behavior. *Crisis, 22*, 27–31.

Horesh, N., & Apter, A. (2006). Self-disclosure, depression, anxiety, and suicidal behavior in adolescent psychiatric inpatients. *Crisis, 27*(2), 66–71. doi:10.1027/0227-5910.27.2.66

Horesh, N., Levi, Y., & Apter, A. (2012). Medically serious versus non-serious suicide attempts: Relationships of lethality and intent to clinical and interpersonal characteristics. *Journal of Affective Disorders, 136*(2), 283–293. doi:10.1016/j.jad.2011.11.035

Horesh, N., Zalsman, G., & Apter, A. (2004). Suicidal behavior and self-disclosure in adolescent psychiatric inpatients. *Journal of Nervous and Mental Disease, 192*(12), 837–842. doi:10.1097/01.nmd.0000146738.78222.e5

Horwitz, A. G., Czyz, E. K., & King, C. A. (2015). Predicting future suicide attempts among adolescent and emerging adult psychiatric emergency patients. *Journal of Clinical Child and Adolescent Psychology, 44*(5), 751–761. doi:10.1080/15374416.2014.910789

Houle, J. N., & Light, M. T. (2014). The home foreclosure crisis and rising suicide rates, 2005 to 2010. *American Journal of Public Health, 104*(6), 1073–1079. doi:10.2105/ajph.2013.301774

Howland, R. H. (2010). Potential adverse effects of discontinuing psychotropic drugs—Part 3: Antipsychotic, dopaminergic, and mood-stabilizing drugs. *Journal of Psychosocial Nursing and Mental Health Services, 48*(8), 11–14.

Hufford, M. R. (2001). Alcohol and suicidal behavior. *Clinical Psychology Review, 21*(5), 797–811.

Isometsä, E. (2014). Suicidal behaviour in mood disorders—Who, when, and why?. *Canadian Journal of Psychiatry, 59*(3), 120–130.

Jacobson, C., Batejan, K., Kleinman, M., & Gould, M. (2013). Reasons for attempting suicide among a community sample of adolescents. *Suicide and Life-Threatening Behavior, 43*(6), 646–662. doi:10.1111/sltb.12047

Jahn, D. R., & Cukrowicz, K. C. (2011). The impact of the nature of relationships on perceived burdensomeness and suicide ideation in a community sample of older adults. *Suicide and Life-Threatening Behavior, 41*(6), 635–649. doi:10.1111/j.1943-278x.2011.00060.x

Jia, C., Wang, L., Xu, A., Dai, A., & Qin, P. (2014). Physical illness and suicide risk in rural residents of contemporary China. *Crisis, 35*(5), 330–337. doi:10.1027/0227-5910/a000271

Jobes, D. A. (2016). *Managing suicidal risk: A collaborative approach.* New York, NY: Guilford.

Jobes, D. A., Comtois, K., Brenner, L., & Gutierrez, P. (2011). Clinical trial feasibility studies of the Collaborative Assessment and Management of Suicidality (CAMS). In R. O'Connor, S. Platt, & J. Gordon (Eds.), *International handbook of suicide prevention: Research, policy, and practice* (pp. 383–400). West Sussex, England: Wiley-Blackwell.

Jobes, D. A., Jacoby, A. M., Cimbolic, P., & Hustead, L. A. T. (1997). Assessment and treatment of suicidal clients in a university counseling center. *Journal of Counseling Psychology, 44*(4), 368–377. doi:10.1037/0022-0167.44.4.368

Jobes, D., & Mann, R. (1999). Reasons for living versus reasons for dying: Examining the internal debate of suicide. *Suicide and Life-Threatening Behavior, 29*, 97–104.

Jobes, D. A., & Nelson, K. N. (2006). Shneidman's contributions to the understanding of suicidal thinking. In T. E. Ellis (Ed.), *Cognition and suicide: Theory, research, and therapy* (pp. 29–49). Washington, DC: American Psychological Association.

Jobes, D. A., Nelson, K. N., Peterson, E. M., Pentiuc, D., Downing, V., Francini, K., & Kiernan, A. (2004). Describing suicidality: An investigation of qualitative SSF responses. *Suicide and Life-Threatening Behavior, 34*(2), 99–112. doi:10.1521/suli.34.2.99.32788

Jobes, D. A., & Shneidman, E. S. (2006). *Managing suicidal risk: A collaborative approach.* New York, NY: Guilford.

Jobes, D. A., Wong, S. A., Conrad, A. K., Drozd, J. F., & Neal-Walden, T. (2005). The collaborative assessment and management of suicidality versus treatment as usual: A retrospective study with suicidal outpatients. *Suicide and Life-Threatening Behavior, 35*(5), 483–497. doi:10.1521/suli.2005.35.5.483

Johnson, J. G., Cohen, P., Gould, M. S., Kasen, S., Brown, J., & Brook, J. S. (2002). Childhood adversities, interpersonal difficulties, and risk for suicide attempts during late adolescence and early adulthood. *Archives of General Psychiatry, 59*(8), 741. doi:10.1001/archpsyc.59.8.741

Joiner, J. T. (1999). The clustering and contagion of suicide. *Current Directions in Psychological Science, 8*(3), 89–92. doi:10.1111/1467-8721.00021

Joiner, T. E. (2005). *Why people die by suicide.* Cambridge, MA: Harvard University Press.

Joiner, T. E., Jr., Brown, J. S., & Wingate, L. R. (2005). The psychology and neurobiology of suicidal behavior. *Annual Review of Psychology, 56*, 287–314.

Joiner, T. E., Jr., Hollar, D., & Van Orden, K. (2006). On buckeyes, gators, Super Bowl Sunday, and the miracle on ice: "Pulling together" is associated with lower suicide rates. *Journal of Social and Clinical Psychology, 25*(2), 179.

Joiner, T. E., Jr., Pettit, J. W., Walker, R. L., & Voelz, Z. R. (2002). Perceived burdensomeness and suicidality: Two studies on the suicide notes of those attempting and those completing suicide. *Journal of Social and Clinical Psychology, 21*(5), 531.

Joiner, T. E., Jr., & Van Orden, K. A. (2008). The interpersonal–psychological theory of suicidal behavior indicates specific and crucial psychotherapeutic targets. *International Journal of Cognitive Therapy, 1*(1), 80–89.

Joiner, T. E., Jr., Van Orden, K. A., Witte, T. K., Cukrowicz, K. C., Braithwaite, S. R., & Selby, E. A. (2010). The interpersonal theory of suicide. *Psychological Review, 117*(2), 575–600. doi:10.1037/a0018697

Joiner, T. E., Jr., Van Orden, K. A., Witte, T. K., Selby, E. A., Ribeiro, J. D., Lewis, R., & Rudd, M. D. (2009). Main predictions of the interpersonal–psychological theory of suicidal behavior: Empirical tests in two samples of young adults. *Journal of Abnormal Psychology, 118*(3), 634–646. doi:10.1037/a0016500

Kabat-Zinn, J. (1990). *Full catastrophe living: Using the wisdom of your body and mind to face stress, pain and illness.* New York, NY: Delacorte.

Kanwar, A., Malik, S., Prokop, L. J., Sim, L. A., Feldstein, D., Wang, Z., & Murad, M. H. (2013). The association between anxiety disorders and suicidal behaviors: A systematic review and meta-analysis. *Depression and Anxiety, 30*(10), 917–929.

Kanzler, K. E., Bryan, C. J., McGeary, D. D., & Morrow, C. E. (2012). Suicidal ideation and perceived burdensomeness in patients with chronic pain. *Pain Practice, 12*(8), 602–609. doi:10.1111/j.1533-2500.2012.00542.x

Kapfhammer, H., & Lange, P. (2012). Suicidal and infanticidal risks in puerperal psychosis of an early onset. *Neuropsychiatrie: Klinik, Diagnostik, Therapie und Rehabilitation, 26*(3), 129–138. doi:10.1007/s40211-012-0023-9

Kashdan, T. B., Ferssizidis, P., Collins, R. L., & Muraven, M. (2010). Emotion differentiation as resilience against excessive alcohol use: An ecological momentary assessment in underage social drinkers. *Psychological Science, 21*(9), 1341–1347. doi:10.1177/0956797610379863

Kassinove, H., & Sukhodolsky, D. G. (1995). Optimism, pessimism and worry in Russian and American children and adolescents. *Journal of Social Behavior and Personality, 10*(1), 157.

Katz, C., Yaseen, Z. S., Mojtabai, R., Cohen, L. J., & Galynker, I. I. (2011). Panic as an independent risk factor for suicide attempt in depressive illness. *Journal of Clinical Psychiatry, 72*(12), 1628–1635. doi:10.4088/jcp.10m06186blu

Keltner, D., & Kring, A. M. (1998). Emotion, social function, and psychopathology. *Review of General Psychology, 2*(3), 320–342. doi:10.1037/1089-2680.2.3.320

Keneally, M., Nathan, S., & Collins, L. (2014, March 18). Designer L'Wren Scott was "embarrassed and millions in debt" when she committed suicide in her Manhattan apartment while "devastated" lover Mick Jagger was on tour in Australia. *Daily Mail.* Retrieved from http://www.dailymail.co.uk/news/article-2582815/Mick-Jaggers-girlfriend-designer-LWren-Scott-commits-suicide.html

Kernberg, O. (1965). Notes on countertransferences. *Journal of the American Psychoanalytic Association, 13*, 38–56.

Kessler, R. C., Borges, G., & Walters, E. E. (1999). Prevalence of and risk factors for lifetime suicide attempts in the National Comorbidity Survey. *Archives of General Psychiatry, 56*(7), 617–626.

Kessler, R. C., Chiu, W. T., Demler, O., & Walters, E. E. (2005). Prevalence, severity, and comorbidity of 12-month DSM-IV disorders in the National Comorbidity Survey replication. *Archives of General Psychiatry, 62*(6), 617. doi:10.1001/archpsyc.62.6.617

Kessler, R. C., Galea, S., Jones, R. T., & Parker, H. A. (2006). Mental illness and suicidality after Hurricane Katrina. *Bulletin of the World Health Organization, 84*(12), 930–939.

King, M., Semlyen, J., Tai, S. S., Killaspy, H., Osborn, D., Popelyuk, D., & Nazareth, I. (2008). A systematic review of mental disorder, suicide, and deliberate self harm in lesbian, gay and bisexual people. *BMC Psychiatry, 8*(1), 70. doi:10.1186/1471-244x-8-70

Kisiel, C. L., & Lyons, J. S. (2001). Dissociation as a mediator of psychopathology among sexually abused children and adolescents. *American Journal of Psychiatry, 158*(7), 1034–1039. doi:10.1176/appi.ajp.158.7.1034

Kitagawa, Y., Shimodera, S., Togo, F., Okazaki, Y., Nishida, A., & Sasaki, T. (2014). Suicidal feelings interferes with help-seeking in bullied adolescents. *PLoS ONE, 9*(9), e106031. doi:10.1371/journal.pone.0106031

Kleber, H., & Gawin, F. (1986). Psychopharmacological trials in cocaine abuse treatment. *American Journal of Drug and Alcohol Abuse, 12*(3), 235–246.

Klein, M. (1935). A contribution to the psychogenesis of manic–depressive states. *International Journal of Psychoanalysis, 16*, 145–174.

Klein, M. (1946). Notes on some schizoid mechanisms. *International Journal of Psychoanalysis, 27*, 99–110.

Kleiman, E. M., Adams, L. M., Kashdan, T. B., & Riskind, J. H. (2013). Gratitude and grit indirectly reduce risk of suicidal ideations by enhancing meaning in life: Evidence for a mediated moderation model. *Journal of Research in Personality, 47*(5), 539–546.

Kleiman, E. M., & Liu, R. T. (2013). Social support as a protective factor in suicide: Findings from two nationally representative samples. *Journal of Affective Disorders, 150*(2), 540–545. doi:10.1016/j.jad.2013.01.033

Klonsky, E. D., & May, A. M. (2014). Differentiating suicide attempters form suicide ideators: A critical frontier for suicidology research. *Suicide and Life Threatening Behavior, 44*(1), 1–5. doi:10.1111/sltb.12068

Knappe, S., Beesdo-Baum, K., Fehm, L., Lieb, R., & Wittchen, H. (2012). Characterizing the association between parenting and adolescent social phobia. *Journal of Anxiety Disorders, 26*(5), 608–616. doi:10.1016/j.janxdis.2012.02.014

Knowlton, D. S., & Hagopian, K. J. (Eds.). (2013). *From entitlement to engagement: Affirming Millennial students' egos in the higher education classroom: New directions for teaching and learning.* San Francisco: John Wiley & Sons.

Koivumaa-Honkanen, H., Honkanen, R., Viinamaeki, H., Heikkilae, K., Kaprio, J., & Koskenvuo, M. (2001). Life satisfaction and suicide: A 20-year follow-up study. *American Journal of Psychiatry, 158*(3), 433–439. doi:10.1176/appi.ajp.158.3.433

Kõlves, K., Värnik, A., Schneider, B., Fritze, J., & Allik, J. (2006). Recent life events and suicide: A case–control study in Tallinn and Frankfurt. *Social Science & Medicine, 62*(11), 2887–2896. doi:10.1016/j.socscimed.2005.11.048

Kramer, A. D. I., Guillory, J. E., & Hancock, J. T. (2014). Experimental evidence of massive-scale emotional contagion through social networks. *Proceedings of the National Academy of Sciences, 111*(24), 8788–8790. doi:10.1073/pnas.1320040111

Krug, E. G., Dahlberg, L. L., Mercy, J. A., Zwi, A. B., & Lozano, R. (2002). *World report on violence and health.* Geneva, Switzerland: World Health Organization.

Labonte, B., & Turecki, G. (2012). Epigenetic effects of childhood adversity in the brain and suicide risk. In Y. Dwivedi (Ed.), *The neurobiological basis of suicide* (pp. 275–296). Boca Raton, FL: Taylor & Francis/CRC Press.

Lamberg, L. (1997). Psychiatrist explores apocalyptic violence in Heaven's Gate and Aum Shinrikyo cults. *JAMA, 278*(3), 191–193. doi:10.1001/jama.278.3.191

Large, M., & Nielssen, O. (2012). Suicide is preventable but not predictable. *Australasian Psychiatry, 20*(6), 532–533. doi:10.1177/1039856212464912

Large, M., Sharma, S., Cannon, E., Ryan, C., & Nielssen, O. (2011). Risk factors for suicide within a year of discharge from psychiatric hospital: A systematic meta-analysis. *Australian and New Zealand Journal of Psychiatry, 45*(8), 619–628. doi:10.3109/00048674.2011.590465

Larkin, G., & Beautrais, A. (2012). *Geospatial mapping of suicide clusters*. Auckland, New Zealand: Te Pou o Te Whakaaro Nui.

Lawrence, D. M., Holman, C. D. J., Jablensky, A. V., & Fuller, S. A. (1999). Suicide rates in psychiatric in-patients: An application of record linkage to mental health research. *Australian and New Zealand Journal of Public Health, 23*(5), 468–470. doi:10.1111/j.1467-842x.1999.tb01300.x

Lawrence, R. E., Oquendo, M. A., & Stanley, B. (2015). Religion and suicide risk: A systematic review. *Archives of Suicide Research, 20*(1), 1–21. doi:10.1080/13811118.2015.1004494

Lazarus, R. S., & Folkman, S. (1984). *Stress, appraisal, and coping*. New York, NY: Springer.

Lecrubier, Y., Sheehan, D., Weiller, E., Amorim, P., Bonora, I., Harnett Sheehan, K., . . . Dunbar, G. (1997). The Mini International Neuropsychiatric Interview (MINI)—A short diagnostic structured interview: Reliability and validity according to the CIDI. *European Psychiatry, 12*(5), 224–231. doi:10.1016/s0924-9338(97)83296-8

Lee, Y., Syeda, K., Maruschak, N. A., Cha, D. S., Mansur, R. B., Wium-Andersen, I. K., . . . McIntyre, R. S. (2016). A new perspective on the anti-suicide effects with ketamine treatment. *Journal of Clinical Psychopharmacology, 36*(1), 50–56. doi:10.1097/jcp.0000000000000441

Leinonen, T., Martikainen, P., Laaksonen, M., & Lahelma, E. (2013). Excess mortality after disability retirement due to mental disorders: Variations by socio-demographic factors and causes of death. *Social Psychiatry and Psychiatric Epidemiology, 49*(4), 639–649. doi:10.1007/s00127-013-0747-2

Lester, D. (1967). Experimental and correlational studies of the fear of death. *Psychological Bulletin, 67*(1), 27–36.

Lester, D. (1997). The role of shame in suicide. *Suicide and Life-Threatening Behavior, 27*(4), 352–361. doi:10.1111/j.1943-278X.1997.tb00514.x

Levi, Y., Horesh, N., Fischel, T., Treves, I., Or, E., & Apter, A. (2008). Mental pain and its communication in medically serious suicide attempts: An "impossible situation." *Journal of Affective Disorders, 111*(2-3), 244–250. doi:10.1016/j.jad.2008.02.022

Levi-Belz, Y., Gvion, Y., Horesh, N., & Apter, A. (2013). Attachment patterns in medically serious suicide attempts: The mediating role of self-disclosure and loneliness. *Suicide and Life-Threatening Behavior, 43*(5), 511–522. doi:10.1111/sltb.12035

Levi-Belz, Y., Gvion, Y., Horesh, N., Fischel, T., Treves, I., Or, E., . . . Apter, A. (2014). Mental pain, communication difficulties, and medically serious suicide attempts: A case–control study. *Archives of Suicide Research, 18*(1), 74–87. doi:10.1080/13811118.2013.809041

Lewis, A. J., Bertino, M. D., Bailey, C. M., Skewes, J., Lubman, D. I., & Toumbourou, J. W. (2014). Depression and suicidal behavior in adolescents: A multi-informant and multi-methods approach to diagnostic classification. *Frontiers in Psychology, 5*, 766. doi:10.3389/fpsyg.2014.00766

Leykin, Y., Roberts, C. S., & DeRubeis, R. J. (2011). Decision-making and depressive symptomatology. *Cognitive Therapy and Research, 35*(4), 333–341.

Libby, A. M., Orton, H. D., & Valuck, R. J. (2009). Persisting decline in depression treatment after FDA warnings. *Archives of General Psychiatry, 66*(6), 633. doi:10.1001/archgenpsychiatry.2009.46

Lim, M., Kim, S., Nam, Y., Moon, E., Yu, J., Lee, S., . . . Park, J. (2014). Reasons for desiring death: Examining causative factors of suicide attempters treated in emergency rooms in Korea. *Journal of Affective Disorders, 168*, 349–356. doi:10.1016/j.jad.2014.07.026

Lim, M., Lee, S., & Park, J. (2014). Difference in suicide methods used between suicide attempters and suicide completers. *International Journal of Mental Health Systems, 8*(1), 54. doi:10.1186/1752-4458-8-54

Lim, S. W., Ko, E. M., Shin, D. W., Shin, Y. C., & Oh, K. S. (2015). Clinical symptoms associated with suicidality in patients with panic disorder. *Psychopathology, 48*(3), 137–144.

Linehan, M. M. (1993a). *Cognitive–behavioral treatment of borderline personality disorder.* New York, NY: Guilford.

Linehan, M. M. (1993b). *Skills training manual for treating borderline personality disorder.* New York, NY: Guilford.

Linehan, M. M., Heard, H., & Armstrong, H. (1993). Naturalistic follow-up of a behavioral treatment for chronically parasuicidal borderline patients. *Archives of General Psychiatry, 50*(12), 971. doi:10.1001/archpsyc.1993.01820240055007

Linehan, M. M., Korslund, K. E., Harned, M. S., Gallop, R. J., Lungu, A., Neacsiu, A. D., . . . Murray-Gregory, A. M. (2015). Dialectical behavior therapy for high suicide risk in individuals with borderline personality disorder. *Journal of the American Medical Association Psychiatry, 72*(5), 475. doi:10.1001/jamapsychiatry.2014.3039

List of suicides. (2016). Retrieved from https://en.wikipedia.org/wiki/List_of_suicides

Litman, R. E., Curphey, T., Shneidman, E. S., Farberow, N. L., & Tabachnik, N. (1963). Investigations of equivocal suicides. *Journal of the American Medical Association, 184*, 924–929. doi:10.1001/jama.1963.03700250060008

Liu, R. T., & Miller, I. (2014). Life events and suicidal ideation and behavior: A systematic review. *Clinical Psychology Review, 34*(3), 181–192. doi:10.1016/j.cpr.2014.01.006

Loas, G. (2007). Anhedonia and suicide: A 6.5-yr. follow-up study of patients hospitalized for a suicide attempt. *Psychological Reports, 100*(1), 183–190. doi:10.2466/pr0.100.1.183-190

Lobera, I. J., Ríos, P. B., & Casals, O. G. (2011). Parenting styles and eating disorders. *Journal of Psychiatric and Mental Health Nursing, 18*(8), 728–735. doi:10.1111/j.1365-2850.2011.01723.x

Locke, T. F., & Newcomb, M. D. (2005). Psychosocial predictors and correlates of suicidality in teenage Latino males. *Hispanic Journal of Behavioral Sciences, 27*(3), 319–336. doi:10.1177/0739986305276745

Lombardo, C., Milne, D., & Proctor, R. (2009). Getting to the heart of clinical supervision: A theoretical review of the role of emotions in professional development. *Behavioural and Cognitive Psychotherapy, 37*(02), 207. doi:10.1017/s135246580900513x

Lundholm, L., Thiblin, I., Runeson, B., Leifman, A., & Fugelstad, A. (2014). Acute influence of alcohol, THC or central stimulants on violent suicide: A Swedish population study. *Journal of Forensic Sciences, 59*(2), 436–440.

Luxton, D. D., June, J. D., & Comtois, K. A. (2013). Can postdischarge follow-up contacts prevent suicide and suicidal behavior? *Crisis, 34*(1), 32–41. doi:10.1027/0227-5910/a000158

Ma, J., Batterham, P. J., Calear, A. L., & Han, J. (2016). A systematic review of the predictions of the interpersonal–psychological theory of suicidal behavior. *Clinical Psychology Review, 46*, 34–45. doi:10.1016/j.cpr.2016.04.008

Machado, D. B., Rasella, D., & Santos, D. N. (2015). Impact of income inequality and other social determinants on suicide rate in brazil. *PLoS One, 10*(4), e0124934. doi:10.1371/journal.pone.0124934

MacLeod, A. K., & Conway, C. (2007). Well-being and positive future thinking for the self versus others. *Cognition & Emotion, 21*(5), 1114–1124. doi:10.1080/02699930601109507

MacLeod, A. K., Pankhania, B., Lee, M., & Mitchell, D. (1997). Brief communication: Parasuicide, depression and the anticipation of positive and negative future experiences. *Psychological Medicine, 27*(4), 973–977.

Maiuro, R. D., O'Sullivan, M. J., Michael, M. C., & Vitaliano, P. P. (1989). Anger, hostility, and depression in assaultive vs. suicide-attempting males. *Journal of Clinical Psychology, 45*(4), 531–541. doi:10.1002/1097-4679(198907)45:43.0.co;2-k

Maltsberger, J. T. (2004). The descent into suicide. *International Journal of Psychoanalysis, 85*(3), 653–667. doi:10.1516/002075704774200799

Maltsberger, J. T., & Buie, M. D. (1974). Countertransference hate in the treatment of suicidal patients. *Archives of General Psychiatry, 30*(5), 625–633. doi:10.1001/archpsyc.1974.01760110049005

Maltsberger, J. T., Hendin, H., Haas, A. P., & Lipschitz, A. (2003). Determination of precipitating events in the suicide of psychiatric patients. *Suicide and Life-Threatening Behavior, 33*(2), 111–119. doi:10.1521/suli.33.2.111.22778

Mancinelli, I., Comparelli, A., Girardi, P., & Tatarelli, R. (2002). Mass suicide: Historical and psychodynamic considerations. *Suicide and Life-Threatening Behavior, 32*(1), 91–100. doi:10.1521/suli.32.1.91.22186

Mann, J. J., Apter, A., Bertolote, J., Beautrais, A., Currier, D., Haas, A., . . . Hendin, H. (2005). Suicide prevention strategies: A systematic review. *Journal of the American Medical Association, 294,* 2064–2074.

Mann, J. J., & Arango, V. A. (1992). Integration of neurobiology and psychopathology in a unified model of suicidal behavior. *Journal of Clinical Psychopharmacology, 12*(2 Suppl.), 2S–7S. doi:10.1097/00004714-199204001-00001

Mann, J. J., Arango, V. A., Avenevoli, S., Brent, D.A., Champagne, F. A., Clayton, P., . . . Wenzel, A. (2009). Candidate endophenotypes for genetic studies of suicidal behavior. *Biological Psychiatry, 65,* 556–563.

Mann, J. J., Waternaux, C., Haas, G. L., & Malone, K. M. (1999). Toward a clinical model of suicidal behavior in psychiatric patients. *American Journal of Psychiatry, 156*(2), 181–189. doi:10.1176/ajp.156.2.181

Marcinko, D., Skocic, M., Popovic-Knapic, V., & Tentor, B. (2008). Countertransference in the therapy of suicidal patients—An important part of integrative treatment. *Psychiatria Danubina, 20,* 402–405.

Martin, G., Bergen, H. A., Richardson, A. S., Roeger, L., & Allison, S. (2004). Sexual abuse and suicidality: Gender differences in a large community sample of adolescents. *Child Abuse & Neglect, 28*(5), 491–503. doi:10.1016/j.chiabu.2003.08.006

Martin, J. A. (2005). Annual summary of vital statistics—2003. *Pediatrics, 115*(3), 619–634. doi:10.1542/peds.2004-2695

Marttunen, M. J., Aro, H. M., & Lonnqvist, J. K. (1993). Adolescence and suicide: A review of psychological autopsy studies. *European Child & Adolescent Psychiatry, 2*(1), 10–18. doi:10.1007/BF02098826

Marzuk, P. M., Hartwell, N., Leon, A. C., & Portera, L. (2005). Executive functioning in depressed patients with suicidal ideation. *Acta Psychiatrica Scandinavica, 112*(4), 294–301.

McAdams, D. P. (2001). The psychology of life stories. *Review of General Psychology, 5*(2), 100.

McGarvey, E. L., Kryzhanovskaya, L. A., Koopman, C., Waite, D., & Canterbury, R. J. (1999). Incarcerated adolescents' distress and suicidality in relation to parental bonding styles. *Crisis, 20*(4), 164–170. doi:10.1027//0227-5910.20.4.16

McIntosh, J. L., & Drapeau, C. W. (2014). *U.S.A. suicide 2011: Official final data.* Washington, DC: American Association of Suicidology. Retrieved from http://www.suicidology.org

McKenzie, N. (2005). Clustering of suicides among people with mental illness. *British Journal of Psychiatry, 187*(5), 476–480. doi:10.1192/bjp.187.5.476

McKenzie, N., & Keane, M. (2007). Contribution of imitative suicide to the suicide rate in prisons. *Suicide and Life-Threatening Behavior, 37*(5), 538–542. doi:10.1521/suli.2007.37.5.538

McKinney, C., Donnelly, R., & Renk, K. (2008). Perceived parenting, positive and negative perceptions of parents, and late adolescent emotional adjustment. *Child and Adolescent Mental Health, 13*(2), 66–73.

McLean, K. C., Pasupathi, M., & Pals, J. L. (2007). Selves creating stories creating selves: A process model of self development. *Personality and Social Psychological Review, 11*, 262–278. doi:10.1177/1088868307301034

Menninger, K. A. (1938). *Man against himself.* New York, NY: Harcourt, Brace.

Mergl, R., Koburger, N., Heinrichs, K., Székely, A., Tóth, M. D., Coyne, J., . . . Hegerl, U. (2015). What are reasons for the large gender differences in the lethality of suicidal acts? An epidemiological analysis in four European countries. *PLoS One, 10*(7), e0129062. doi:10.1371/journal.pone.0129062

Merrall, E. L. C., Kariminia, A., Binswanger, I. A., Hobbs, M. S., Farrell, M., Marsden, J., . . . Bird, S. M. (2010). Meta-analysis of drug-related deaths soon after release from prison. *Addiction, 105*(9), 1545–1554. doi:10.1111/j.1360-0443.2010.02990.x

Mesoudi, A. (2009). The cultural dynamics of copycat suicide. *PLoS One, 4*(9), e7252. doi:10.1371/journal.pone.0007252

Miller, A. B., Esposito-Smythers, C., Weismoore, J. T., & Renshaw, K. D. (2013). The relation between child maltreatment and adolescent suicidal behavior: A systematic review and critical examination of the literature. *Clinical Child and Family Psychology Review, 16*(2), 146–172. doi:10.1007/s10567-013-0131-5

Miller, K. E., King, C. A., Shain, B. N., & Naylor, M. W. (1992). Suicidal adolescents' perceptions of their family environment. *Suicide and Life-Threatening Behavior, 22*, 226–239.

Miller, L. (2006). Suicide by cop: Causes, reactions, and practical intervention strategies. *International Journal of Emergency Mental Health, 8*(3), 165–174.

Miller, M., Azrael, D., & Barber, C. (2012). Suicide mortality in the United States: The importance of attending to method in understanding population-level disparities in the burden of suicide. *Annual Review of Public Health, 33*(1), 393–408. doi:10.1146/annurev-publhealth-031811-124636

Miller, M., Azrael, D., & Hemenway, D. (2006). Belief in the inevitability of suicide: Results from a national survey. *Suicide and Life-Threatening Behavior, 36*(1), 1–11. doi:10.1521/suli.2006.36.1.1

Miller, M., Barber, C., Young, M., Azrael, D., Mukamal, K., & Lawler, E. (2012). Veterans and suicide: A reexamination of the National Death Index–linked National Health Interview Survey. *American Journal of Public Health, 102*(Suppl. 1), S154–S159. doi:10.2105/ajph.2011.300409

Miranda, R., Gallagher, M., Bauchner, B., Vaysman, R., & Marroquín, B. (2012). Cognitive inflexibility as a prospective predictor of suicidal ideation among young adults with a suicide attempt history. *Depression and Anxiety, 29*, 180–186.

Modestin, J. (1987). Counter-transference reactions contributing to completed suicide. *British Journal of Medical Psychology, 60*(4), 379–385. doi:10.1111/j.2044-8341.1987.tb02757.x

Mohamed, F., Perera, A., Wijayaweera, K., Kularatne, K., Jayamanne, S., Eddleston, M., . . . Gunnell, D. (2010). The prevalence of previous self-harm amongst self-poisoning patients in Sri Lanka. *Social Psychiatry and Psychiatric Epidemiology, 46*(6), 517–520. doi:10.1007/s00127-010-0217-z

Mojtabai, R., & Olfson, M. (2008). National trends in psychotherapy by office-based psychiatrists. *Archives of General Psychiatry, 65*(8), 962. doi:10.1001/archpsyc.65.8.962

Montgomery, S. A. (2008). Tolerability of serotonin norepinephrine reuptake inhibitor antidepressants. *CNS Spectrums, 13*(Suppl. 11), 27–33. doi:10.1017/s1092852900028297

Morrison, R., & O'Connor, R. C. (2008). A systematic review of the relationship between rumination and suicidality. *Suicide & Life-Threatening Behavior, 38*(5), 523–538.

Mortensen, P. B., & Juel, K. (1993). Mortality and causes of death in first admitted schizo-phrenic patients. *British Journal of Psychiatry, 163*(2), 183–189. doi:10.1192/bjp.163.2.183

Mościcki, E. K. (1997). Identification of suicide risk factors using epidemiologic studies. *Psychiatric Clinics of North America, 20*(3), 82–84.

Mościcki, E. K. (2001). Epidemiology of completed and attempted suicide: Toward a framework for prevention. *Clinical Neuroscience Research, 1*(5), 310–323. doi:10.1016/s1566-2772(01)00032-9

Murphy, S. M., & Tyrer, P. (1991). A double-blind comparison of the effects of gradual with-drawal of lorazepam, diazepam and bromazepam in benzodiazepine dependence. *British Journal of Psychiatry, 158*(4), 511–516.

Murrough, J. W., Perez, A. M., Pillemer, S., Stern, J., Parides, M. K., Aan het Rot, M., Collins, K. A., . . . Iosifescu, D. V. (2013). Rapid and longer-term antidepressant effects of repeated ketamine infusions in treatment-resistant major depression. *Biological Psychiatry, 74*(4), 250–256. doi:10.1016/j.biopsych.2012.06.022

Müller-Oerlinghausen, B., & Lewitzka, U. (2010). Lithium reduces pathological aggression and suicidality: A mini-review. *Neuropsychobiology, 62*(1), 43–49. doi:10.1159/000314309

Naito, A. (2007). Internet suicide in Japan: Implications for child and adolescent men-tal health. *Clinical Child Psychology and Psychiatry, 12*(4), 583–597. doi:10.1177/1359104507080990

Najmi, S., Wegner, D. M., & Nock, M. K. (2007). Thought suppression and self-injurious thoughts and behaviors. *Behavior Research and Therapy, 45*(8), 1957–1965.

Nam, Y. Y., Kim, C. H., & Roh, D. (2016). Comorbid panic disorder as an independent risk factor for suicide attempts in depressed outpatients. *Comprehensive Psychiatry, 67*, 13–18.

Nanayakkara, S., Misch, D., Chang, L., & Henry, D. (2013). Depression and exposure to suicide predict suicide attempt. *Depression and Anxiety, 30*(10), 991–996. doi:10.1002/da.22143

Nasseri, K., & Moulton, L. H. (2009). Patterns of death in the first and second generation immigrants from selected Middle Eastern countries in California. *Journal of Immigrant and Minority Health, 13*(2), 361–370. doi:10.1007/s10903-009-9270-7

Nesse, R. (2000). Is Depression an Adaptation? *Archive General Psychiatry, 1*, 14–20. doi:10.1001/archpsyc.57.1.14

Newport, D. J., Carpenter, L. L., McDonald, W. M., Potash, J. B., Tohen, M., & Nemeroff, C. B. (2015). Ketamine and other NMDA antagonists: Early clinical trials and possible mecha-nisms in depression. *American Journal of Psychiatry, 172*(10), 950–966. doi:10.1176/appi.ajp.2015.15040465

Newport, D. J., Schatzberg, A. F., & Nemeroff, C. B. (2016). Whither ketamine as an antide-pressant: Panacea or toxin? *Depression and Anxiety, 33*(8), 685–688. doi:10.1002/da.22535

Niederkrotenthaler, T., Voracek, M., Herberth, A., Till, B., Strauss, M., Etzersdorfer, E., . . . Sonneck, G. (2010). Role of media reports in completed and prevented suicide: *Werther v. Papageno* effects. *British Journal of Psychiatry, 197*(3), 234–243. doi:10.1192/bjp.bp.109.074633

Nielsen, A., Alberdi, F., & Rosenbaum, B. (2011). Collaborative assessment and management of suicidality method shows effect. *Danish Medical Bulletin, 58*(8), A4300.

Nielsen, L., & Kaszniak, A. W. (2006). Awareness of subtle emotional feelings: A compari-son of long-term meditators and nonmeditators. *Emotion, 6*(3), 392–405. doi:10.1037/1528-3542.6.3.392

Nishimura, A., Shioiri, T., Nushida, H., Ueno, Y., Ushiyama, I., Tanegashima, A., . . . Nishi, K. (1999). Changes in choice of method and lethality between last attempted and completed suicides: How did suicide attempters carry out their desire? *Legal Medicine, 1*(3), 150–158. doi:10.1016/s1344-6223(99)80028-5

Nivoli, A., Nivoli, F., Nivoli, G., & Lorettu, L. (2011). Therapist's reactions on the treatment of suicidal patients. *Rivista di Psichiatria, 46*(1), 57–65.

Nock, M. K., & Kazdin, A. E. (2002). Examination of affective, cognitive, and behavioral factors and suicide-related outcomes in children and young adolescents. *Journal of Clinical Child & Adolescent Psychology, 31*(1), 48–58. doi:10.1207/s15374424jccp3101_07

Nock, M. K., Park, J. M., Finn, C. T., Deliberto, T. L., Dour, H. J., & Banaji, M. R. (2010). Measuring the suicidal mind: Implicit cognition predicts suicidal behavior. *Psychological Science, 21*(4), 511–517. doi:10.1177/0956797610364762

Nock, M. K., Stein, M. B., Heeringa, S. G., Ursano, R. J., Colpe, L. J., Fullerton, C. S., . . . Kessler, R. C. (2014). Prevalence and correlates of suicidal behavior among soldiers: Results from the Army Study to Assess Risk and Resilience in Service Members (Army STARRS). *Journal of the American Medical Association Psychiatry, 71*(5), 514–522.

Nordentoft, M., Breum, L., Munck, L. K., Nordestgaard, A. G., Hunding, A., & Laursen Bjaeldager, P. A. (1993). High mortality by natural and unnatural causes: A 10 year follow up study of patients admitted to a poisoning treatment centre after suicide attempts. *BMJ, 306*(6893), 1637–1641. doi:10.1136/bmj.306.6893.1637

Nordentoft, M., Mortensen, P. B., & Pedersen, C. B. (2011). Absolute risk of suicide after first hospital contact in mental disorder. *Archives of General Psychiatry, 68*(10), 1058–1064.

Nordentoft, M., Pedersen, C. B., & Mortensen, P. B. (2012). 15:00 Absolute risk of suicide following first hospital contact with mental disorder. *Schizophrenia Research, 136*, S73–S74. doi:10.1016/s0920-9964(12)70268-2

Novick, D. M., Swartz, H. A., & Frank, E. (2010). Suicide attempts in bipolar I and bipolar II disorder: A review and meta-analysis of the evidence. *Bipolar Disorders, 12*(1), 1–9.

Nummenmaa, L., Hirvonen, J., Parkkola, R., & Hietanen, J. K. (2008). Is emotional contagion special? An fMRI study on neural systems for affective and cognitive empathy. *NeuroImage, 43*(3), 571–580. doi:10.1016/j.neuroimage.2008.08.014

O'Connor, E., Gaynes, B. N., Burda, B. U., Soh, C., & Whitlock, E. P. (2013). Screening for and treatment of suicide risk relevant to primary care: A systematic review for the U.S. Preventive Services Task Force. *Annals of Internal Medicine, 158*(10), 741. doi:10.7326/0003-4819-158-10-201305210-00642

O'Connor, R. C. (2003). Suicidal behavior as a cry of pain: Test of a psychological model. *Archives of Suicide Research, 7*(4), 297–308. doi:10.1080/713848941

O'Connor, R. C. (2007). The relations between perfectionism and suicidality: A systematic review. *Suicide and Life-Threatening Behavior, 37*(6), 698–714.

O'Connor, R. C. (2011). The integrated motivational–volitional model of suicidal behavior. *Crisis, 32*(6), 295–298. doi:10.1027/0227-5910/a000120

O'Connor, R. C., Armitage, C. J., & Gray, L. (2006). The role of clinical and social cognitive variables in parasuicide. *British Journal of Clinical Psychology, 45*, 465–481

O'Connor, R. C., Connery, H., & Cheyne, W. M. (2000). Hopelessness: The role of depression, future directed thinking and cognitive vulnerability. *Psychology, Health and Medicine, 5*(2), 155–161.

O'Connor, R. C., & Forgan, G. (2007). Suicidal thinking and perfectionism: The role of goal adjustment and behavioral inhibition/activation systems (BIS/BAS). *Journal of Rational-Emotive & Cognitive-Behavior Therapy, 25*(4), 321–341.

O'Connor, R. C., O'Carroll, R. E., Ryan, C., & Smyth, R. (2012). Self-regulation of unattainable goals in suicide attempters: A two year prospective study. *Journal of Affective Disorders, 142*, 248–255.

O'Connor, R. C., & O'Connor, D. B. (2003). Predicting hopelessness and psychological distress: The role of perfectionism and coping. *Journal of Counseling Psychology, 50*(3), 362–372. doi:10.1037/0022-0167.50.3.362

O'Connor, R. C., O'Connor, D. B., O'Connor, S. M., Smallwood, J. M., &. Miles, J. (2004). Hopelessness, stress and perfectionism: The moderating effects of future thinking. *Cognition and Emotion, 18*, 1099–1120.

O'Connor, R. C., Rasmussen, S., & Hawton, K. (2009). Predicting deliberate self-harm in adolescents: A six month prospective study. *Suicide and Life-Threatening Behavior, 39*, 364–375.

O'Connor, R. C., Rasmussen, S., & Hawton, K. (2014). Adolescent self-harm: A school-based study in Northern Ireland. *Journal of Affective Disorders, 159*, 46–52. doi:10.1016/j.jad.2014.02.015

O'Connor, R. C., Smyth, R., Ferguson, E., Ryan, C., & Williams, J. M. (2013). Psychological processes and repeat suicidal behavior: A four-year prospective study. *Journal of Consulting and Clinical Psychology, 81*(6), 1137–1143. doi:10.1037/a0033751

O'Connor, R. C., Smyth, R., & Williams, J. M. G. (2015). Intrapersonal positive future thinking predicts repeat suicide attempts in hospital-treated suicide attempters. *Journal of Consulting and Clinical Psychology, 83*(1), 169–176. doi:10.1037/a0037846

Office for National Statistics. (2016). *Suicides in the United Kingdom: 2014 registrations.* Retrieved from https://www.ons.gov.uk/peoplepopulationandcommunity/birthsdeathsandmarriages/deaths/bulletins/suicidesintheunitedkingdom/2014registrations

Öhman, A., & Mineka, S. (2001). Fear, phobias and preparedness: Toward an evolved module of fear and fear learning. *Psychological Review, 108*, 483–522.

Olfson, M., & Marcus, S. C. (2008). A case–control study of antidepressants and attempted suicide during early phase treatment of major depressive episodes. *Journal of Clinical Psychiatry, 69*(3), 425–432. doi:10.4088/jcp.v69n0313

Oquendo, M. A. (2015). Suicidal behavior: Measurement and mechanism. *Journal of Clinical Psychiatry, 76*(12), 1675. doi:10.4088/jcp.15f10520

Oquendo, M. A., Barrera, A., Ellis, S. P., Li, S., Burke, A. K., Grunebaum, M., . . . Mann, J. J. (2004). Instability of symptoms in recurrent major depression: A prospective study. *American Journal of Psychiatry, 161*(2), 255–261. doi:10.1176/appi.ajp.161.2.255

Oquendo, M. A., Currier, D., Liu, S. M., Hasin, D. S., Grant, B. F., & Blanco, C. (2010). Increased risk for suicidal behavior in comorbid bipolar disorder and alcohol use disorders: Results from the National Epidemiologic Survey on Alcohol and Related Conditions (NESARC). *Journal of Clinical Psychiatry, 71*(7), 902–909.

Oquendo, M. A., Perez-Rodriguez, M. M., Poh, E., Sullivan, G., Burke, A. K., Sublette, M. E., . . . Galfalvy, H. (2014). Life events: A complex role in the timing of suicidal behavior among depressed patients. *Molecular Psychiatry, 19*(8), 902–909. doi:10.1038/mp.2013.128

Orbach, I. (1996). The role of the body experience in self-destruction. *Clinical Child Psychology and Psychiatry, 1*(4), 607–619. doi:10.1177/1359104596014012

Orbach, I. (2003a). Suicide and the suicidal body. *Suicide and Life-Threatening Behavior, 33*(1), 1–8. doi:10.1521/suli.33.1.1.22786

Orbach, I. (2003b). Mental pain and suicide. *Israeli Journal of Psychiatry and Related Science, 40*(3), 191–201.

Ortega L. A., & Karch D. (2010). Precipitating circumstances of suicide among women of reproductive age in 16 U.S. states, 2003–2007. *Journal of Women's Health, 19*(1), 5–7. doi:10.1089/jwh.2009.1788

Orth, M., Handley, O. J., Schwenke, C., Dunnett, S. B., Craufurd, D., . . . Tabrizi, J. (2010). Observing Huntington's disease: The European Huntington's Disease Network's registry. *PLoS Currents, 2*, RRN1184. doi:10.1371/currents.RRN1184

Osterman, L. L., & Brown, R. P. (2011). Culture of honor and violence against the self. *Personality and Social Psychology Bulletin, 37*(12), 1611–1623. doi:10.1177/0146167211418529

Owens, D., Horrocks, J., & House, A. (2002). Fatal and non-fatal repetition of self-harm: Systematic review. *British Journal of Psychiatry, 181*, 193–199.

Ozturk, E., & Sar, V. (2008). Somatization as a predictor of suicidal ideation in dissociative disorders. *Psychiatry and Clinical Neuroscience, 62*(6), 662–668. doi:10.1111/j.1440-1819.2008.01865.x.

Pals, J. L. (2006). Narrative identity processing of difficult life experiences: Pathways of personality development and positive self-transformation in adulthood. *Journal of Personality, 74*(4), 1079–1110. doi:10.1111/j.1467-6494.2006.00403.x

Pan, Y., Stewart, R., & Chang, C. (2013). Socioeconomic disadvantage, mental disorders and risk of 12-month suicide ideation and attempt in the National Comorbidity Survey Replication (NCS-R) in US. *Social Psychiatry and Psychiatric Epidemiology, 48*(1), 71–79. doi:10.1007/s00127-012-0591-9

Parker, G. (1981). Parental reports of depressives. *Journal of Affective Disorders, 3*(2), 131–140. doi:10.1016/0165-0327(81)90038-0

Parker, G. (1989). The Parental Bonding Instrument: Psychometric properties reviewed. *Psychiatric Development, 7*(4), 317–335.

Parker, G., Tupling, H., & Brown, L. B. (1979). A parental bonding instrument. *British Journal of Medical Psychology, 52*, 1–10.

Patten, S. B. (2003). Recall bias and major depression lifetime prevalence. *Social Psychiatry and Psychiatric Epidemiology, 38*(6), 290–296.

Patterson, W. M., Dohn, H. H., Bird, J., & Patterson, G. A. (1983). Evaluation of suicidal patients: The SAD PERSONS scale. *Psychosomatics, 24*(4), 343–349. doi:10.1016/s0033-3182(83)73213-5

Paykel, E. S., Myers, J. K., Lindenthal, J. J., & Tanner, J. (1974). Suicidal feelings in the general population: A prevalence study. *British Journal of Psychiatry, 124*(5), 460–469. doi:10.1192/bjp.124.5.460

Penttinen, J. (1995). Back pain and risk of suicide among Finnish farmers. *American Journal of Public Health, 85*, 1452–1453.

Pettit, J. W., Temple, S. R., Norton, P. J., Yaroslavsky, I., Grover, K. E., Morgan, S. T., & Schatte, D. J. (2009). Thought suppression and suicidal ideation: Preliminary evidence in support of a robust association. *Depression and Anxiety, 26*(8), 758–763.

Philipsen, A., Schmahl, C., & Lieb, K. (2004). Naloxone in the treatment of acute dissociative states in female patients with borderline personality disorder. *Pharmacopsychiatry, 37*(5), 196–199.

Phillips, M. R., Yang, G., Zhang, Y., Wang, L., Ji, H., & Zhou, M. (2002). Risk factors for suicide in China: A national case–control psychological autopsy study. *Lancet, 360*(9347), 1728–1736. doi:10.1016/s0140-6736(02)11681-3

Pirkis, J., & Nordentoft, M. (2011). Media influences on suicide and attempted suicide. *International Handbook of Suicide Prevention: Research, Policy and Practice*, 531–544. doi:10.1002/9781119998556.ch30

Plunkett, A., O'Toole, B., Swanston, H., Oates, R. K., Shrimpton, S., & Parkinson, P. (2001). Suicide risk following child sexual abuse. *Ambulatory Pediatrics, 1*(5), 262–266.

Pokorny, A. D. (1983). Prediction of suicide in psychiatric patients. *Archives of General Psychiatry, 40*(3), 249. doi:10.1001/archpsyc.1983.01790030019002

Pollock, L. R., & Williams, J. M. G. (1998). Problem solving and suicidal behavior. *Suicide and Life-Threatening Behavior, 28,* 375–387.

Pollock, L. R., & Williams, J. M. G. (2001). Effective problem solving in suicide attempters depends on specific autobiographical recall. *Suicide and Life-Threatening Behavior, 31,* 386–396.

Pomerantsev, P. (2014). *Nothing is True and Everything is Possible: The Surreal Heart of the New Russia.* Santa Barbara, CA, United States: PublicAffairs, U.S.

Pompili, M., Innamorati, M., Szanto, K., Di Vittorio, C., Conwell, Y., Lester, D., . . . Amore, M. (2011). Life events as precipitants of suicide attempts among first-time suicide attempters, repeaters, and non-attempters. *Psychiatry Research, 186*(2-3), 300–305. doi:10.1016/j.psychres.2010.09.003

Pompili, M., Serafini, G., Innamorati, M., Lester, D., Shrivastava, A., Girardi, P., & Nordentoft, M. (2011). Suicide risk in first episode psychosis: A selective review of the current literature. *Schizophrenia Research, 129*(1), 1–11. doi:10.1016/j.schres.2011.03.008

Price, J. S., Sloman, L., Gardner, R., Jr., Gilbert, P., & Rohde, P. (1994). The social competition hypothesis of depression. *British Journal of Psychiatry, 164,* 309–315. doi:10.1192/bjp.164.3.309

Prigerson, H. G., Maciejewski, P. K., & Rosenheck, R. A. (1999). The effects of marital dissolution and marital quality on health and health service use among women. *Medical Care, 37*(9), 858–873. doi:10.1097/00005650-199909000-00003

Qin, P., Agerbo, E., & Mortensen, P. B. (2002). Suicide risk in relation to family history of completed suicide and psychiatric disorders: A nested case–control study based on longitudinal registers. *Lancet, 360*(9340), 1126–1130. doi:10.1016/s0140-6736(02)11197-4

Qin, P., Hawton, K., Mortensen, P. B., & Webb, R. (2014). Combined effects of physical illness and comorbid psychiatric disorder on risk of suicide in a national population study. *British Journal of Psychiatry, 204*(6), 430–435. doi:10.1192/bjp.bp.113.128785

Qin, P., Mortensen, P. B., & Pedersen, C. B. (2009). Frequent change of residence and risk of attempted and completed suicide among children and adolescents. *Archives of General Psychiatry, 66*(6), 628. doi:10.1001/archgenpsychiatry.2009.20

Qin, P., & Nordentoft, M. (2005). Suicide risk in relation to psychiatric hospitalization: Evidence based on longitudinal registers. *Archives of General Psychiatry, 62*(4), 427–432. doi:10.1001/archpsyc.62.4.427

Quan, H., Arboleda-Flórez, J., Fick, G. H., Stuart, H. L., & Love, E. J. (2002). Association between physical illness and suicide among the elderly. *Social Psychiatry and Psychiatric Epidemiology, 37*(4), 190–197. doi:10.1007/s001270200014

Rahe, R. H., & Arthur, R. J. (1978). Life change and illness studies: Past history and future directions. *Journal of Human Stress, 4*(1), 3–15. doi:10.1080/0097840x.1978.9934972

Randall, J. R., Walld, R., Chateau, D., Finlayson, G., Sareen, J., & Bolton, J. M. (2014). Risk of suicide and suicide attempts associated with physical disorders: A population-based, balancing score-matched analysis. *Psychological Medicine, 45*(3), 495–504. doi:10.1017/s0033291714001639

Rappaport, L. M., Moskowitz, D. S., Galynker, I., & Yaseen, Z. S. (2014). Panic symptom clusters differentially predict suicide ideation and attempt. *Comprehensive Psychiatry, 55*(4), 762–769.

Rasmussen, K. A., Slish, M. L., Wingate, L. R. R., Davidson, C. L., & Grant, D. M. M. (2012). Can perceived burdensomeness explain the relationship between suicide and perfectionism? *Suicide and Life-Threatening Behavior, 42*(2), 121–128. doi:10.1111/j.1943-278x.2011.00074.x

Reeves, A., McKee, M., & Stuckler, D. (2014). Economic suicides in the great recession in Europe and North America. *British Journal of Psychiatry, 205*(3), 246–247. doi:10.1192/bjp.bp.114.144766

Reger, M. A., Gahm, G. A., Kinn, J. T., Luxton, D. D., Skopp, N. A., & Bush, N. E. (2011). *Department of Defense Suicide Event Report (DoDSER) calendar year 2010 annual report.* Tacoma, WA: National Center for Telehealth and Technology.

Rehkopf, D. H., & Buka, S. L. (2006). The association between suicide and the socio-economic characteristics of geographical areas: A systematic review. *Psychological Medicine, 36*(2), 145. doi:10.1017/s003329170500588x

Rew, L., Thomas, N., Horner, S. D., Resnick, M. D., & Beuhring, T. (2001). Correlates of recent suicide attempts in a triethnic group of adolescents. *Journal of Nursing Scholarship, 33*(4), 361–367. doi:10.1111/j.1547-5069.2001.00361.x

Reyes, A. D., Henry, D. B., Tolan, P. H., & Wakschlag, L. S. (2009). Linking informant discrepancies to observed variations in young children's disruptive behavior. *Journal of Abnormal Child Psychology, 37*(5), 637–652. doi:10.1007/s10802-009-9307-3

Reyes, A. D., Thomas, S. A., Goodman, K. L., & Kundey, S. M. (2013). Principles underlying the use of multiple informants' reports. *Annual Review of Clinical Psychology, 9*(1), 123–149. doi:10.1146/annurev-clinpsy-050212-185617

Ribeiro, J. D., Bender, T. W., & Buchman, J. M. (2015). An investigation of the interactive effects of the capability for suicide and acute agitation on suicidality in a military sample. *Depression and Anxiety, 32*(1), 25–31. doi:10.1002/da.22240.

Ribeiro, J. D., Silva, C., & Joiner, T. E. (2014). Over arousal interacts with a sense of fearlessness about death to predict suicide risk in a sample of clinical outpatients. *Psychiatry Research, 218*(1-2), 106–112. doi:10.1016/j.psychres.2014.03.036

Rihmer, Z., & Akiskal, H. (2006). Do antidepressants t(h)reat(en) depressives? Toward a clinically judicious formulation of the antidepressant–suicidality FDA advisory in light of declining national suicide statistics from many countries. *Journal of Affective Disorders, 94*(1), 3–13.

Rogers, M. L., Ringer, F. B., & Joiner, T. E. (2016). A meta-analytic review of the association between agitation and suicide attempts. *Clinical Psychology Review, 48*, 1–6.

Roos, L., Sareen, J., & Bolton, J. M. (2013). Suicide risk assessment tools, predictive validity findings and utility today: Time for a revamp? *Neuropsychiatry, 3*(5), 483–495. doi:10.2217/npy.13.60

Rosenberg, H. J., Jankowski, M. K., Sengupta, A., Wolfe, R. S., Wolford, G. L., & Rosenberg, S. D. (2005). Single and multiple suicide attempts and associated health risk factors in New Hampshire adolescents. *Suicide and Life-Threatening Behavior, 35*(5), 547–557. doi:10.1521/suli.2005.35.5.547

Roth, R. (2009). *Suicide and euthanasia—A biblical perspective.* Retrieved from http://www.acu-cell.com/suicide.html

Routley, V. H., & Ozanne-Smith, J. E. (2012). Work-related suicide in Victoria, Australia: A broad perspective. *International Journal of Injury Control and Safety Promotion, 19*(2), 131–134. doi:10.1080/17457300.2011.635209

Rubanzana, W., Hedt-Gauthier, B. L., Ntaganira, J., & Freeman, M. D. (2014). Exposure to genocide and risk of suicide in Rwanda: A population-based case–control study. *Journal of Epidemiology and Community Health, 69*(2), 117–122. doi:10.1136/jech-2014-204307

Rudd, M. D. (2006). Fluid vulnerability theory: A cognitive approach to understanding the process of acute and chronic suicide risk. In T. E. Ellis (Ed.), *Cognition and suicide: Theory, research, and therapy* (pp. 355–368). Washington, DC: American Psychological Association.

Rudd, M. D., Berman, A. L., Joiner, T. E., Jr., Nock., M. K., Silverman, M. M., . . . Witte, T. (2006). Warning signs for suicide: Theory, research, and clinical application. *Suicide and Life Threatening Behavior, 36*(3), 255–262.

Rudd, M. D., Rajab, M. H., & Dahm, P. F. (1994). Problem-solving appraisal in suicide ideators and attempters. *American Journal of Orthopsychiatry, 64*(1), 136–149. doi:10.1037/h0079492

Runeson, B., Tidemalm, D., Dahlin, M., Lichtenstein, P., & Langstrom, N. (2010). Method of attempted suicide as predictor of subsequent successful suicide: National long term cohort study. *BMJ, 341,* c3222. doi:10.1136/bmj.c3222

Russell, S. T., & Joyner, K. (2001). Adolescent sexual orientation and suicide risk: Evidence from a national study. *American Journal of Public Health, 91*(8), 1276–1281. doi:10.2105/ajph.91.8.1276

Ryan, R. M., & Deci, E. L. (2000). Self-determination theory and the facilitation of intrinsic motivation, social development, and well-being. *American Psychologist, 55*(1), 68–78.

Rycroft, C. (1995). *Dictionary of psychoanalysis.* London, England: Penguin.

Sakinofsky, I. (2000). Repetition of suicidal behaviour. In K. Hawton & K. Van Heeringen (Eds.), *The international handbook of suicide and attempted suicide* (pp. 385–404). Chichester, England: Wiley.

Santa Mina, E. E., & Gallop, R. M. (1998). Childhood sexual and physical abuse and adult self-harm and suicidal behaviour: A literature review. *Canadian Journal of Psychiatry, 43,* 793–800.

Sati handprints. (2016). Retrieved from http://www.atlasobscura.com/places/sati-handprints

Schaffer, A., Sinyor, M., Kurdyak, P., Vigod, S., Sareen, J., Reis, C., . . . Cheung, A. (2016). Population-based analysis of health care contacts among suicide decedents: Identifying opportunities for more targeted suicide prevention strategies. *World Psychiatry, 15*(2), 135–145. doi:10.1002/wps.20321

Schechter, M., Goldblatt, M. J., Ronningstam, E., Herbstman, B., & Maltsberger, J. T. (2016). Post discharge suicide: A psychodynamic understanding of subjective experience and its importance in suicide prevention. *Bulletin of the Menninger Clinic, 80*(1), 80–96. doi:10.1521/bumc.2016.80.1.80

Schilling, E. A., Aseltine, R. H., Glanovsky, J. L., James, A., & Jacobs, D. (2009). Adolescent alcohol use, suicidal ideation, and suicide attempts. *Journal of Adolescent Health, 44*(4), 335–341. doi:10.1016/j.jadohealth.2008.08.006

Schneidman, E. S. (1998). *The suicidal mind.* New York, NY: Oxford University Press.

Schotte, D. E., & Clum, G. A. (1987). Problem-solving skills in suicidal psychiatric patients. *Journal of Consulting and Clinical Psychology, 55*(1), 49–54. doi:10.1037/0022-006x.55.1.49

Segal Z. V., Williams J. M. G., & Teasdale J. D. (2002). *Mindfulness-based cognitive therapy for depression: A new approach to preventing relapse.* New York, NY: Guilford.

Selby, E. A., Anestis, M. D., Bender, T. W., Ribeiro, J. D., Nock, M. K., Rudd, M. D., . . . Joiner, T. E., Jr. (2010). Overcoming the fear of lethal injury: Evaluating suicidal behavior in the military through the lens of the interpersonal–psychological theory of suicide. *Clinical Psychology Review, 30,* 298–307. doi:10.1016/j.cpr.2009.12.004

Serby, M. J., Brody, D., Amin, S., & Yanowitch, P. (2006). Eviction as a risk factor for suicide. *Psychiatric Services, 57*(2), 273–274. doi:10.1176/appi.ps.57.2.273-b

Shaffer, D., Gould, M., & Hicks, R. C. (1994). Worsening suicide rate in Black teenagers. *American Journal of Psychiatry, 151*(12), 1810–1812. doi:10.1176/ajp.151.12.1810

Shiratori, Y., Tachikawa, H., Nemoto, K., Endo, G., Aiba, M., Matsui, Y., & Asada, T. (2014). Network analysis for motives in suicide cases: A cross-sectional study. *Psychiatry and Clinical Neurosciences, 68*(4), 299–307. doi:10.1111/pcn.12132

Shneidman, E. (1993). Suicide as psychache. *Journal of Nervous and Mental Disease, 181*, 147–149.

Shpigel, M. S., & Diamond, G. M. (2012). Changes in parenting behaviors, attachment, depressive symptoms, and suicidal ideation in attachment-based family therapy for depressive and suicidal adolescents. *Journal of Marital and Family Therapy, 38*, 271–283. doi:10.1111/j.1752-0606.2012.00295.x

Siddaway, A. P., Taylor, P. J., Wood, A. M., & Schulz, J. (2015). A meta-analysis of perceptions of defeat and entrapment in depression, anxiety problems, posttraumatic stress disorder, and suicidality. *Journal of Affective Disorders, 184*, 149–159.

Simon, R. I. (2006). Imminent suicide: The illusion of short-term prediction. *Suicide and Life-Threatening Behavior, 36*(3), 296–301.

Simon, T. R., Swann, A. C., Powell, K. E., Potter, L. B., Kresnow, M. J., & O'Carroll, P. W. (2002). Characteristics of impulsive suicide attempts and attempters. *Suicide and Life-Threatening Behavior, 32*(Suppl. 1), 49–59.

Singhal, A., Ross, J., Seminog, O., Hawton, K., & Goldacre, M. J. (2014). Risk of self-harm and suicide in people with specific psychiatric and physical disorders: Comparisons between disorders using English national record linkage. *Journal of the Royal Society of Medicine, 107*(5), 194–204. doi:10.1177/0141076814522033

Smith, E. G., Kim, H. M., Ganoczy, D., Stano, C., Pfeiffer, P. N., & Valenstein, M. (2013). Suicide risk assessment received prior to suicide death by Veterans Health Administration patients with a history of depression. *Journal of Clinical Psychiatry, 74*(03), 226–232. doi:10.4088/jcp.12m07853

Smith, J. C., Mercy, J. A., & Conn, J. M. (1988). Marital status and the risk of suicide. *American Journal of Public Health, 78*(1), 78–80. doi:10.2105/ajph.78.1.78

Snowden, M., Steinman, L., Frederick, J., & Wilson, N. (2009). Screening for depression in older adults: Recommended instruments and considerations for community-based practice. *Clinical Geriatrics, 17*(9), 26–32.

Solomon, R. L., & Corbit, J. D. (1974). An opponent-process theory of motivation: Temporal dynamics of affect. *Psychological Review, 81*(2), 119–145. doi:10.1037/h0036128

Soole, R., Kõlves, K., & De Leo, D. (2014). Factors related to childhood suicides: Analysis of the Queensland Child Death Register. *Crisis, 35*, 292–300.

Spada, M. M., Caselli, G., Manfredi, C., Rebecchi, D., Rovetto, F., Ruggiero, G. M., . . . Sassaroli, S. (2011). Parental overprotection and metacognitions as predictors of worry and anxiety. *Behavioural and Cognitive Psychotherapy, 40*(3), 287–296. doi:10.1017/s135246581100021x

Spiegel, B., Schoenfeld, P., & Naliboff, B. (2007). Systematic review: The prevalence of suicidal behaviour in patients with chronic abdominal pain and irritable bowel syndrome. *Alimentary Pharmacology & Therapeutics, 26*(2), 183–193. doi:10.1111/j.1365-2036.2007.03357.x

Stack, S., & Wasserman, I. (1993). Marital status, alcohol consumption, and suicide: An analysis of national data. *Journal of Marriage and the Family, 55*(4), 1018–1024. doi:10.2307/352781

Stanley, B., Brown, G., Brent, D. A., Wells, K., Poling, K., Curry, J., . . . Hughes, J. (2009). Cognitive–behavioral therapy for suicide prevention (CBT-SP): Treatment model, feasibility, and acceptability. *Journal of the American Academy of Child & Adolescent Psychiatry, 48*(10), 1005–1013. doi:10.1097/chi.0b013e3181b5dbfe

Stark, C., Riordan, V., & O'Connor, R. (2011). A conceptual model of suicide in rural areas. *Rural Remote Health, 11*(2), 1622.

Stepp, S. D., Morse, J. Q., Yaggi, K. E., Reynolds, S. K., Reed, L. I., & Pilkonis, P. A. (2008). The role of attachment styles and interpersonal problems in suicide-related behaviors. *Suicide and Life-Threatening Behavior, 38*(5), 592–607. doi:10.1521/suli.2008.38.5.592

Stone, A. A., Schwartz, J. E., Broderick, J. E., & Deaton, A. (2010). A snapshot of the age distribution of psychological well-being in the United States. *Proceedings of the National Academy of Sciences, 107*(22), 9985–9990. doi:10.1073/pnas.1003744107

Stop bullying. (2016). Retrieved from http://www.stopbullying.gov

Sublette, M. E., Carballo, J. J., Moreno, C., Galfalvy, H. C., Brent, D. A., Birmaher, B., . . . Oquendo, M. A. (2009). Substance use disorders and suicide attempts in bipolar subtypes. *Journal of Psychiatric Research, 43*(3), 230–238.

Sue, D., Sue, D., Sue, S., & Sue, D. (2013). *Cengage advantage books: Essentials of understanding abnormal behavior.* Belmont, CA: Wadsworth.

Surrence, K., Miranda, R., Marroquín, B. M., & Chan, S. (2009). Brooding and reflective rumination among suicide attempters: Cognitive vulnerability to suicidal ideation. *Behaviour Research and Therapy, 47*, 803–808.

Sy, T., Côté, S., & Saavedra, R. (2005). The contagious leader: Impact of the leader's mood on the mood of group members, group affective tone, and group processes. *Journal of Applied Psychology, 90*(2), 295–305. doi:10.1037/0021-9010.90.2.295

Takeshima, M., & Oka, T. (2013). A comprehensive analysis of features that suggest bipolarity in patients with a major depressive episode: Which is the best combination to predict soft bipolarity diagnosis? *Journal of Affective Disorders, 147*, 150–155.

Tanaka, E., Sakamoto, S., Ono, Y., Fujihara, S., & Kitamura, T. (1998). Hopelessness in a community population: Factorial structure and psychosocial correlates. *Journal of Social Psychology, 138*(5), 581–590. doi:10.1080/00224549809600413

Tang, N. K., & Crane, C. (2006). Suicidality in chronic pain: A review of the prevalence, risk factors and psychological links. *Psychological Medicine, 36*(5), 575. doi:10.1017/s0033291705006859

Tanriverdi, D., Cuhadar, D., & Ciftci, S. (2014). Does the impairment of functional life increase the probability of suicide in cancer patients? *Asian Pacific Journal of Cancer Prevention, 15*(21), 9549–9553. doi:10.7314/apjcp.2014.15.21.9549

Tavernise, S. (2016, April 22). U.S. suicide rate surges to a 30-year high. *The New York Times.* Retrieved from http://www.nytimes.com/2016/04/22/health/us-suicide-rate-surges-to-a-30-year-high.html?_r=0

Taylor, P. J., Gooding, P., Wood, A. M., & Tarrier, N. (2011). The role of defeat and entrapment in depression, anxiety and suicide. *Psychological Bulletin, 137*(3), 391–420. doi:10.1037/a0022935

Taylor, P. J., Wood, A. M., Gooding, P. A., Johnson, J., & Tarrier, N. (2009). Are defeat and entrapment best defined as a single construct? *Personality and Individual Differences, 47*, 795–797. doi:10.1016/j.paid.2009.06.011

Terra, M. B., Figueira, I., & Barros, H. M. T. (2004). Impact of alcohol intoxication and withdrawal syndrome on social phobia and panic disorder in alcoholic inpatients. *Revista do Hospital das Clínicas, 59*(4), 187–192.

Thibodeau, M. A., Welch, P. G., Sareen, J., & Asmundson, G. J. (2013). Anxiety disorders are independently associated with suicide ideation and attempts: Propensity score matching in two epidemiological samples. *Depression and Anxiety, 30*(10), 947–954. doi:10.1002/da.22203

Thomas, K., Jiang, Y., & McCombs, J. (2015). Clozapine revisited: Impact of clozapine vs. olanzapine on health care use by schizophrenia patients on Medicaid. *Annals of Clinical Psychiatry, 27*, 90–99.

Thompson, A. H., Dewa, C. S., & Phare, S. (2012). The suicidal process: Age of onset and severity of suicidal behavior. *Social Psychiatry and Psychiatry Epidemiology, 47*(8), 1263–1269. doi:10.1007/s00127-011-0434-0

Thompson, R., Proctor, L. J., English, D. J., Dubowitz, H., Narasimhan, S., & Everson, M. D. (2012). Suicidal ideation in adolescence: Examining the role of recent adverse experiences. *Journal of Adolescence, 35*(1), 175–186. doi:10.1016/j.adolescence.2011.03.003

Tondo, L., Hennen, J., & Baldessarini, R. J. (2001). Lower suicide risk with long-term lithium treatment in major affective illness: A meta-analysis. *Acta Psychiatrica Scandinavica, 104*(3), 163–172. doi:10.1034/j.1600-0447.2001.00464.x

Townsend, E. (2007). Suicide terrorists: Are they suicidal? *Suicide and Life-Threatening Behavior, 37*(1), 35–49. doi:10.1521/suli.2007.37.1.35

Treadway, M. T., & Zald, D. H. (2011). Reconsidering anhedonia in depression: Lessons from translational neuroscience. *Neuroscience and Biobehavioral Reviews, 35*(3), 537–555.

Troister, T., & Holden, R. R. (2010). Comparing psychache, depression, and hopelessness in their associations with suicidality: A test of Shneidman's theory of suicide. *Personality and Individual Differences, 49*, 689–693. doi:10.1016/j.paid.2010.06.006

Troister, T., & Holden, R. R. (2012). A two-year prospective study of psychache and its relationship to suicidality among high-risk undergraduates. *Journal of Clinical Psychology, 68*(9), 1019–1027. doi:10.1002/jclp.21869

Tsai, A. C., Lucas, M., & Kawachi, I. (2015). Association between social integration and suicide among women in the United States. *Journal of the American Medical Association Psychiatry, 72*(10), 987–993.

Tucker, R. P., O'Connor, R. C., & Wingate, L. R. (2016). An investigation of the relationship between rumination styles, hope, and suicide ideation through the lens of the integrated motivational–volitional model of suicidal behavior. *Archives in Suicide Research, 20*(4), 553–566. doi:10.1080/13811118.2016.1158682

Tugade, M. M., Fredrickson, B. L., & Barrett, L. F. (2004). Psychological resilience and positive emotional granularity: Examining the benefits of positive emotions on coping and health. *Journal of Personality, 72*(6), 1161–1190. doi:10.1111/j.1467-6494.2004.00294.x

US Food and Drug Administration. (2007). *FDA proposes new warnings about suicidal thinking, behavior in young adults who take antidepressant medications* [Press release]. Retrieved from http://www.fda.gov/NewsEvents/Newsroom/PressAnnouncements/2007/ucm108905.htm

US Public Health Service. (1999). *The Surgeon General's call to action to prevent suicide.* Washington, DC: Author.

Valtonen, H. M., Suominen, K., & Haukka, J. (2008). Differences in incidence of suicide attempts during phases of bipolar I and II disorders. *Bipolar Disorders, 10*, 588–596.

Valtonen, H. M., Suominen, J., Sokero, P., Mantere, O., Arvilommi, P., . . . Isomesta, E. T. (2009). How suicidal bipolar patients are depends on how suicidal ideation is defined. *Journal of Affective Disorders, 118*(1-3), 48–54. doi:10.1016/j.jad.2009.02.008

Van der Does, W. (2005). Thought suppression and cognitive vulnerability to depression. *British Journal of Clinical Psychology, 44*(1), 1–14.

Van Geel, M., Vedder, P., & Tanilon, J. (2014). Relationship between peer victimization, cyberbullying, and suicide in children and adolescents. *Journal of the American Medical Association Pediatrics, 168*(5), 435. doi:10.1001/jamapediatrics.2013.4143

Van Orden, K. A., Witte, T. K., James, L. M., Castro, Y., Gordon, K. H., Braithwaite, S. R., . . . Joiner, T. E. (2008). Suicidal ideation in college students varies across semesters: The mediating role of belongingness. *Suicide and Life-Threatening Behavior, 38*(4), 427–435. doi:10.1521/suli.2008.38.4.427

Van Os, J., & Kapur, S. (2009). Schizophrenia. *Lancet, 374*(9690), 635–645.

Van Wagoner, S. L., Gelso, C. J., Hayes, J. A., & Diemer, R. A. (1991). Countertransference and the reputedly excellent therapist. *Psychotherapy: Theory, Research, Practice, Training, 28*(3), 411–421. doi:10.1037/0033-3204.28.3.411

Varghese, F., & Kelly, B. (1999). Countertransference and assisted suicide. In G. Gabbard (Ed.), *Countertransference issues in psychiatric treatment* (pp. 85–116). Washington DC: American Psychiatric Press.

Värnik, P. (2012). Suicide in the world. *International Journal of Environmental Research and Public Health, 9*(3), 760–771. doi:10.3390/ijerph9030760

Veilleux, J. C. (2011). Coping with client death: Using a case study to discuss the effects of accidental, undetermined, and suicidal deaths on therapists. *Professional Psychology: Research and Practice, 42*(3), 222–228. doi:10.1037/a0023650

Viguera, A. C., Baldessarini, R. J., Hegarty, J. D., van Kammen, D. P., & Tohen, M. (1997). Clinical risk following abrupt and gradual withdrawal of maintenance neuroleptic treatment. *Archives of General Psychiatry, 54*(1), 49–55.

Virtual hope box. (n.d.). Retrieved from http://t2health.dcoe.mil/apps/virtual-hope-box

Vishnuvardhan, G., & Saddichha, S. (2012). Psychiatric comorbidity and gender differences among suicide attempters in Bangalore, India. *General Hospital Psychiatry, 34*(4), 410–414. doi:10.1016/j.genhosppsych.2012.03.017

Vita, A., De Peri, L., & Sacchetti, E. (2011). Antipsychotics, antidepressants, anticonvulsants, and placebo on the symptom dimensions of borderline personality disorder: A meta-analysis of randomized controlled and open-label trials. *Journal of Clinical Psychopharmacology, 31*(5), 613–624.

Voshaar, R. C. O., Couvée, J. E., Van Balkom, A. J., Mulder, P. G., & Zitman, F. G. (2006). Strategies for discontinuing long-term benzodiazepine use. *British Journal of Psychiatry, 189*(3), 213–220.

Waldrop, A. E., Hanson, R. F., Resnick, H. S., Kilpatrick, D. G., Naugle, A. E., & Saunders, B. E. (2007). Risk factors for suicidal behaviors among a national sample of adolescents: Implications for prevention. *Journal of Traumatic Stress, 20*(5), 869–879. doi:10.1002/jts.20291

Walsh, S. L., Stoops, W. W., Moody, D. E., Lin, S. N., & Bigelow, G. E. (2009). Repeated dosing with oral cocaine in humans: Assessment of direct effects, withdrawal, and pharmacokinetics. *Experimental and Clinical Psychopharmacology, 17*(4), 205–216. doi:10.1037/a0016469

Wang, S., Fuh, J., Juang, K., & Lu, S. (2009). Migraine and suicidal ideation in adolescents aged 13 to 15 years. *Neurology, 72*(13), 1146–1152. doi:10.1212/01.wnl.0000345362.91734.b3

Wang, Y., Bhaskaran, J., Sareen, J., Wang, J., Spiwak, R., & Bolton, J. (2015). Predictors of Future Suicide Attempts Among Individuals Referred to Psychiatric Services in the Emergency Department. *The Journal Of Nervous And Mental Disease, 203*(7), 507-513. http://dx.doi.org/10.1097/nmd.0000000000000320

Warburton, K., & Lazarus, J. (1991). Tendency-distance models of social cohesion in animal groups. *Journal of Theoretical Biology, 150*(4), 473–488. doi:10.1016/s0022-5193(05)80441-2

Warner, C. H., Bobo, W., Warner, C., Reid, S., & Rachal, J. (2006). Antidepressant discontinuation syndrome. *American Family Physician, 74*(3), 449–456.

Watkins, E. R. (2008). Constructive and unconstructive repetitive thought. *Psychological Bulletin, 134*, 163–206.

Wegner, D. M. (1989). *White bears and other unwanted thoughts: Suppression, obsession, and the psychology of mental control.* New York, NY: Viking/Penguin.

Wegner, D. M., Schneider, D. J., Carter, S. R., & White, T. L. (1987). Paradoxical effects of thought suppression. *Journal of Personality and Social Psychology, 53*(1), 5–13.

Wegner, D. M., & Zanakos, S. (1994). Chronic thought suppression. *Journal of Personality, 62*(4), 616–640.

Weissman, M. M., Klerman, G. L., Markowitz, J. S., & Ouellette, R. (1989). Suicidal ideation and suicide attempts in panic disorder and attacks. *New England Journal of Medicine, 321*(18), 1209–1214. doi:10.1056/nejm198911023211801

Weng, S. C., Chang, J. C., Yeh, M. K., Wang, S. M., & Chen, Y. H. (2016). Factors influencing attempted and completed suicide in postnatal women: A population-based study in Taiwan. *Scientific Reports, 6*, 25770. doi:10.1038/srep25770

Wenzel, A., & Beck, A. T. (2008). A cognitive model of suicidal behavior: Theory and treatment. *Applied and Preventive Psychology, 12*, 189–201.

Williams, J. M. G. (1997). *Cry of pain: Understanding suicide and self-harm.* Harmondsworth, England: Penguin.

Williams, J. M. G., Barnhofer, T., Crane, C., & Beck, A. T. (2005). Problem solving deteriorates following mood challenge in formerly depressed patients with a history of suicidal ideation. *Journal of Abnormal Psychology, 114*, 421–431.

Williams, J. M. G., Barnhofer, T., Crane, C., Herman, D., Raes, F., Watkins, E., & Dalgleish, T. (2007). Autobiographical memory specificity and emotional disorder. *Psychological Bulletin, 133*(1), 122–148. doi:10.1037/0033-2909.133.1.122

Williams, J. M. G., & Pollock, L. R. (2001). Psychological aspects of the suicidal process. In K. van Heeringen (Ed.), *Understanding suicidal behaviour.* Chichester, England: Wiley.

Windfuhr, K., & Kapur, N. (2011). Suicide and mental illness: A clinical review of 15 years findings from the UK National Confidential Inquiry into Suicide. *British Medical Bulletin, 100*(1), 101–121. doi:10.1093/bmb/ldr042

Wise, R. A. (1980). The dopamine synapse and the notion of "pleasure centers" in the brain. *Trends in Neuroscience, 3*, 91–95.

Witte, T. K., Gordon, K. H., Smith, P. N., & Van Orden, K. A. (2012). Stoicism and sensation seeking: Male vulnerabilities for the acquired capability for suicide. *Journal of Research in Personality, 46*(4), 384–392. doi:10.1016/j.jrp.2012.03.004

Witte, T. K., Merrill, K. A., Stellrecht, N. E., Bernert, R. A., Hollar, D. L., Schatschneider, C., & Joiner, T. E., Jr. (2008). "Impulsive" youth suicide attempters are not necessarily all that impulsive. *Journal of Affective Disorders, 107*, 107–116.

Woike, B., & Polo, M. (2001). Motive-related memories: content, structure, and affect. *Journal of Personality, 69*(3), 391–415. doi:10.1111/1467-6494.00150

Wojnar, M., Ilgen, M. A., Jakubczyk, A., Wnorowska, A., Klimkiewicz, A., & Brower, K. J. (2008). Impulsive suicide attempts predict post-treatment relapse in alcohol-dependent patients. *Drug and Alcohol Dependence, 97*(3), 268–275.

Wong, M. M., Brower, K. J., & Craun, E. A. (2016). Insomnia symptoms and suicidality in the National Comorbidity Survey—Adolescent supplement. *Journal of Psychiatric Research*, *81*, 1–8. doi:10.1016/j.jpsychires.2016.06.004

Woznica, J. G., & Shapiro, J. R. (1990). An analysis of adolescent suicide attempts: The expendable child. *Journal of Pediatric Psychology*, *15*, 789–796. doi:10.1093/jpepsy/15.6.789

Wrosch, C., Scheier, M. F., Miller, G. E., Schulz, R., & Carver, C. S. (2003). Adaptive self-regulation of unattainable goals: Goal disengagement, goal Reengagement, and subjective well-being. *Personality and Social Psychology Bulletin*, *29*(12), 1494–1508. doi:10.1177/0146167203256921

Wyder, M., Ward, P., & De Leo, D. (2009). Separation as a suicide risk factor. *Journal of Affective Disorders*, *116*(3), 208–213. doi:10.1016/j.jad.2008.11.007

Yamaguchi, T., Fujii, C., Nemoto, T., Tsujino, N., Takeshi, K., & Mizuno, M. (2015). Differences between subjective experiences and observed behaviors in near-fatal suicide attempters with untreated schizophrenia: A qualitative pilot study. *Annals of General Psychiatry*, *14*(17). doi:10.1186/s12991-015-0055-1x

Yaseen, Z. S., Briggs, J., Kopeykina, I., Orchard, K. M., Silberlicht, J., Bhingradia, H., . . . Gaylnker, I. I. (2013). Distinctive emotional responses of clinicians to suicide-attempting patients: A comparative study. *BMC Psychiatry*, *13*, 230. doi:10.1186/1471-244x-13-230

Yaseen, Z. S., Chartrand, H., Mojtabai, R., Bolton, J., & Galynker, I. I. (2013). Fear of dying in panic attacks predicts suicide attempt in comorbid depressive illness: Prospective evidence from the National Epidemiological Survey on Alcohol and Related Conditions. *Depression and Anxiety*, *30*(10), 930–939. doi:10.1002/da.22039

Yaseen, Z. S., Fisher, K., Morales, E., & Galynker, I. I. (2012). Love and suicide: The structure of the Affective Intensity Rating Scale (AIRS) and its relation to suicidal behavior. *PLoS One*, *7*(8), e0044069. doi:10.1371/journal.pone.0044069

Yaseen, Z. S., Galynker, I. I., Briggs, J., Freed, R. D., & Gabbay, V. (2016). Functional domains as correlates of suicidality among psychiatric inpatients. *Journal of Affective Disorders*, *203*, 7–83. doi:10.1016/j.jad.2016.05.066.

Yaseen, Z. S., Galynker, I. I., Cohen, L. J., & Briggs, J. (2016). Clinicians' conflicting emotional responses to high-risk suicidal patients predict short-term suicidal behavior: A prospective analysis. Submitted for publication.

Yaseen, Z. S., Gilmer, E., Modi, J., Cohen, L. J., & Galynker, I. I. (2012). Emergency room validation of the revised Suicide Trigger Scale (STS-3): A measure of a hypothesized suicide trigger state. *PLoS One*, *7*(9), e45157. doi:10.1371/journal.pone.0045157

Yaseen, Z., Katz, C., Johnson, M. S., Eisenberg, D., Cohen, L. J., & Galynker, I. I. (2010). Construct development: The suicide trigger scale (STS-2), a measure of a hypothesized suicide trigger state. *BMC Psychiatry*, *10*(1). doi:10.1186/1471-244x-10-110

Yaseen, Z. S., Kopeykina, I., Gutkovich, Z., Bassirnia, A., Cohen, L. J., & Galynker, I. I. (2014). Predictive validity of the Suicide Trigger Scale (STS-3) for post-discharge suicide attempt in high-risk psychiatric inpatients. *PLoS One*, *9*(1), e86768. doi:10.1371/journal.pone.0086768

Yaseen, Z., Galynker, I., Cohen, L., & Briggs, J. (in press). Clinicians' conflicting emotional responses to high suicide-risk patients—association with short-term suicide behaviors: A prospective pilot study. *Comprehensive Psychiatry*.

Ying, Y., & Chang, K. (2009). A study of suicide and socioeconomic factors. *Suicide and Life-Threatening Behavior*, *39*(2), 214–226. doi:10.1521/suli.2009.39.2.214

Zanarini, M. C., Frankenburg, M. D., Wedig, M. M., & Fitzmaurice, G. M. (2013). Cognitive experiences reported by patients with borderline personality disorder and Axis II comparison subjects: A 16-year prospective follow-up study. *American Journal of Psychiatry, 170*(6), 671–679.

Zayas, L. H., Bright, C. L., Álvarez-Sánchez, T., & Cabassa, L. J. (2009). Acculturation, familism and mother–daughter relations among suicidal and non-suicidal adolescent Latinas. *Journal of Primary Prevention, 30*(3-4), 351–369. doi:10.1007/s10935-009-0181-0

Zero suicide. (2015). Retrieved from http://www.zerosuicide.sprc.org

Zhang, J., & Lester, D. (2008). Psychological tensions found in suicide notes: A test for the strain theory of suicide. *Archives of Suicide Research, 12*(1), 67–73.

Zhang, J., Li, N., Tu, X., Xiao, S., & Jia, C. (2011). Risk factors for rural young suicide in China: A case–control study. *Journal of Affective Disorders, 129*(1-3), 244–251. doi:10.1016/j.jad.2010.09.008

Zhang, J., & Ma, Z. (2012). Patterns of life events preceding the suicide in rural young Chinese: A case–control study. *Journal of Affective Disorders, 140*(2), 161–167. doi:10.1016/j.jad.2012.01.010.

Zhang, J., & Xu, H. (2007). The effects of religion, superstition, and perceived gender inequality on the degree of suicide intent: A study of serious attempters in China. *OMEGA, 55*(3), 185–197.

Zisook, S., Trivedi, M. H., Warden, D., Lebowitz, B., Thase, M. E., Stewart, J. W., . . . Rush, A. J. (2009). Clinical correlates of the worsening or emergence of suicidal ideation during SSRI treatment of depression: An examination of citalopram in the STAR*D study. *Journal of Affective Disorders, 117*(1), 63–73.

Index

Note: Page numbers followed by *f* and *t* indicate figures and tables, respectively.

age, 62, 221
  goal losses with, 106
  and history of suicide attempts, 40
  and suicide risk, 29, 36–37
aggression, 22
  in activation syndrome, 88
  alcohol-related, 91–92
  impulsive, 19, 21, 27, 28
  turned inward, suicide as, 11
agitation, 13, 170–172
  in activation syndrome, 88, 156
  assessment of, 170, 176, 181,
    187, 192, 227
    test case, 198–199
  case examples, 171–172, 181, 187, 192
  definition of, 170
  in depressive turmoil, 155
  drug initiation/withdrawal and, 88
  and frantic anxiety, overlap of, 171
  and short-term suicide risk, 3, 170
  and suicidality, 170
  in suicide crisis syndrome, 144, 170–172
agoraphobia, 148
akathisia, 170
  in activation syndrome, 88
  antipsychotic-related, 87
Alaska, 37, 222
Alaskan Natives, 37
  alcohol use by, 92
alcohol
  abuse, 141
    and short-term suicide risk, 2t
  addiction, emotional pain and anhedonia
    in, 159
  dependence, 38
  to facilitate suicide, 91–92
  intoxication, 91–93, 224
  withdrawal, 93–94, 224
alcohol use disorder, 39, 165, 222, 224
  case example, 92–93, 94–95
  comorbidity with, and suicidality, 91
  severity subclassifications, 91
  and suicidality, 90–91, 92–93
alexithymia, 101
alienation
  case examples, 117–118
  and suicidality, 96–97, 113–114
allosteric shift, 159

alternative uses test, 17
American Association of Suicidology, ten
    suicide warning signs, 142
American Indians, 37
  alcohol use by, 92
anesthetic agents, 261
anger
  clinician's, toward patient, 204–206
  in depressive turmoil, 155
anguish
  clinician's, about patient's suicide, 220
  and suicidality, 110
anguished turmoil, 155
anhedonia, 6, 141, 143
  acute, 154–155, 159–160, 164
    assessment of, 175, 179–180, 185–186,
      191, 227
    case examples, 161–162, 163–164,
      179–180, 185–186, 191
    test case, 197
  cocaine withdrawal and, 94
  consummatory, 159, 162
  definition of, 159
  drug/alcohol withdrawal and, 93
  motivational, 159, 162
  neurophysiology of, 159
  and short-term suicide risk, 2t, 3
  in suicide crisis syndrome, 144, 154–155,
    159–160
  as transdiagnostic syndrome, 159
antidepressants. See also activation
    syndrome
  adverse effects and side
    effects of, 87, 170
  depressive mixed state induced by, 88
  discontinuation of, 88–89, 224
  initiation of, suicide danger zone
    with, 87–88
antipsychotic(s), 167
  adverse effects and side effects of, 87, 170
  atypical, 260
  discontinuation of, 88, 224
antisocial personality disorder, 39, 94–95
anxiety, 6, 13, 143–144, 154–155. See also
    depressive turmoil
  in activation syndrome, 88
  alcohol-related, 92
  antidepressant discontinuation and, 89

clinician's
    about patient, 204–206
    elicited by suicidal patient, 202
cocaine withdrawal and, 94
drug/alcohol withdrawal and, 93
entrapment and, 150
frantic (extreme). *See* frantic anxiety
opiate withdrawal and, 94
as predictor of suicidal behavior, 157
psychic, 141
and short-term suicide risk, 2*t*, 3, 141
situational, 156
SSRI-related, 87
state, 28
suicidal, 156
and suicidality, 110
in suicide crisis syndrome, 144, 156–157
anxiety disorders
    parental overcontrol and, 41
    recent diagnosis, and suicidality, 78
    and suicide risk, 38–39
app-based interventions, 264–265
Arab countries, 36
arousal, disturbance in
    assessment of, 227
    in suicide crisis syndrome, 143–144,
        170–172
arrested flight model. *See* cry of pain/
    arrested flight model (Williams)
arthritis, 76
Asia
    pesticide ingestion in, 84
    rates of suicide attempts in, 83
    rural, rates of suicide attempts in, 83
Asian Americans, alcohol use by, 92
Asian families
    cultural attitudes in, 45
    parent–child conflict and, 67
Asian immigrants, suicidality in, 83–84
    case example, 83–84
Asians/Pacific Islanders, 37
asphyxiation, 48, 84
assessment. *See also* trait vulnerability,
        assessment
    comprehensive, 9, 122
        outline for, 221–228, 235, 236
    of imminent suicide risk, 4–5
    multimodal, 5–6

one-informant *vs.* multi-informant, 6–7
of suicide crisis syndrome, 172–176
assessment instruments, 230–235. *See also*
    specific instrument
    shortcomings of, 3–4, 4*t*
asthma, 76
attachment-based family therapy, 263
attachment style, 42–43, 222
    dismissing, 42–43
    fearful, 42–43
    preoccupied, 42–43
    secure, 42–43
attachment theory (Bowlby), 42
attention, biases, in suicidal
        individuals, 16–17
attentional fixation, 20–21
attention-deficit/hyperactivity disorder, 69
attitudes toward suicide, interview questions
        about, 49
AUA. *See* acute use of alcohol
AUD. *See* alcohol use disorder
automatic thoughts, negative, 14–15
autonomic–limbic arousal, 14*f*, 15
aversion, in countertransference hate,
        208–209
avoidant-dependent personality disorder, 39

back pain, chronic, and suicidality, 77, 224
barbiturates
    abuse, 94
    withdrawal symptoms, 94
        case example, 94–95
Baumeister, escape theory of suicide, 12–13, 143
BDI. *See* Beck Depression Inventory
Beck Depression Inventory, 3, 4*t*, 145, 230
Beck Hopelessness Scale, 3, 4*t*, 230
Beck Suicide Intent Scale, 3, 4*t*
belongingness. *See also* thwarted
        belongingness
    assessment of, 125
benzodiazepines
    discontinuation of, 88
    withdrawal, 88–89
betrayal, romantic, *case example,* 85
BHS. *See* Beck Hopelessness Scale
binge drinking, and suicide risk in
        children, 69
biological therapeutics, 260–261

patients' sensitivity to, 220
as predictor of patient suicide, 202,
206, 213
and therapeutic outcome, 201–202
emotions "forbidden" to, 204. *See also*
countertransference
feelings about patient's suicide, 220
guilty response to suicidal patient,
diagnostic value of, 215
as independent informants, 7
language used by, in interview, 122
objective assessment *vs.* subjective
opinion of patient, 7
overinvolvement with patient, 205,
209, 213
patient's testing of, 205, 208–209
use of psychiatric terminology, 122
clonidine, for opiate withdrawal-related
anxiety, 94
clozapine, 260
cocaine withdrawal, 94
cognitive-behavioral therapy for suicidal
patients, 21, 262
phases of, 21
cognitive control, loss of, 154
assessment of, 167–170, 173, 175–176,
180–181, 186–187, 191–192, 227
test case, 197–198
case examples, 167–170, 180–181,
186–187, 191–192
in suicide crisis syndrome, 143–144
symptoms of, 164
cognitive distortion, and
self-destructiveness, 13
cognitive disturbances
alcohol-related, 92
drug initiation/withdrawal and, 88
cognitive rigidity
assessment of, 166, 175, 180–181, 186,
192, 227
test case, 198
case examples, 168, 169, 180–181,
186, 192
characteristics of, 165–166
of stress–diathesis model, 17
and suicidality, 16, 17, 19, 26, 164,
165–166, 168
in suicide crisis syndrome, 144

cognitive style, maladaptive, 5, 19–20, 26,
30, 43. *See also* perfectionism
cognitive vulnerability model
(Schotte & Clum), 17, 26
Collaborative Assessment and Management
of Suicidality, 262–263
college student suicide, 98
completed suicide
methods, 48
psychiatric diagnoses and, 141
comprehensive narrative-crisis model. *See*
narrative-crisis model of suicide
comprehensive short-term risk assessment
interview, 235–237, 237f
case example, 237–246
concentration, diminished, 141
confidentiality, app-based interventions
and, 265
congenital heart disease, 76
consent, in multi-informant
assessment, 6–7
COPD. *See* chronic obstructive pulmonary
disease
coping strategies, 264
countertransference. *See also* clinician(s),
emotional response to suicidal patients
definition of, 208
mixed, assessment of, 215
negative, 202
countertransference hate, 202, 208–209,
213–215, 228, 245–246. *See also* denial;
reaction formation
and clinician's denial, 211–212
countertransference love, 207–208,
213–215
case example, 207–208
and clinician's denial, 211–212
crisis-driven suicide, 33, 256
Croatia, 92
cry of pain/arrested flight model (Williams),
12, 15–17, 16f, 24, 26, 149–150
cults, 46
cultural acceptability, of suicide, 44–48, 110,
222–223
assessment
in expanded MARIS interview, 252
in MARIS interview, 248
cultural attitudes, 44–45, 222

culture
  interview questions about, 49
  and maternal affectionless control, 41
cutting, 48, 84

day of the week, and post-discharge
    suicide, 79
DBT. *See* dialectical behavior therapy
"death by distress," 157, 162
death wish, 11
defeat, 26, 31, 97, 122, 150. *See also* personal
    defeat; social defeat
  attentional bias to, 16
  and depression, 150–151
  and entrapment, overlap of, 119, 150–151
  humiliating personal or social (phase 4 of
      suicidal narrative), 109–112, 225
    assessment of, 123–124, 125
    case examples, 111–112
defense mechanisms, used by clinicians
  case examples, 215–219
  clinician's self-assessment of, 213–215
  against "forbidden" emotions, 204,
      209–213, 214–215
delirium, agitated, 170
dementia, 76
denial
  as defense, 211
  used by clinicians, 245–246
    case example, 217–218
    clinician's own assessment of, 214–215
    against "forbidden" emotions, 204,
        211–212, 213, 228
depression, 5, 43, 86, 143–144. *See also*
    depressive turmoil
  alcohol-related, 92
  and alcohol use disorder, 91
  as anger turned inward, 210
  antidepressant discontinuation and, 89
  cannabis withdrawal and, 94
  cocaine withdrawal and, 94
  and comorbid medical illness, 75
  defeat and, 150–151
  drug/alcohol withdrawal and, 93
  entrapment and, 150–151
  in honor states, 46
  and hypersensitivity to defeat, 16
  improvement, and suicide, 39

  and long-term suicide risk, 3
  and panic attacks, 157–159
  parental overcontrol and, 42
  and post-discharge suicide, 79
  and psychache, 12
  recent diagnosis, and suicidality, 78
  relapsing-remitting, and suicidality, 86
  religion and, 45
  social defeat and, 109–110
  social-rank theories of, 119
  state, 28
  and suicidality, 110
  and suicide in children, 69
  and suicide in elderly, 36
  and suicide risk, 38, 69
depressive mixed state. *See* syndrome of
    depressive mixed state
depressive schema, 20
depressive turmoil, 143–144, 152, 154, 164
  assessment of, 174, 178, 185, 190, 226
    test case, 196
  case examples, 160, 162–163, 178,
      185, 190
  definition of, 155
despair, 6, 142
desperation
  assessment of, 173–174, 177–178, 184,
      190, 226
    test case, 195
  case examples, 152–154, 177–178,
      184, 190
  definition of, 150, 151
  and hopelessness, 152
  and suicidality, 110, 116, 142
diabetes mellitus, 75, 76
*Diagnostic and Statistical Manual of Mental
    Disorders,* criteria for suicide crisis
    syndrome, 143–144, 154–155, 164,
    170, 228
dialectical behavior therapy, 203, 204,
    261–262
diathesis–stress model (Beck), 5, 19–21,
    20*f*, 28, 43
disgrace, 155disinhibition,
    alcohol-related, 92
displacement, used by clinicians, against
    "forbidden" emotions, 210
divorce, and suicide risk in adolescents, 69

DMX. *See* syndrome of depressive
  mixed state
domestic violence, 66
Down's syndrome, 76
dread, clinician's, about patient, 204–206
drivers, of suicidality, 30–31, 262–263
drowning, 48, 84–85
drug(s)
  acute use of, 224
  illicit. *See* street drugs
  overdose, 48, 84
  recent use of, 224
  withdrawal, 93–94, 224
drug addiction, emotional pain and
  anhedonia in, 159
drug dependence, 38
  and drug-related death after hospital
  discharge, 80
drug treatment, 260–261
drug use disorder, 39, 222
  and alcohol use disorder, 91
  and suicidality, 90–91, 224
dysthymia, 39

eating disorders, 165
  parental overcontrol and, 42
economic crises, 62
economic hardship, 62–63, 223
eczema, 76
eerie calm, of suicidal patient, 256–259
elderly
  events precipitating suicide in, 36
  and history of suicide attempts, 40
  past suicide attempts, as risk factor for
  future suicide, 82
  perceived burdensomeness in, 116
  suicidality in, medical illness and,
  74, 76–77
emerging adulthood, 70, 103
emotion(s)
  clinicians', after patients' suicide, 220
  "forbidden" to clinicians, 204
  negative, 202–203
  clinicians', 204
  positive, 202
  rapid changes in, in suicide crisis
  syndrome, 144
  and suicidal ideation, 142

and thoughts, differentiation of, 203
  as warning signs, 142
emotional awareness, 203
emotional contagion, 204
emotional dynamic, between suicidal patient
  and therapist, *case example,* 204–206
emotional pain, 15, 32, 143, 154–155
  assessment of, 174, 178–180, 184–185,
  190, 226
  test case, 196
  case examples, 160, 162, 178–180,
  184–185, 190
  entrapment and, 151
  comparison of, 155
  incongruously quick resolution in
  psychiatric inpatients, 80–81
  in suicide crisis syndrome, 144
emotional response. *See* clinician(s),
  emotional response to suicidal patients
emotion differentiation, 202–203
  definition of, 202–203
encephalopathy, 76
entrapment, 14, 15–16, 26, 31, 32, 43, 63,
  97, 119, 122, 142. *See also* frantic
  hopelessness
  assessment of, 150, 152–153, 173, 177,
  184, 189–190, 226
  test case, 195
  case examples, 119–121, 152–153, 177,
  184, 189–190
  and defeat, overlap of, 119, 150–151
  and depression, 150–151
  and emotional pain, 151
  comparison of, 155
  external, 150
  internal, 150
  perceived, assessment of, 124, 125–126
  and short-term sucide risk, 151
  subclasses of, 150
  in suicide crisis syndrome, 143–144,
  149–151
environment, 21, 48
epigenetics, 28
epilepsy, 76
escape theory, of suicide (Baumeister),
  12–13, 143
escitalopram, discontinuation of, 89
ethanol withdrawal syndrome, 93

medication(s) (*cont.*)

    initiation. *See also* activation syndrome

        and suicidality, 224

    nonadherence

        and suicidality, 224

        syndromes induced by, 88

    withdrawal syndromes, 88–89

memory, overgeneral, 19, 26, 30

memory retrieval, alterations in, 16–17

men

    age of, and suicidality, 107

    completed suicide rates, 79

    gay, suicide risk in, 38

    genital disorders, 76

    marital status of, and suicidality, 66

    suicide after discharge from inpatient

        unit, 79

    suicide attempts

        failed, and re-use of method, 84–85

        history of, 40

        intimate partner violence and, 66

        past, as risk factor for future suicide, 82

        rates of, 79

    suicide rate for, 36, 37

    unemployed, 62–63

Menninger, Karl, 11

mental health services, clients, suicide

    clusters in, 47

mental illness, 61–62. *See also specific*

    disorder

    acute episodes, and suicidality, 86–87

    comorbidity, 39

    and comorbid medical illness, 74–75, 80

    and eviction, and suicide risk, 64

    exacerbation, and suicidality, 86–87, 224

    family history of, 46–47, 100–101

    history of, and suicide risk, 29, 38–40, 222

    recent diagnosis, and suicidality,

        78–79, 224

    reduction in level of care for, and

        suicidality, 101

    relapsing-remitting, and suicidality, 86

    and suicidality, 78–90, 141

    and suicidal narrative, 98

    and suicide risk, 265

        economic hardship and, 62

    and suicide risk in children, 69

MEPS. *See* means-end problem solving test

method(s), of suicide

    gender differences in, 37

    lethality, variations, 48

    regional differences in, 48

Middle Eastern immigrants,

    suicidality in, 83

migraine, 76

military suicide, 24, 44, 48, 62, 65

    after discharge from hospital, 80

    interview questions about, 50

    rates of, 80

millennials, and entitlement to happiness,

    103–104

mindfulness

    clinicians' capacity for, 203–204

    clinicians' use of, 203–204, 214–215

    definition of, 203

    therapeutic uses of, 203

mindfulness-based cognitive therapy,

    203, 204

mindfulness-based stress reduction, 203

mindfulness meditation, 264–265

model(s), of suicidal behavior, 10. *See also*

    suicide crisis; *specific model*

    affective, 26

    cognitive, 5, 19–21, 26, 28

    first-generation, 10

    predictive value of, 10

    psychodynamic, 10

    second-generation, 10, 97

    third-generation, 10

Modular Assessment of Risk for Imminent

    Suicide, 232–235. *See also* interview(s),

    expanded MARIS; interview(s), MARIS

Montana, 37

mood

    cocaine withdrawal and, 94

    drug/alcohol withdrawal and, 93

    drug initiation/withdrawal and, 88

    sudden brightening, as warning

        sign, 39–40

mood disorders, 86, 141

    substance-induced, 210

mood stabilizers, discontinuation of, 88, 224

mood swings. *See also* depressive turmoil

    in suicide crisis syndrome, 144

moral objections to suicide, 45, 222

moratorium (in millennials' life), 103

moves, frequent, and suicide risk in
adolescents, 69
MSPS. *See* SAD PERSONS scale, modified
murder–suicide, 48

narcissism, unfulfilled, 98
narcissistic personality disorder, 39, 194
narrative-crisis model of suicide, 5, 27,
28–35, 34f
flexibility, 33
overview of, 29–30
suicidal narrative component. *See*
suicidal narrative
suicide crisis component. *See*
suicide crisis
trait vulnerability component. *See* trait
vulnerability
narrative identity, theory of, 30, 31, 96
National Epidemiologic Survey on Alcohol
and Related Conditions, 38
near-psychotic somatization, 14–15
near-term suicide risk, 1, 27, 35
clinician's optimism about patient
and, 207
need(s), Shneidman's classification of, 12
neglect. *See* abuse/neglect
NESARC. *See* National Epidemiologic
Survey on Alcohol and Related
Conditions
New Jersey, 37
New York, 37
nightmares, 170
night terrors, 170
norepinephrine, 5, 21, 27, 28, 43

obsessive-compulsive disorder, 165
olanzapine, 260
older adults. *See also* elderly
goal disengagement and re-engagement
by, 106
opiate(s)
unintended overdose, 224
withdrawal, 93–94
opiate use disorder, 210
opponent processes, and capability for
suicide, 22–24, 23f
optimism, clinician's, about patient
and near-term suicide risk, 207

as reaction formation, 213
osteoporosis, 76
overarousal. *See* agitation; hyperarousal;
insomnia
overdose
accidental, misidentification of, 77
unintentional, 80, 144, 224
overvalued ideas, 167

pain
chronic
non-arthritic, 77
and perceived burdensomeness, 116
and suicidality, 77, 224
emotional. *See* emotional pain
psychic, 13, 32, 160
psychological, 11–13. *See also*
psychache
and suicidality, 224
painful engagement, 107–108
pain insensitivity, 44, 222
interview questions about, 50
panic attacks
in activation syndrome, 88
antidepressant discontinuation and, 89
depression-associated, 157–159
drug/alcohol withdrawal and, 93
with fear of dying, 157–158
opiate withdrawal and, 94
and short-term suicide risk, 2t, 3,
158–159
signs and symptoms, 158
and suicidality, 110, 141, 157, 158
in suicide crisis syndrome, 144
and suicide risk, 15, 38–39, 158–159
panic disorder, 39, 133–136, 165
panic–dissociation, 32, 151, 154–155,
158–159, 164
assessment of, 174, 179, 185, 191, 227
test case, 196–197
case examples, 161, 163, 179, 185, 191
characteristics of, 158
definition of, 143, 158
paranoia, of cocaine withdrawal, 94
parent(s)
in conflict with children, 67–68, 223
death of, and suicide risk in
adolescents, 69

parent(s) (*cont.*)
    as informants in clinical evaluation
        of adolescents, 6
    suicidal behavior, and suicide risk in
        offspring, 46–47, 194, 200
parental separation, and suicide risk in
    children/adolescents, 69
parent–child conflict(s), 62, 67–70, 223
    case example, 68
    and child suicides, 36
parenting style (parental bonding), 41–42
    affectionless control, 41, 68, 74, 222
    authoritarian ("helicopter"), 41, 104
    authoritative, 69
    maladaptive, 29
    neglectful, 41
    overcontrolling, 41–42
    with protective effect, 69
    rejecting-neglecting, 69
    and suicide risk, 222
paroxetine, discontinuation of, 89
PAS. *See* Physical Anhedonia Scale
paternalized child, 100
paternal suicidal behavior, and suicide risk
    in children, 47
peptic ulcer, 75
perceived burdensomeness, 5, 22–23, 23*f*,
    26, 31, 97, 112–115, 116, 122, 124
    assessment of, 124, 125
    case examples, 113–115, 117–118
    as phase5 of suicidal narrative,
        112–115, 225
perfectionism
    assessment of, 125
    predictive value of, 43
    socially prescribed, 19, 26, 43, 98–99
    and suicidality, 19, 26, 43–44, 97, 98–99
        perceived burdensomeness and, 113
    and suicide risk, 222
    trait, and unrealistic life goals, 98
personal defeat, 97, 117–118
    and suicidality, 110
personality, as vulnerability factor,
    19–20, 26, 30
personality disorders, 38, 61, 222
    and drug withdrawal symptoms, 89
    externalizing, 39
    internalizing, 39

personality traits
    externalizing, 44
    internalizing, 44
pessimism, 27, 43
    as cultural phenomenon, 102
    and suicide risk, 222
pesticide ingestion, 48–49, 84
physical abuse
    of adult women, and suicide, 66
    and sexual abuse, simultaneous, and
        youth suicidal behavior, 71–72
    and youth suicidal behavior, 71
Physical Anhedonia Scale, 4*t*
physical disability, and suicide in
    elderly, 36
physical illness, 62
physician(s), suicide rates in, 44
physician-assisted suicide, 201
planned behavior, Ajzen's theory of, 24
podcasts, 265
poisoning, 48, 84
    in Asia, 83
    deliberate, of self, 82
    in pain patients, 77
    suicide by, demographics of, 37
policemen, 48
postpartum psychosis, 87
post-traumatic stress disorder, 165
    war-related, 92
practicing, of suicidal behavior, 46–47, 223
precipitating events, 201
preparatory behavior, 48
prisons, suicide clusters in, 47
problem solving, impaired, 16, 17, 19, 30
projection, used by clinicians, against
    "forbidden" emotions, 211
prostatic disorder, 75, 76
protective factors, 45, 61, 66, 69, 103, 115,
    222, 265
provocation
    direct, by patient, 208
    indirect, by patient, 208
psoriasis, 76
psychache, 13, 143
    Shneidman's theory of, 11–12, 12*f*
psychiatric disorders. *See* mental illness;
    specific disorder
psychiatric inpatients

high-risk, clinicians' conflicted emotional response to, as predictor of imminent risk, 213

incongruously quick resolution of emotional pain, 80–81

near-term suicidal behavior, prediction, 14

post-discharge suicidal behavior, 32–33, 39, 45, 79–82, 257

entrapment subscale of SCI and, 151

SCS intensity in, 33

self-report, dishonest, 80–81

suicide among, 39

suicide clusters in, 47

psychiatric treatment, and suicide risk, 265

psychoanalytical theories, of suicide, 11

psychobabble, 122

psychopaths, 44

psychosis, 141, 165

and comorbid medical illness, 75

exacerbation, and suicidality, 86–87

postpartum, 87

puerperal, 87

ruminative flooding and, 167

puerperal psychosis, 87

race/ethnicity, 221

and alcohol use in suicide, 92

and child suicide, 68

of immigrants, and suicidality, 45, 83

and suicide risk, 29, 36–37

rage, 155

rapport building, 125, 172, 236

interview questions for, 238

rationalization

definition of, 212

in medical field, 212

in suicide risk assessment, 212–213

case example, 218–219

reaction formation, 209, 213, 228

case example, 215–216

used by clinicians, 249–250

clinician's self-assessment of, 214–215

rejection

attentional bias to, 16

and suicidality, case example, 73–74

of suicidal patient, by clinician, 213

relationship conflict, 62, 223

case example, 65

religion

interview questions about, 49

as protective factor, 45, 222

repetitive negative thinking, 165

repression, used by clinicians

case example, 217–218

against "forbidden" emotions, 204, 210

rescue fantasy, 209, 213

case example, 204–206

residence, change of, and suicide risk in adolescents, 69

retirement, goal disengagement and re-engagement after, 106

risk assessment, 1, 265

British guidelines for, 232

comprehensive, outline for, 221–228, 235, 236

explicit

in comprehense interview, 243–244

in expanded MARIS interview, 252–253

in MARIS interview, 248–249

final risk formulation in, 228, 245–246, 249, 256

instruments for, 230–235

preliminary risk formulation in, 228, 244–245, 249, 253, 255

risk assessment interview(s), 8. See also interview(s)

comprehensive, 235–246, 237f

modules, 235–237

question order in, 236

time needed for, 235

strategies for, 235–256

time needed for, 235–236

risk factors, 2–3, 2t, 10, 141, 201, 265

acute, 19

chronic, 19

demographic, 29, 36–38, 221

dynamic, 10, 29

long-term, 2–3, 2t, 221–223

SAD PERSONS acronym for, 230

short-term, 2–3, 2t, 40

state, 29

static, 10, 29. See also trait vulnerability

vs. dynamic, 29

suicide-specific, 141–142

trait vs. state, 28

vs. warning signs, 3

risk formulation. *See* risk assessment

risperidone, withdrawal symptoms,
    case example, 89–90

RNT. *See* repetitive negative thinking

romantic rejection, 65, 223
    case example, 65, 85, 107–108

ruminations, 19, 26
    assessment of, 175, 180, 186, 191–192, 227
        test case, 197–198
    brooding, 165
    case examples, 167, 169, 180, 186, 191–192
    definition of, 165
    simple, *vs.* ruminative flooding, 14
    and suicidality, 165
    in suicide crisis syndrome, 144, 164–165

ruminative flooding
    assessment of, 175–176, 181, 186–187, 192, 227
        test case, 198
    case examples, 168, 169, 181, 186–187, 192
    characteristics of, 164–165
    definition of, 143, 166–167
    and suicidality, 14–15, 32, 151, 154,
        166–167, 168–170
    in suicide crisis syndrome, 143–144, 164

rural communities, 46

SAD PERSONS scale, 3, 230–231
    modified, 231
    predictive power of, acute use of alcohol
        and, 91

safety plan, 263–264

Safety Planning Intervention, 263–264

Sati Handprints, 44

Saudi Arabia, 36

Scale for Suicidal Ideation, 145, 230

schema
    definition of, 20
    depressive, 20
    suicide, 20

schizoaffective disorder, 100–101, 146
    postpartum exacerbations, 87

schizoid personality disorder, 39

schizophrenia, 38, 222
    anhedonia in, 159
    exacerbation, and suicidality, 86–87
    recent diagnosis, and suicidality, 78–79

schizotypal personality disorder, 39

schools, suicide clusters in, 47

SCI. *See* Suicidal Crisis Inventory

SCS. *See* suicide crisis syndrome

seasonal affective disorder, 39

security, app-based interventions and, 265

selective norepinephrine reuptake
    inhibitors, withdrawal, 89

selective serotonin reuptake inhibitors
    anxiety related to, 87
    initiation, 87, 224
    withdrawal, 89

self-care, 265

self-destructiveness, as biological drive, 11

self-determination theory, 113, 116

self-harm, 40. *See also* self-injury
    deliberate, behavioral definition of, 82
    history of, and post-discharge suicide, 79

self-injury, 82. *See also* self-harm
    as escape from mental pain, 159
    as risk factor for future suicide, 82
    case example, 83–84

self-report
    dishonest/misleading, 229–230
        interview strategy to avoid, 172
        in psychiatric inpatients, 80–81
    limitations of, 228–230
    in Modular Assessment of Risk for
        Imminent Suicide, 232–234
    poor predictive validity of, 229
    in risk assessment, 228–230
    of suicidal ideation, 4–5, 124–125, 145,
        147, 228–230

sensory disturbances. *See also*
    panic–dissociation
    assessment of, 174
        test case, 196–197

Seppuku, 44

serotonin, 5, 21, 27, 28, 43

sex/sex differences. *See also* men; women
    in past suicide attempts as risk factor for
        future suicide, 82
    in suicide after discharge from inpatient
        unit, 79
    in suicide risk, 29, 221
        bullying and, 72
        childhood maltreatment and, 72
        in children, 69

sexual abuse
    of adult women, and suicide, 66
    age of onset, 72
    childhood

and adult suicide, 40–41, 66
  effects of, sex differences in, 70–72
  and suicidality, 70–71
  and childhood and adolescent
    suicidality, 70–74
  contact *vs.* noncontact, 72
  ongoing, and suicide risk, 223
sexual attraction, to patient, clinicians'
    defenses against, 204, 214
sexual orientation. *See* LGBT persons
shame, 155
  and child suicide, 69, 70
sharp objects, use of, suicide by,
    demographics of, 37
Shneidman, E., theory of psychache,
    11–12, 12*f*
short-term suicide risk, 1, 2–3, 2*t*, 35, 141
  assessment instruments, 230–232
  entrapment and, 151
  expectation of happiness and, 102–103
  increased, factors in, 40
sickle cell anemia, 76
SIS. *See* Suicide Intent Scale
SKA- 2, 4*t*
skin, feeling of having no, 156
"skin thickness," 156
smoking, 22
  and suicide risk in children, 69
social contacts, 264, 265
social defeat, 97, 117–118, 119
  assessment of, 123–124
  consequences of, 110
  definition of, 109
  and depression, 109–110
  magnitude of, objective *vs.* perceived, 110
  and suicidality, 110
social isolation, 23, 46, 113–114, 116
socializations, 264
social networks, and transmission of suicide
    contagion, 47
social phobia, 39, 165
  parental overcontrol and, 41
social rank theory, 109
social support, low, 116
socioeconomic status, 62
  and suicide risk, 29
Soviet Union (former), 36
SPI. *See* Safety Planning Intervention
spinal fracture, 76

SPS. *See* SAD PERSONS scale
Sri Lanka, 36
  rates of suicide attempts in, 83
SSF. *See* Suicide Status Form
SSI. *See* Scale for Suicidal Ideation
SSRI. *See* selective serotonin reuptake
    inhibitors
state, definition of, 28
stimulants, adverse effects and side
    effects of, 87
Stockholm syndrome, 209
street drugs
  intoxication with, 89
  withdrawal symptoms, 89
stress, 5, 17
  causes of, 61
stress–diathesis models of suicide, 5, 17, 24
  Mann's, 21–22, 22*f*, 27, 28
stressful life events, 61–95, 223–224
  assessment of, interview questions for,
    239–240, 253–254
  case example, 63, 64
  and suicide risk in children, 69
  summary, 240–241, 254
stressor(s), 97
  interpersonal, 29
  Mann's definition of, 21
  socioeconomic, 29
stroke, 76
STS. *See* Suicide Trigger Scale
substance misuse, recent, and suicidality,
    90–95, 224
substance use disorder, 22
  case example, 94–95, 104–105
  recent diagnosis, and suicidality, 78
  and suicidality, 90–91
suffocation, 84, 92–93
  suicide by, demographics of, 37
suicidal behavior
  of family/friends
    adolescents' exposure to, 46–47
    interview questions about, 50
  history of, and suicide risk, 29
Suicidal Crisis Inventory, 15, 30, 32, 158
suicidal desire, 5
suicidal ideation, 141, 142
  assessment of, 173, 226
  case examples, 146–149, 176–177,
    183–184, 189

suicidal ideation (*cont.*)
  test case, 194
  defeat and, 119
  definition of, 145
  entrapment and, 119
  first, and suicide attempt, average time
    interval between, 116
  in gay men, 38
  in interpersonal theory of suicide
    (Joiner), 116
  and long-term suicide risk, 2*t*, 3
  panic symptoms and, 158
  perceived burdensomeness and, 112–113
  prediction, IMV model and, 26
  prevalence of, 2
  self-report of, 4–5, 124–125, 145, 147,
    228–230
  stages of, in O'Connor's IMV model,
    24–26, 25*f*
  in suicide crisis syndrome, 144–145
suicidal narrative, 5, 29–30, 30–32, 32*f*. *See
  also* narrative-crisis model of suicide
  common themes in, 31
  constructing, 121–124, 126, 225–226,
    241–242, 254–255
  test case, 136–140
  and imminent suicide risk, 5
  intensity, and suicide risk, 98
  phases of, 96–98, 122. *See also*
    specific phase
    summary of, 225
  summary, 242, 255
The Suicidal Narrative, how to use, 8
suicidal narrative interview, 121–122
  algorithm for, 124–136
suicidal narrative risk assessment table, 140
suicidal process
  evolution of, 27
  stages of, 24–27, 25*f*
suicide
  conscious and planned, 144
  unconscious or unplanned, 144
suicide attempt(s)
  aborted, 224
  age at, as risk factor for future suicide, 82
  alcohol-involved, 91–92
  vs. deliberate self-harm, 82
  eerie calm after, 256–259
  failed, 224

lethality, 48, 84
  perceived burdensomeness and, 113
  and re-use of method, 84–85
future, prediction of, 145
by gay men, 38
gender differences in, 37
history of, 40, 141
  and long-term suicide risk, 2*t*, 222
  predictive power of, 145
interrupted, 224
intimate partner violence and, 66
lethality, 48, 84–85, 224, 229
  alcohol use and, 92
  and degree of suicide intent, 146
  perceived burdensomeness and, 113
  Suicide Intent Scale and, 146
methods, 48, 84–85
number of, as risk factor for future
  suicide, 82
panic symptoms and, 158
perceived burdensomeness and, 112–113
predictive factors for, 15
rates, 2
recent, 40
  as risk factor for suicide, 82–84, 224
remote, 40
  as risk factor for future suicide, 82
stress and, 61
thwarted belongingness and, 112, 116
unpredictability of, 4
suicide bombing, 92
suicide clusters, 47–48
  interview questions about, 50–51
suicide contagion
  interview questions about, 50–51
  transmission of, 47
suicide crisis, 27, 32–33, 168–170
  definition of, 143
  Hendin's concept of, 13–14, 143
  intensity, and imminent suicide risk,
    5, 14, 32
  signal of, 6
  summary of, 226–228
suicide crisis assessment algorithm, 172–176
Suicide Crisis Inventory, 80
suicide crisis syndrome, 3, 13–15, 27, 30,
  32–33, 96, 143–144
  affective symptoms in, 143. *See also*
    affective disturbance